Introduction Public Health

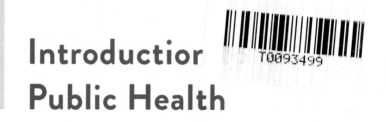

Raymond L. Goldsteen, DrPH, is professor emeritus of Family, Population and Preventive Medicine, at the Health Sciences Center, Stony Brook University, where he was founding director of the Master of Public Health (MPH) program. Formerly, he was founding director of the MPH program and professor of Family and Community Medicine, School of Medicine and Health Sciences at the University of North Dakota. He received his doctoral degree from the Columbia University School of Public Health. Dr. Goldsteen has an extensive background in health care and was director of health policy research centers at the University of Illinois in Urbana-Champaign, University of Oklahoma College of Public Health, and the West Virginia University School of Medicine. He has authored numerous publications in academic journals including the *American Journal of Public Health*; *Journal of Rural Health*; *Journal of Health Politics, Policy, and Law*; and *Journal of Aging and Health*. He is coauthor of the *Introduction to Public Health*, first and second editions, and the highly acclaimed *Jonas' Introduction to the U.S. Health Care System*, now in its 10th edition.

Karen Goldsteen, PhD, MPH, is affiliated research associate professor of Family, Population and Preventive Medicine at the Health Sciences Center, Stony Brook University. Formerly, she was research associate professor of Family and Community Medicine in the Master of Public Health program and the Center for Rural Health, School of Medicine and Health Sciences at the University of North Dakota. She received her MPH from the Columbia University School of Public Health and a PhD in Community Health from the University of Illinois at Urbana-Champaign. She was a Pew Health Policy Fellow at the University of California, San Francisco. Dr. Goldsteen is coauthor of the *Introduction to Public Health*, first and second editions, and the highly acclaimed *Jonas' Introduction to the U.S. Health Care System*, now in its 10th edition.

Terry Dwelle, MD, MPHTM, CPH, is founder and president of the North Dakota Public Health Training Network. He received his MD degree from St. Louis University and completed a pediatric residency and pediatric infectious disease fellowship at Cardinal Glennon Hospital for Children in St. Louis. He received an MPHTM from Tulane University where he also completed a preventive medicine residency specializing in international health and tropical medicine. He served as a clinical director in the Indian Health Service, assistant professor of pediatrics at University of North Dakota School of Medicine, clinician at the Centre Medical Evangelique in northeastern Zaire, regional director for Medical Ambassadors International's faith-based community engagement programs in East Africa, State Health Officer for North Dakota, chair of the National Board of Public Health Examiners, and public health consultant for the Turtle Mountain Band of Chippewa Indians.

Introduction to Public Health: Promises and Practices

Third Edition

Raymond L. Goldsteen, DrPH

Karen Goldsteen, PhD, MPH

Terry Dwelle, MD, MPHTM, CPH

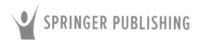 SPRINGER PUBLISHING

First Springer Publishing edition: 9780826141521 (2010); subsequent edition: 2014.

Springer Publishing Company, LLC
902 Carnegie Center/Suite 140, Princeton, NJ 08540
www.springerpub.com
connect.springerpub.com

Acquisitions Editor: David D'Addona
Production Editor: Ashley Hannen
Compositor: S4Carlisle Publishing Services

ISBN: 978-0-8261-8614-0
ebook ISBN: 978-0-8261-8615-7
DOI: 10.1891/9780826186157

SUPPLEMENTS:

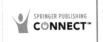

A robust set of instructor resources designed to supplement this text is located at
http://connect.springerpub.com/content/book/**978-0-8261-8615-7**. Qualifying
instructors may request access by emailing **textbook@springerpub.com**.

Instructor Materials:
LMS Common Cartridge (All Instructor Resources and Instructions for Use) ISBN: 978-0-8261-3977-1
Instructor Manual ISBN: 978-0-8261-8616-4
Test Bank ISBN: 978-0-8261-8617-1
PowerPoints ISBN: 978-0-8261-8618-8
Syllabus ISBN: 978-0-8261-8619-5

24 25 26 27 / 5 4 3 2 1

The author and the publisher of this Work have made every effort to use sources believed to be reliable
to provide information that is accurate and compatible with the standards generally accepted at the
time of publication. Because medical science is continually advancing, our knowledge base continues
to expand. Therefore, as new information becomes available, changes in procedures become necessary.
We recommend that the reader always consult current research and specific institutional policies before
performing any clinical procedure or delivering any medication. The author and publisher shall not be
liable for any special, consequential, or exemplary damages resulting, in whole or in part, from the readers'
use of, or reliance on, the information contained in this book. The publisher has no responsibility for the
persistence or accuracy of URLs for external or third-party Internet websites referred to in this publication
and does not guarantee that any content on such websites is, or will remain, accurate or appropriate.

Library of Congress Cataloging-in-Publication Data

Names: Goldsteen, Raymond L., author. | Goldsteen, Karen, author. | Dwelle, Terry L., author.
Title: Introduction to public health : promises and practices / Raymond L.
   Goldsteen, DrPH, Karen Goldsteen, PhD, MPH, Terry Dwelle, MD, MPHTM, CPH.
Identifiers: LCCN 2023032052 (print) | LCCN 2023032053 (ebook) | ISBN
   9780826186140 (paperback) | ISBN 9780826186157 (ebook)
Subjects: LCSH: Public health.
Classification: LCC RA425 .G58 2024 (print) | LCC RA425 (ebook) | DDC
   362.1—dc23/eng/20231016
LC record available at https://lccn.loc.gov/2023032052
LC ebook record available at https://lccn.loc.gov/2023032053

Contact sales@springerpub.com to receive discount rates on bulk purchases.

Printed in the United States of America by Gasch Printing.

This book is dedicated to public health professionals everywhere who care deeply about the people they serve and strive daily to make the conditions in which they live healthful, which they demonstrated so poignantly during the turmoil of the COVID-19 pandemic.

Contents

Preface

This book describes the public health system in broad strokes in order to focus the reader on basic public health goals, principles, structures, and practices. The context in which public health is practiced today has changed considerably since its historic roots in the Industrial Revolution of the 18th and 19th centuries. However, the overarching goal of public health systems remains the same—to ensure through collective action a healthful environment for all people. The 21st century offers incredible challenges to public health. The disparity in access to healthy environments is widening, and the threats to the foundations of health—including adequate and nutritious food, clean and sufficient water, and shelter—persist. Moreover, these are global problems that touch every country to some extent and threaten to affect all countries within our lifetimes. This fact was made particularly clear by the COVID-19 pandemic.

In order to meet these challenges, our aim in the coming years will be to embrace how, when, and where to improve the quality and value of public health received by the populations served. There will be more emphasis on transparent decision-making, fully integrated information technology and computational expertise, and a systems orientation toward population health improvement. In addition, we will need to mobilize public support for public health—our goals and methods—which was shown during the COVID-19 pandemic. The scientific basis of public health and the nature of science especially need emphasis. Science needs to be shown as "a candle in the dark" within "the demon-haunted world," as Carl Sagan wrote in 1996. The war against science and the resulting voodoo public health have arisen from partisanship that must be counteracted. All of these actions will allow us to provide a healthy environment for all people.

An Instructor Manual, Test Bank, and PowerPoint slides are available to supplement this text. To obtain an electronic copy of these materials, contact Springer Publishing Company at textbook@springerpub.com

Raymond L. Goldsteen, DrPH
Karen Goldsteen, PhD, MPH
Terry Dwelle, MD, MPHTM, CPH

Acknowledgments

Raymond and Karen Goldsteen wish to acknowledge the continuing support of their colleagues at Stony Brook University's Program in Public Health, including Lisa Benz Scott, director, Lauren Hale, Jaymie Meliker, and Norman Edelman. We also acknowledge the contribution of Benjamin Goldsteen, who wrote very creatively in Chapter 2 about the origins of the *International Statistical Classification of Diseases* (*ICD*) and its importance to modern public health. Finally, we thank Helen Sullinger and Sarah Lake for their important contributions to the case studies in public health. Terry Dwelle would like to acknowledge David Hesselgrave, Stan Rowland, Ron Heifetz, Marty Linsky, Steve Farber, the Bush Foundation, and Governors John Hoeven and Jack Dalrymple, who provided support and the many practical concepts and ideas for leadership and truly engaging communities that are included in this work.

Springer Publishing Resources

 A robust set of instructor resources designed to supplement this text is located at http://connect.springerpub.com/content/book/978-0-8261-8615-7. Qualifying instructors may request access by emailing textbook@springerpub.com.

Instructor Resources:

- LMS Common Cartridge With All Instructor Material
- Instructor Manual
- Test Bank
- Chapter-Based PowerPoint Presentations

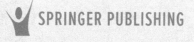 SPRINGER PUBLISHING

Visit https://connect.springerpub.com/ and look for the "**Show Supplementary**" button on the **book homepage**.

1   What Is Public Health?

LEARNING OBJECTIVES

Students will learn . . .

1. How the fields of medicine and public health are different and complementary.
2. How health is defined, theoretically and in practice.
3. The multiple determinants of health and the impact of each.
4. The models that have been used to integrate the determinants of health.
5. How public health interventions have changed over the past century.

THE PROMISE OF PUBLIC HEALTH

Every year since 1873, the American Public Health Association (APHA) has held an annual meeting—a huge event attended by thousands of people, containing hundreds of sessions, over a period of nearly a week. The meeting expresses the public health priorities for that year and gives forum to the full range of current public health issues and activities. Current scientific and educational programs represent all sections, special interest groups, and caucuses. In the 2021 APHA Annual Meeting in Denver, a typical recent year, the 32 sections, three special primary interest groups (SPIGs), and 17 caucuses were represented.

Among the sections were the following:

- Aging and Public Health;
- Maternal and Child Health;
- Alcohol, Tobacco, and Other Drugs;
- Integrative, Complementary, and Traditional Health Practices;
- Occupational Health and Safety;
- Chiropractic Health Care;
- Physical Activity;
- Disability;

- Public Health Education and Promotion;
- Food and Nutrition;
- Law; and
- Ethics.

Some of the caucuses represented were:

- Academic and Practice Linkages in Public Health Caucus;
- American Indian, Alaska Native, and Native Hawaiian Caucus;
- Asian and Pacific Islander Caucus for Public Health;
- Black Caucus of Health Workers;
- Caucus on Homelessness;
- Caucus on Public Health and the Faith Community;
- Caucus on Refugee and Immigrant Health;
- Community-Based Public Health Caucus; and
- Family Violence Prevention Caucus.

The theme of the 2021 APHA Annual Meeting was *Strengthening Social Connectedness Across the Racial Divide,* and sessions spanned a wide array of topics, including this sampling from among the hundreds of presentations:

- Social and Community Context of Homelessness;
- Social Connection, Isolation, Loneliness, and Mental Health;
- Social Connectedness in Occupational Health and Safety;
- Building Community Resilience and Addressing Social Vulnerability;
- Communicating for Connection: Strengthening Injury and Violence Prevention;
- Preventing Social Isolation Across the Lifespan;
- Creating Food Justice Through Community Networks; and
- Engaging Fathers to Strengthen Family Social Connectedness and Improve Perinatal Outcomes.

This small sample of topics at one meeting indicates the diversity and abundance of subjects that concern public health professionals. In reviewing the topics and noting their scope and variety, we may be motivated to ask questions such as, "What does creating food justice have to do with thirdhand smoke research?" "How is social connectedness related to waste and environmental justice?" "How is engaging fathers to strengthen family social connectedness linked to occupational health and safety?" Similarly, when we examine the composition of the public health workforce through job postings at the APHA Annual Meeting and other public health employment sites, we see positions as different as sanitarian, community organizer, health educator, environmental safety specialist, infectious disease manager, epidemiologist, microbiologist, data analyst, and reproductive health specialist. Again, we may ask, "What is the common thread that connects these disparate types of employment?"

The answer to these questions lies in the following statement written in 1988 by the Institute of Medicine's (IOM) Committee for the Study of the Future of Public Health:

> The broad mission of public health is to "fulfill society's interest in assuring conditions in which people can be healthy." (p. 1)

This statement was intended to capture the essence of the historical and present work of public health, and it binds us together by identifying our common bond. It asserts that we, in the field of public health, are engaged in a great societal endeavor to create the circumstances that make health possible. We may have little in common on a day-to-day basis with our fellow public health professionals, and our knowledge base and skills may vary widely from others in our field. However, our mission is the same, and each of us contributes to that mission in some important way, which we will begin to explicate in the coming pages. Before proceeding, though, we need to examine this statement more closely to understand its assumptions and implications. By examining these, we understand our commonalities with other professionals focused on health—particularly the clinical professions such as medicine, nursing, dentistry, physical therapy, and others.

First, the idea of ensuring health for all people—the entire population—is embedded in the mission statement. Although public health will focus on different populations within the larger population when planning services, we are obligated to ensure health-producing conditions for all people—not just the poor, not just the rich, but people of all incomes; not only the young or the old, but people of all ages; not exclusively Whites, Hispanics, Asians, or Blacks, but people of all races and ethnicities.

Second, the belief that a society benefits from having a healthy populace is clear in the public health mission's phrase "to fulfill society's interest." The work of public health is a societal effort with a societal benefit. Public health takes the view held by many professions and societies throughout human history that healthy people are more productive and creative, and these attributes create a strong society. Healthy people lead to better societies. For the welfare of the society, as a whole, it is better for people to be healthy than sick. There will be less dependence, less lost time from productive work, and a greater pool of productive workers—teachers, entrepreneurs, soldiers, and others needed to accomplish society's goals. Thus, as public health professionals, we believe that society has an interest in the health of the population; it benefits the society, as a whole, when people are healthy.

Third, the public health mission acknowledges that health is not guaranteed. The mission states that "people *can* (not *will*) be healthy." Health is a possibility, although we intend through our actions to make it highly probable. However, not everyone will be healthy, even if each individual exists in health-producing conditions. Public health efforts will not result in every person being healthy—although we certainly would not object to that kind of success. Rather, public health creates conditions in which people can be healthy. Whether any single individual is healthy, we acknowledge, will vary.

The fourth and fifth assumptions differentiate public health from the healing, or clinical, professions—medicine, nursing, dentistry, physical therapy, and others—that we will refer to for simplicity throughout the remainder of this book as the clinical professions. All clinical professions believe in the obligation of their practitioners to care for all people in need of their services. Further, they accept the fallibility of their professions; not every patient will be "cured" regardless of the effort expended by the practitioner to bring about this outcome. Finally, all health care professions believe that improving health is a benefit, not only to the individuals treated, but also to the society as a whole.

These beliefs are evident in the widely referenced Physician's Pledge adopted by the World Medical Association Declaration of Geneva (1948 and amended most recently at the *WMA General Assembly, Chicago, United States, October 2017*):

As a member of the medical profession:

- I solemnly pledge to dedicate my life to the service of humanity;
- The health and well-being of my patient will be my first consideration;
- I will respect the autonomy and dignity of my patient;
- I will maintain the utmost respect for human life;
- I will not permit considerations of age, disease or disability, creed, ethnic origin, gender, nationality, political affiliation, race, sexual orientation, social standing, or any other factor to intervene between my duty and my patient;
- I will respect the secrets that are confided in me, even after the patient has died;
- I will practice my profession with conscience and dignity and in accordance with good medical practice;
- I will foster the honor and noble traditions of the medical profession;
- I will give to my teachers, colleagues, and students the respect and gratitude that is their due;
- I will share my medical knowledge for the benefit of the patient and the advancement of health care;
- I will attend to my own health, well-being, and abilities in order to provide care of the highest standard;
- I will not use my medical knowledge to violate human rights and civil liberties, even under threat;
- I make these promises solemnly, freely, and upon my honor.

Thus, public health shares with the clinical professions a fundamental caring for humanity through concern for health. For these reasons, public health is sometimes viewed as a type of clinical profession.

Prevention: The Cornerstone of Public Health

However, if we examine the public health mission closely, we find that public health is complementary to the clinical professions, but not subsumed by them. The critical differences between public health and the clinical professions relate to their strategies for creating a healthy populace. The fourth and fifth assumptions embedded in the public health mission are that prevention is the preferred strategy, and to be successful, prevention must address the "conditions," that is, environment, in the fullest sense, in which people live. The classic and defining public health strategy is to prevent poor health by "assuring conditions in which people can be healthy."

The choice of an environment-based prevention strategy (as opposed to an individual-based strategy) clearly distinguishes public health from the clinical professions. The clinical professions focus on diagnosing individuals and treating them when they have health problems detectable by clinical methods—history, physical examinations, laboratory tests, imaging, and so forth. Here, an understanding of the different types of prevention—primary, secondary, and tertiary— is necessary to differentiate between public health and the clinical professions.

Primary, Secondary, and Tertiary Prevention

There are three types of prevention: primary, secondary, and tertiary. Fos and Fine (2000) define primary, secondary, and tertiary prevention as follows:

> Primary prevention is concerned with eliminating risk factors for a disease. Secondary prevention focuses on early detection and treatment of disease (subclinical and clinical). Tertiary prevention attempts to eliminate or moderate disability associated with advanced disease. (pp. 108–109)

Primary prevention is intended to prevent the development of disease and the occurrence of injury, and thus, to reduce their incidence in the population. Primary prevention includes the historic public health emphases on ensuring clean drinking water, safe housing and workplaces, and nutritious and uncontaminated food. Primary prevention also includes promoting healthy behaviors such as using automobile seat belts, protecting skin from ultraviolet light, and refraining from smoking.

Secondary prevention is concerned with injury or disease after they have occurred and their prompt and effective treatment. Early detection is emphasized, especially screening before signs and symptoms of disease are apparent. Secondary prevention activities are intended to identify the presence of disease early so that prompt treatment can mitigate chronic adverse outcomes. Examples include screening for breast cancer, diabetes, and hypertension.

Tertiary prevention focuses on the optimum treatment of clinically apparent and clearly identified disease to reduce adverse health outcomes to the greatest possible degree. Tertiary prevention often involves limiting disability that occurs if disease and injury are not effectively treated. "Tertiary prevention concerns managing disease post diagnosis to slow or stop disease progression through measures such as chemotherapy, rehabilitation, and screening for complications" (Centers for Disease Control and Prevention [CDC], 2022, para. 3).

Since the central focus of clinical professions is to restore health or prevent exacerbation of health problems, health care is primarily concerned with secondary and tertiary prevention: (a) early detection, diagnosis, and treatment of conditions that can be cured or stopped from progressing (secondary prevention); and (b) treatment of chronic diseases and other conditions to prevent exacerbation and minimize future complications and disability (tertiary prevention). The health care system undoubtedly has its smallest impact on primary prevention, once again that group of interventions that focus on preventing disease, illness, and injury from occurring. Moreover, as Evans and Stoddart (1994) argued in 1994, other than for immunization, the major focus of the health care system's primary prevention activities is on the behavioral determinants of health, rather than structural or policy factors:

> The focus on individual risk factors and specific diseases has tended to lead not away from but back to the health care system itself. Interventions, particularly those addressing personal life-styles, are offered in the form of "provider counseling" for smoking cessation, seat belt use, or dietary modification. These in turn are subsumed under a more general and rapidly growing set of interventions attempting to modify risk factors through transactions between clinicians and individual patients.
>
> The "product line" of the health care system is thus extended to deal with a more broadly defined set of "diseases": unhealthy behaviors. The boundary becomes blurred between, e.g., heart disease as manifest in symptoms, or in elevated serum cholesterol measurements, or in excessive consumption of fats. All are "diseases" and represent a "need" for health care intervention. . . . The behaviors of large and powerful organizations, or the effects of economic and social policies, public and private, [are] not brought under scrutiny. (pp. 43–44)

Another often-quoted modern version of the Hippocratic Oath written by Lasagna (1962) in *The Doctor's Dilemma* provides an example of the difference between the clinical professional, whose improvement strategy is based on diagnosis and treatment of individuals, and the public health professional.

I swear to fulfill, to the best of my ability and judgment, this covenant:

- I will respect the hard-won scientific gains of those physicians in whose steps I walk, and gladly share such knowledge as is mine with those who are to follow.
- I will apply, for the benefit of the sick, all measures [that] are required, avoiding those twin traps of overtreatment and therapeutic nihilism.

- I will remember that there is art to medicine as well as science, and that warmth, sympathy, and understanding may outweigh the surgeon's knife or the chemist's drug.

- I will not be ashamed to say "I know not," nor will I fail to call in my colleagues when the skills of another are needed for a patient's recovery.

- I will respect the privacy of my patients, for their problems are not disclosed to me that the world may know. Most especially must I tread with care in matters of life and death. If it is given me to save a life, all thanks. But it may also be within my power to take a life; this awesome responsibility must be faced with great humbleness and awareness of my own frailty. Above all, I must not play at God.

- I will remember that I do not treat a fever chart, a cancerous growth, but a sick human being, whose illness may affect the person's family and economic stability. My responsibility includes these related problems, if I am to care adequately for the sick.

- I will prevent disease whenever I can, for prevention is preferable to cure.

- I will remember that I remain a member of society, with special obligations to all my fellow human beings, those sound of mind and body as well as the infirm.

- If I do not violate this oath, may I enjoy life and art, respected while I live and remembered with affection thereafter. May I always act so as to preserve the finest traditions of my calling and may I long experience the joy of healing those who seek my help.

Although *The Doctor's Dilemma* contains one statement about the importance of primary prevention—"I will prevent disease whenever I can"—it is clear that the physician is viewed as a healer of individuals. The idea conveyed by this statement is that the physician uses clinical tools to treat health problems that have already begun, which is very different from the public health professional whose main goal is primary prevention of health problems employing strategies based on improving the circumstances in which people live.

Today, medicine and public health work together more closely than in the past. Particularly primary care physicians contribute to public health-oriented practices, accepting the ideas of population health. They have always been active in tertiary prevention by providing vaccinations and disease screening. There is a general recognition among physicians that disease, disability, and premature death result from a variety of factors outside of medicine's purview and that impacting them to prevent health problems is the preferable course of action.

Secondary and Tertiary Prevention and Public Health

The public health emphasis on primary prevention does not mean that public health has no role or interest in secondary and tertiary prevention. On the contrary, public health professionals are vitally interested and involved in secondary and tertiary prevention. However, public health professionals' focus is on ensuring access to effective clinical care, rather than on providing the care itself. Preventing long-term consequences of health problems and limiting the progression of illness, disability, and disease are dependent on access to excellent medical care. Thus, ensuring that all people have health insurance has been an important issue for public health in the United States, as has health care reform that improves the quality and efficiency of health care. Access to primary care and the specialties has historically been a target of public health initiatives. Other issues that impact on people's ability to access and use health care appropriately are important, as well. These include such concerns as transportation to health care providers, cultural competence of health care providers, health literacy of patients, and the efficiency and effectiveness of health care delivery.

An example of public health's interest in secondary and tertiary prevention is the development of Medically Underserved Areas (MUAs), Medically Underserved Populations (MUPs), and Health Professional Shortage Areas (HPSAs), which are designated by the federal Health Resources and Services Administration (HRSA):

> Medically Underserved Areas/Populations are areas or populations designated by HRSA as having too few primary care providers, high infant mortality, high poverty or a high elderly population. Health Professional Shortage Areas (HPSAs) are designated by HRSA as having shortages of primary medical care, dental or mental health providers and may be geographic (a county or service area), population (e.g., low income or Medicaid eligible) or facilities (e.g., federally qualified health center or other state or federal prisons). (U.S. Department of Health and Human Services & Health Resources and Services Administration, 2022, para. 1)

Through designation of areas and populations as medically underserved, programs responding to their medical needs have been developed. These programs address the concerns about access to quality medical care in specific populations and geographic areas, which is necessary for secondary and tertiary prevention. Public health is vitally interested and involved in the identification of MUPs and MUAs, as well as in the development of programs to address these needs.

If we were to apply the language of the clinical professions to public health, we might say that classic public health "diagnoses" and "treats" the circumstances in which people live, and the success of public health is measured by the health of the populations living in the "treated" circumstances. However, the languages of epidemiology and ecology are preferred to describe the work of public health professionals, as we explore later in this chapter. In summary, public health is proactive, rather than curative: Do not wait until people get sick and then treat them. Rather, go out and create conditions that promote health and prevent disease, injury, and disability.

Box 1.1. Collaboration to Prevent Disease Outbreak

An infectious disease outbreak provides an example of the complementary roles played by public health and clinical professionals. In 2009, the PulseNet staff at the Centers for Disease Control and Prevention (CDC) identified a multistate cluster of *Escherichia coli*, or *E. coli*, mainly from physicians who had diagnosed and treated patients with the disease. The CDC's OutbreakNet team then worked with state and local partners, including physicians, to gather epidemiologic information about persons in the cluster to determine if any of the individuals who had become ill had been exposed to the same food source(s). They found that most ill persons had consumed beef, many in restaurants. At least some of the illnesses appeared to be associated with products subject to a recent U.S. Department of Agriculture's Food Safety and Inspection Service (FSIS) recall. Public health officials continued to work with FSIS officials to determine the source of the infection and how to prevent recurrence in others. Thus, CDC officials collaborated with local physicians, the FSIS, and local public health staff to address the circumstances in which the *E. coli* infection developed so that others would be spared the illness resulting from exposure to the pathogen (CDC, 2010a).

Summary

The control of an infectious disease outbreak in **Box 1.1** is an example of the promise of public health—collective action that prevents the occurrence of disease, disability, and premature death by "assuring conditions in which people can be healthy." Because of public health, people will have the opportunity, to the best of our knowledge and capabilities, to be healthy. Public health, as a field and as a collection of practicing professionals, will ensure that the environment in which people lead their lives promotes health.

Underlying this mission is a commitment to social justice because it assumes that all people are deserving of healthy conditions in which to live—not just the rich, but people of all incomes; not only the young or the old, but people of all ages; not exclusively the majority race or ethnicity, but people of all races and ethnicities. Public health is a leader and plays an integral role in carrying out this societal obligation. For this reason, public health is often associated with advocating and providing services for the structurally disadvantaged—those with the least power in their social circumstances. As Krieger and Birn (1998) argue powerfully:

> Social justice is the foundation of public health. This powerful proposition—still contested—first emerged around 150 years ago during the formative years of public health as both a modern movement and a profession. It is an assertion that reminds us that public health is indeed a public matter, that societal patterns of disease and death, of health and well-being, of bodily integrity and disintegration, intimately reflect the

workings of the body politic for good and for ill. It is a statement that asks us, pointedly, to remember that worldwide dramatic declines—and continued inequalities—in mortality and morbidity signal as much the victories and defeats of social movements to create a just, fair, caring, and inclusive world as they do the achievements and unresolved challenges of scientific research and technology. To declare that social justice is the foundation of public health is to call upon and nurture that invincible human spirit that led so many of us to enter the field of public health in the first place: a spirit that has a compelling desire to make the world a better place, free of misery, inequity, and preventable suffering, a world in which we all can live, love, work, play, ail and die with our dignity intact and our humanity cherished. (p. 1603)

The cornerstone of public health is prevention, particularly primary prevention. Prevention is public health's historic and ideal approach to promoting health, and the distinguishing public health prevention strategy is to influence the "conditions" (i.e., the environment, in the fullest sense) in which people live. The classic and defining public health strategy to prevent poor health is to ensure "conditions in which people can be healthy." A commitment to social justice underlies the public health mission to achieve health-promoting conditions for all. How public health has attempted to ensure conditions that promote health is the story of the practice of public health, which we will introduce next.

THE PRACTICE OF PUBLIC HEALTH

What is entailed in "ensuring conditions in which people can be healthy"? In the answer to this question lies the source of the varied interests, knowledge, and skills that differentiate public health professionals from each other. The causes of poor health are many and complex, and, therefore, solutions are complex and diverse, as well. Public health conceptualizes and organizes this complexity by applying the concepts and principles of ecology, which views individuals as embedded within their environment, or context. The ecological approach to understanding how health is either fostered or undermined is fundamental to public health practice.

However, before we can discuss the practice of public health, that is, the ways that public health professionals attempt to influence context and promote health, we will discuss how we define health and conceptualize the complex set of factors that affect health, called the determinants of health.

How Do We Define Health?

The most famous and influential definition of health is the one developed by the World Health Organization (WHO) and enshrined in the Preamble of its Constitution of 1948: "Health is a state of complete physical, mental and social well-being and not merely the absence of disease or infirmity." And although the Constitution has been amended since 1946, this opening statement defining health has not been changed (WHO, 2022a, para. 2). Many subsequent definitions have taken an equally broad view of health, including that of the Association of Teachers of Preventive Medicine (Stokes et al., 1982): "A state characterized by anatomical, physiological, and psychological integrity; ability to perform personally valued family, work, and community roles; ability to deal with physical, biological, psychological, and social stress; a feeling of well-being; and freedom from the risk of disease and untimely death" (p. 34).

Both definitions exemplify the tendency over the second half of the 20th century to enlarge the definition of health beyond morbidity, disability, and premature mortality to include sense of well-being, ability to adapt to change, and social functioning. This is perhaps due to criticisms such as those of Smith (2008) that defining health exclusively as disease and disability, and treating them singularly, places almost everyone in the "unhealthy" category. Conversely, "Health may become so inclusive that virtually all human endeavors, including the pursuit of happiness, are considered within its domain" (Young, 1998, p. 2).

However, in practice, the more limited view of health as diagnosable morbidity, mortality, and disability usually guides public health efforts to improve health status. As Young wrote in 1998 and is still true in 2022, "Indeed, the WHO definition is 'honored in repetition, rarely in application'" (Young, 1998, p. 2). This is partially a practical matter for public health professionals, as data needed to assess health need, develop public health strategies, and evaluate public health effectiveness are often most readily available in the form of morbidity, mortality, and disability. In this book, as in general public health practice, the term *health* will refer to the more restricted definition—diagnosable morbidity, disability, and premature mortality.

The Determinants of Health

There are many influences on individual and population health. It is generally accepted that the **determinants of health** include the physical environment—natural and built—and the social environment, as well as individual behavior, genetic inheritance, and health care (Evans & Stoddart, 1994). As the WHO puts it:

> Many factors combine together to affect the health of individuals and communities. Whether people are healthy or not, is determined by their circumstances and environment. To a large extent, factors such as where we live, the state of our environment, genetics, our income and education level, and our relationships with friends and family all have considerable impacts on health, whereas the more commonly considered factors such as access and use of health care services often have less of an impact. (WHO, 2022b, para. 1)

The awareness that health is a product of the individual's physical and social environment, as well as genetic and behavioral characteristics, justifies public health's focus on the conditions that produce health status:

> The context of people's lives determine their health, and so blaming individuals for having poor health or crediting them for good health

is inappropriate. Individuals are unlikely to be able to directly control many of the determinants of health. (WHO, 2022b, para. 3)

Note that although we talk about the "determinants of health," they are usually discussed in terms of how they relate to poor health—the determinants of poor health. A brief overview of the determinants of health follows.

Physical Environment

Physical environment includes both the natural and built environments. The natural environment is defined by the features of an area that include its topography, weather, soil, water, animal life, and other such attributes; the built environment is defined by the structures that people have created for housing, commerce, transportation, government, recreation, and so forth. Health threats arise from both the physical and built environments. Common health threats related to the natural environment include weather-related disasters such as tornados, hurricanes, and earthquakes, as well as exposure to infectious disease agents that are endemic in a region, such as *Plasmodium falciparum*, the microbe that causes malaria and is endemic in Africa.

Health threats related to the built environment include exposure to toxins and unsafe conditions, particularly in occupational and residential settings where people spend most of their time. Many occupations expose workers to disease-causing substances, high risk of injury, and other physical risks. For example, the greatest health threats to U.S. farm workers are injuries from farm machinery and falls that result in sprains, strains, fractures, and abrasions (Myers, 2001).

In addition, they are subject to "work-related lung diseases, noise-induced hearing loss, skin diseases, and certain cancers associated with chemical use and prolonged sun exposure" (National Institute of Occupational Safety and Health, 2018). There are well-documented health threats to office workers from indoor air pollution, found by research beginning in the 1970s, including passive exposure to tobacco smoke, nitrogen dioxide from gas-fueled cooking stoves, formaldehyde exposure, "radon daughter" exposure, and other health problems encountered in sealed office buildings (Samet et al., 1987; U.S. Environmental Protection Agency, 2006). In residential settings, exposure to pollutants from nearby industrial facilities, power plants, toxic waste sites, or a high volume of traffic presents hazards for many. In the United States, these threats are increasingly known to have a disproportionately heavy impact on low-income and minority communities (CDC, 2003; IOM, 1999).

KEY IDEA

Both the natural and built environments impact the health of individuals living within them—for better or worse.

Social Environment

The **social environment**, as the name implies, is the context defined by our relationships with other people—our social relationships. These relationships occur at all levels of social interaction from societal, to community, to familial, to occupation, and so forth. The formal and informal "rules" that govern our social interactions at each level reflect the values, beliefs, and norms of the group—be it societal, community, family, occupation, or other. These formal and informal rules—and the values, beliefs, and norms they reflect—have historical roots, and they affect how individuals live and behave, their relationships with others, and what resources and opportunities individuals have.

Of particular importance to public health is the role of the social environment in affecting health status and producing health disparities. The CDC defines health disparities as follows:

> Health disparities are preventable differences in the burden of disease, injury, violence, or opportunities to achieve optimal health that are experienced by socially disadvantaged populations. (CDC, 2020, para. 1)

Some people are systematically disadvantaged because of their place in the social environment. In a social setting that values certain characteristics, people with those characteristics are advantaged (e.g., paid more, have greater access to resources, have higher status) compared to those without them.

Socioeconomic status—an attribute conferred to individuals within a social context—provides an example of the social environment's effect on health. In the United States and other Western countries, this aspect is often indicated by a combination of education, occupation, and income/wealth. Persistent and substantial health differences exist between groups defined by socioeconomic status. Socioeconomic status is associated with significant variations in health status and risk for health problems for those with lower status compared to higher status individuals. There is a large literature demonstrating the relationship between socioeconomic status and health, including a gradient in which the higher the socioeconomic status, the better the health (Lynch et al., 2000).

Box 1.2. The Whitehall Study

The famous Whitehall Study of English civil servants in the 1970s was one of the first and most influential to demonstrate the relationship between socioeconomic status and health. In this ingenious study design, participants were chosen to be similar in all but a modest socioeconomic gradient. They were relatively similar in ethnicity, and they were all employed in stable office-based jobs—not subject to industrial hazards, unemployment, or extreme poverty or wealth. They all lived and worked in Greater London and adjoining areas. The study found that within this relatively homogeneous population, there was a gradient in mortality—"each group experiencing a higher mortality than the one above it in the hierarchy. The difference in mortality between the highest and lowest grades was threefold" (Marmot et al., 1995, p. 173).

Similarly, much research indicates that disparities in health status exist between racial and ethnic groups in the United States. Minority Americans, including African Americans, Hispanics/Latinos, Native Americans, and Pacific Islanders, generally have poorer health outcomes than do Whites. The preventable and treatable conditions for which disparities between majority and minority Americans have been shown include diabetes, hypertension, obesity, asthma, and heart disease (CDC, 2011, 2023). Racial disparities in health are linked to racism and the policies and practices within the social environment that express it. These policies and practices prevent or inhibit racial equity in health (Krieger, 2000; Mays et al., 2007).

The CDC explains it this way:

> Racism is a system—consisting of structures, policies, practices, and norms—that assigns value and determines opportunity based on the way people look or the color of their skin. This results in conditions that unfairly advantage some and disadvantage others throughout society.
>
> Racism—both interpersonal and structural—negatively affects the mental and physical health of millions of people, preventing them from attaining their highest level of health, and consequently, affecting the health of our nation. (CDC, 2023, paras. 1 and 2)

Nonphysical occupational factors also affect health. For example, a great deal of research demonstrates the relationship between poor health outcomes and the psychosocial work environment. The demand–control model is one well-known theory, hypothesizing that employees with the highest psychological demands and the lowest decision-making latitude are at the highest risk for poor health outcomes (Karasek et al., 1981, 1998; Theorell, 2000). In addition, job loss and threat of job loss also have a negative impact on health. Evidence suggests that transitions from employment to unemployment adversely affect physical health and psychological well-being among working-age persons (Dooley et al., 1996; Kasl & Jones, 2000; Kasl et al., 1998).

Another large body of research on the social environment and health focuses on social integration, social networks, and social support (Berkman & Glass, 2000). For example, numerous studies over the past 20 years have found that people who are isolated or disengaged from others have a higher risk of premature death. In addition, research has found that survival of cardiovascular disease events and stroke is higher among people with close ties to others, particularly emotional ties. Social relations have been found to predict compliance with medical care recommendations, adaptation to adverse life events such as death of a loved one or natural disaster, and coping with long-term difficulties such as caring for a dependent parent or a disabled child.

A great deal of research in the area of social support was conducted during the 1960s and 1970s. A seminal review article published in 1977 by Kaplan et al. identified methodological issues that needed to be addressed. Since then, there has been further specification of the relationship between social support and health to explain the relationship. For example, Cohen (2004) discusses three factors that indicate different aspects of social relationships: social integration, negative interaction, and social support, each influencing health through different mechanisms. Thoits (1982) reanalyzed data to test the hypothesis that disadvantaged sociodemographic groups such as low-income women are more vulnerable to the effects of life events because they experience more negative events and have fewer psychological resources to cope with them. Although the relationship between social support and health is still not well understood, it is found over and over again in health studies.

KEY IDEA

The social environment encompasses the full range of social relationships from the societal-level to the interpersonal, and its effect is structured by the "rules" that govern social relationships, both formal and informal.

Genetic Inheritance

Our knowledge about the effects of genetic inheritance on health is growing rapidly. Genetic diseases are caused by changes to the normal DNA sequence, in whole or in part. Although genetic disorders can be inherited from family members, others are random occurrences or caused by damage to the genome from environmental exposures (National Human Genome Research Institute, 2018a). It is understood that, with few exceptions, disease processes "are determined both by environmental and by genetic factors. These usually interact, and individuals with a particular set of genes may be either more or less likely, if exposed, to be at risk of developing a particular disease. These effects can be measured by showing that the relative risk of exposure to an environmental factor is significantly greater (or lesser) for the subgroup with the abnormal gene, than the risk in those without" (Pencheon et al., 2001, p. 544).

The Human Genome Project (HGP), which began in 1990, advanced our understanding of biology and disease in order to improve health. "In the years since the HGP's completion there has been much excitement about the potential for so-called 'personalized medicine' to reach the clinic" (National Human Genome Research Institute, 2018b, para. 2). In 2011, a National Academy of Sciences report called for the adoption of "precision medicine"—based on genomics, epigenomics, environmental exposure, and other data—to guide individual diagnosis.

KEY IDEA

An understanding of the role of genetics in the development of disease is another tool in the public health toolbox for preventing and treating health problems.

Health Behavior

The term *health behavior* can refer to behaviors that are beneficial to health. However, the term is generally used in the negative to refer to behaviors that harm health, including smoking, abusing alcohol or other substances, failing to use seat belts or practicing other unsafe behaviors, making unhealthy food choices, and not engaging in adequate physical activity.

The effect of health behaviors on health status has been widely studied and found to be an important determinant of health. Consider the 10 leading causes of death in the United States in 2019 (pre-COVID), as characterized by diagnosed diseases or conditions in the general population (Heron, 2021):

- Diseases of the heart;
- Malignant neoplasms (cancer);
- Unintentional injuries (accidents);
- Chronic lower respiratory diseases
- Cerebrovascular diseases (stroke);
- Alzheimer disease;
- Diabetes mellitus;
- Nephritis, nephrotic syndrome, and nephrosis;
- Influenza and pneumonia; and
- Intentional self-harm (suicide).

These 10 causes accounted for about 75% of all deaths, and the first two accounted for approximately half of all deaths. Moreover, health behaviors including poor nutrition, physical inactivity, tobacco use, unsafe motor vehicle use, alcohol and drug use, failure to vaccinate, and others contributed substantially to these figures. In one way or another, personal health behavior has an impact on the occurrence in any given individual of most of the diseases and conditions on this list.

Looking at the cause of death in a different way (i.e., by major contributing cause of the disease to which the death was attributed rather than by the disease itself), in the first study of its kind, McGinnis and Foege (1993) showed that, as of 1990, the leading factors were tobacco use, dietary patterns, sedentary lifestyle, alcohol consumption, microbial agents, toxic agents, firearms, sexual behavior, motor vehicles, and use of illicit drugs. As of 2002, the situation remained the same (McGinnis et al., 2002)—making the case for more active policy attention to health promotion.

Examining premature mortality by race and ethnicity adds information about the impact of health behaviors on health. In the United States, premature mortality is death before age 75 years, the approximate average age of death in the population. Studies of premature mortality in the 21st century indicate that it is significantly associated with health behaviors related to substance abuse. Further, two race/ethnicity groups are particularly affected at the present time:

Though increases in total U.S. mortality trends are recent, pronounced heterogeneity in death rates has been documented across age and racial/ethnic groups for the last two decades. Premature mortality rates among Hispanic, non-Hispanic Black/African American (i.e., Black) and Asian/Pacific Islander (API) men and women declined steadily during the 21st century. In contrast, notable increases have occurred among young and middle-age non-Hispanic White (i.e., White) and American Indian/Alaska Natives (AIANs) during the same time period. (Best et al., 2018, p. 2)

These increases in mortality rates are explained by increases in accidental deaths, suicide, and chronic liver disease/cirrhosis deaths.

- Increases in accidental deaths result from unintentional drug poisonings, as motor vehicle accident deaths have declined.

- Opioid overdoses are a major contributor to the increases in drug poisonings, including prescription opioids, heroin, and fentanyl, despite recent policies to curb the opioid epidemic (Best et al., 2018).

Figure 1.1 illustrates these trends in mortality rates for men and women, ages 25 to 64.

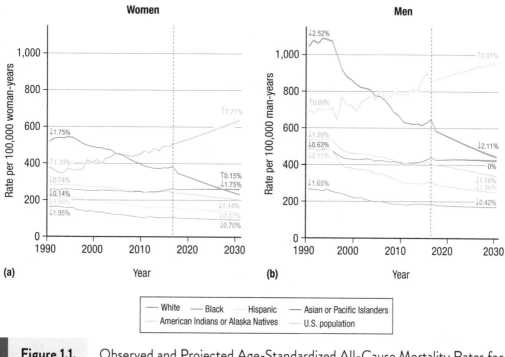

Figure 1.1.   Observed and Projected Age-Standardized All-Cause Mortality Rates for Those Aged 25 to 64 Years

Source: Best, A. F., Haozous, E. A., Berrington de Gonzalez, A., Chernyavskiy, P., Freedman, N. D., Hartge, P., Thomas, D., Rosenberg, P. S., & Shiels, M. S. (2018). Premature mortality projections in the USA through 2030: A modelling study. *The Lancet, 3*(8), E374–E384. https://www.thelancet.com/pdfs/journals/lanpub/PIIS2468 -2667(18)30114-2.pdf

KEY IDEA

Unhealthy behaviors exert a negative impact on mortality, morbidity, and disability and continue to focus public health prevention efforts.

Health Care as a Determinant of Health

If we argue that health is the product of multiple factors including genetic inheritance, the physical environment, and the social environment, as well as an individual's behavioral and biologic response to these factors, we see that health care has an impact late in the causal chain leading to disease, illness, and injury. Often by the time the individual interacts with the health care system, the determinants of health have had their impact on their health status, for better or for worse. Thus, the need for health care may be seen as a failure to prevent the determinants of health from adversely affecting the individual patient.

The success of any health care system is affected by the other determinants of health. Genetic predisposition to breast cancer may limit the long-term success rates of cancer treatment. Continued exposure to toxins in the environment or at work may decrease the likelihood that the physician can stabilize an individual with allergies. Health behaviors, such as smoking or substance abuse, may stymie the best health care system when treating an individual with lung disease. The lack of support at home for changes in behaviors or adherence to medical regimens may undermine the ability of the health care system to successfully treat an individual with diabetes. Poverty, race, and ethnicity often limit access to health care, and therefore, the ability of physicians to diagnose and treat health problems effectively (Smedley et al., 2003). We recognize that health, as well as health care, exist within a biological, physical, and social context, and all of these factors influence the probability of a health care system's success.

KEY IDEA

Health care is only one determinant of health, the need for which can be reduced by prevention efforts focused on the other health determinants—the social and physical environments, genetic predisposition, and health behavior.

Relationships Among the Determinants of Health

The determinants of health do not act independently of each other. They are interconnected, and the concepts of ecology provide the framework for understanding how to model their interconnectedness. In the most general sense, the ecological approach means that the person is viewed as embedded in the environment—both social and physical—and is both influenced by and influences that environment. Stokols (1996) outlines the history of ecology, and social ecology, which are fundamental to the public health perspective and its practice:

> The term ecology refers to the study of the relationships between organisms and their environments. Early ecological analyses of the relations between plant and animal populations and their natural habitats were later extended and applied to the study of human communities and environments within the fields of sociology, psychology, and public health. The field of social ecology, which emerged during the mid-1960s and early 1970s, gives greater attention to the social, institutional, and cultural contexts of people–environment relations than did earlier versions of human ecology, which focused primarily on biologic processes and the geographic environment. (p. 285)

Stokols (1996) identifies core principles of social ecology that make it an appropriate overarching paradigm for public health. First, ecological models may include all aspects of the environment that impact health, including physical, social, and cultural aspects. Second, ecological models include characteristics of individuals, and, for example, can incorporate their genetic heritage, psychological attributes, and behavioral practices. Third, concepts from systems theory are used to understand the interplay between environmental and individual characteristics and their mutual influence on health.

> For instance, people–environment transactions are characterized by cycles of mutual influence, in which the physical and social features of settings directly influence occupants' health and, concurrently, the participants in settings modify the healthfulness of their surroundings through their individual and collective actions. (p. 286)

Fourth, the ecological perspective emphasizes the interdependence of all factors contributing to health, including the nearby and distant factors, as well as those in different domains such as family, work, neighborhood, and community.

> Thus, efforts to promote human health must take into account the interdependencies that exist among immediate and more distant environments (e.g., the "spill-over" of workplace and commuting stress to residential environments, and the influence of state and national ordinances on the healthfulness of occupational settings). (Stokols, 1996, p. 286)

Fifth, the ecological perspective is interdisciplinary. With the multitude of factors that affect human health, many disciplines are required to understand the interplay among them and their effect on health and to bring about health improvement. "Thus, ecologically based health research incorporates multiple levels of analysis and diverse methodologies . . . for assessing the healthfulness of settings and the well-being of persons and groups" (Stokols, 1996, p. 286). Thus, the interdisciplinary perspective is required for public health practice.

The classic 1959 book, *Mirage of Health*, by René Dubos provides an example of how the ecological approach is applied to understanding human health. Dubos describes the causes of the tuberculosis epidemic in the tenements of 1900 New York City and other U.S. cities at that time. He recounts:

> The story of the roundabout way in which a microscopic fungus proba- bly native to Central America destroyed the potato crop in Ireland and exerted thereby a dramatic influence on the destiny of the Irish people, illustrating the complexity of the interplay between the external envi- ronment and the affairs of man. (pp. 96–97)

Dubos's description of the factors contributing to the development of the tu- berculosis epidemic includes international exploration and trade by Europeans subsequent to the 15th century that transported a native plant, the wild potato, from the Andes to Ireland and elsewhere in Europe; the improvement of the wild potato in Europe for large yields, which made the plant more susceptible to in- fection than the wild varieties; a fungus that accompanied the potato to Europe and was benign until it was enabled by unusually wet weather conditions to proliferate and destroy the potato crop in 1845 and 1846 in Ireland; the growth of the Irish population from 3.5 to 8 million between 1700 and 1840; the de- pendence on the potato for sustenance among the burgeoning Irish population; the political and economic dependence of Ireland on England that resulted in the food shortage following the destruction of the 1845 and 1846 potato crops; the disaster that followed in which a million Irish died of starvation and many more became susceptible to disease; and finally, the mass emigration from Ireland to the United States in the middle of the 19th century, when the immigrants took up residence in the crowded and unhealthy conditions of the tenements of indus- trial cities along the Atlantic coast.

> The profound upheaval in their way of life made them ready victims to all sorts of infection. The sudden and dramatic increase of tuberculosis mortality in the Philadelphia, New York, and Boston areas around 1850 can be traced in large part to the Irish immigrants who settled in these cities at that time. (Dubos, 1959, p. 100)

Dubos's account included many determinants of health, including aspects of the social environment, the physical environment, and individual behavior. Interest- ingly, he does not mention health care, nor its absence, as a factor leading to the tuberculosis epidemic, but then there was little that medicine offered at that time for the treatment of tuberculosis. His analysis of events incorporated the "causes of causes," which were political, economic, and cultural. These included the im- petus among Europeans to explore and trade that caused the transport of the wild potato from Central America to Europe; the application of scientific princi- ples to farming that caused the improvement of the potato; the political and eco- nomic relationships between Ireland and England that caused the dependence of the Irish on the potato for food; and so forth. We understand the disease, not only in terms of immediate individual actions, for example, sanitary habits of the individuals with tuberculosis, but in terms of societal attributes that reach back into history and relate to political and economic events and policies of the times.

Dubos's account exemplifies the ecological approach to understanding the causes of poor health—in this case, tuberculosis—which is the foundation of the public health orientation. Dubos's account links the determinants of health in a causal chain that ends in illness, disability, and premature death in the tenements of 19th-century American cities.

ECOLOGICAL MODELS AND PUBLIC HEALTH PRACTICE

The environment, or context, influences the way people live and their health outcomes, for better or for worse. That is, context can have positive or negative impacts on the health of individuals.

KEY IDEA

As a field, public health attempts to maintain or create healthy contexts in which people live and prevent or dismantle unhealthy contexts—to promote health and reduce morbidity, disability, and premature mortality.

The way in which public health attempts to affect contexts is the story of public health practice, and public health practice reflects public health ecological models. However, the ecological models in use change over time to respond to the health problems predominant in their day and incorporate the knowledge, beliefs, values, and resources of that time and place.

For example, in times and places where infectious diseases are predominant, models reflect the issues required to understand their spread and control. A classic public health model that uses the ecological approach for understanding and preventing disease is the epidemiologic triangle with its agent–host–environment triad. The epidemiologic triangle (see **Figure 1.2**) was developed and is used to understand infectious disease transmission and to provide a model for preventing transmission, and thus, infectious disease outbreaks. The three points of the triangle are the agent, host, and environment. The agent is the microbial organism that

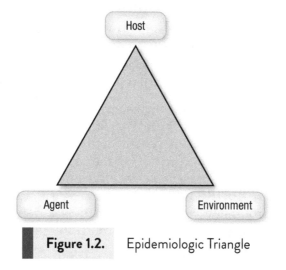

Figure 1.2.   Epidemiologic Triangle

causes the infectious disease—virus, bacterium, protozoan, or fungus; the host is the organism that harbors the agent; and the environmental aspects included in an epidemiologic triangle are those factors that facilitate transmission of the agent to the host. These could be aspects of the natural environment, the built environment, or the social environment, including policies. Time is considered in the triangle as the period between exposure to the agent and when the illness occurs; the period that it takes to recover from illness; or the period it takes an outbreak to subside. Prevention measures are those that disrupt the relationship between at least two of the factors in the triangle—agent, host, and environment.

Although there are no explicitly specified environmental factors included in the epidemiologic triangle, the environment is central to conceptualizing disease transmission among individuals at risk (the hosts). The environment is the total of factors that enable the agent to infect the host. The environmental factors specified in the model can include, depending upon the disease itself, an array of social and physical attributes that permit the agent to infect the host. For example, Friis and Sellers (1996) have written:

- The external environment is the sum total of influences that are not part of the host and comprises physical, climatologic, biologic, social, and economic components.
- The physical environment includes weather, temperature, humidity, geologic formations, and similar physical dimensions.
- The social environment is the totality of the behavioral, personality, attitudinal, and cultural characteristics of a group of people.
- Both physical and social environments impact agents of disease and potential hosts because the environment may either increase or decrease the survival of disease agents and bring agent and host into contact.

Because infectious diseases have a single agent, the epidemiological triangle works well as a model for understanding the development of these diseases. In the case of other kinds of diseases or health problems, it is not as helpful because of its emphasis on a single agent, its isolation of the agent from the environment, and its conceptually unspecified environment.

The wheel of causation is another model exemplifying the ecological approach (see Figure 1.3). It has also been used, but not as extensively as the epidemiological triangle, for explaining infectious disease transmission. However, it has some advantages over the epidemiological triangle, as Peterson (1995) notes:

> Although it is not used as often as the epidemiological triangle model, it has several appealing attributes. . . . For instance, the wheel contains a hub with the host at its center. For our use, humans represent the host. Also, surrounding the host is the total environment divided into the biological, physical, and social environments. These divisions, of course, are not true divisions—there are considerable interactions among the environment types. Although it is a general model, the wheel of causation does illustrate the multiple etiological factors of human infectious diseases. (p. 147)

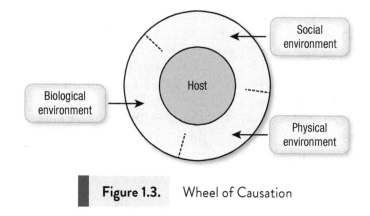

Figure 1.3.   Wheel of Causation

In general, every ecological model explaining the development of health (or poor health) contains a set of distal causes related to the environment—physical and/or social—and a set of proximal causes related to the individual—primarily behavioral. One of the major issues in developing public health models is where to place the emphasis and, thus, where to intervene to improve health. Is it at the individual level or at the environmental level? This issue is at the heart of public health practice.

Therefore, in the simplest conceptualization of prevention strategies, we have two choices: We can focus our efforts on changing individual behavior directly or on changing the environment in which individual behavior occurs. For example, after examining Dubos's description of the development of the tuberculosis epidemics of the 1850s in the northeastern cities of the United States, we might decide that tuberculosis should have been prevented by focusing on the sanitary habits of the Irish immigrants, which would have reduced the spread of disease from person to person. These habits might have included handwashing, housekeeping, food preparation practices, and so forth. Changing behavior might have taken the form of encouraging compliance through education or coercing compliance through surveillance and laws.

On the other hand, we might decide that the tuberculosis epidemics should have been prevented by changing the social, political, or physical environments. For instance, if the cities to which the Irish emigrated had provided more healthful housing and working conditions, the Irish immigrants would not have been as susceptible to illness, including tuberculosis. We might have targeted the crowding and other relevant conditions in the neighborhoods where the immigrants came to live. Thus, instead of motivating individuals to change their behavior— through education—we might argue that we could have changed the physical environment to reduce the spread of tuberculosis.

Alternatively, stepping further back in the causal chain, we might decide that the political environment in Ireland should have been the focus of intervention. If England had provided aid to the Irish during the potato blight, the Irish would not have perished in such numbers, and survivors, poor and already weakened by famine, would not have been motivated to emigrate to the United States where they were highly susceptible to tuberculosis. On the other hand, going back even further, we might decide that the undiversified diet of the Irish should have been the subject of intervention. If the Irish food supply had been diversified, the potato blight would not have become a crisis for the people of that country. Again, this was a political decision on the part of the English. Thus, political strategies might be proposed that would have changed the environment, and, thus, prevented the tuberculosis epidemics of the 1850s in the United States.

The general ecological model is extremely flexible and can assume many different forms. The model becomes differentiated when a specific health problem is identified for intervention in a particular time and place. The ecological models developed beginning in the 1960s in response to the increased importance of chronic diseases made a significant departure from the classic models such as the epidemiologic triangle and the wheel of causation (see Figure 1.3) used for infectious disease control and prevention. Let us explain.

Health Promotion and the Ecological Models in Public Health Since 1960

Beginning in the 1960s, the models explaining health status became increasingly limited to the behavioral determinants of health such as smoking, sedentary lifestyle, poor dietary habits, unprotected sexual activity, and failure to use seat belts, which placed the focus of public health interventions on changing individuals rather than their context. The watchwords of this trend were health promotion and disease prevention. As Green (1999) states, 1974 was a turning point when health promotion was accepted as a significant component of health policy. In a classic review of the rise in importance of health promotion, McLeroy et al. (1988) summarized the events and initiatives characterizing the ascendance during the 1970s and 1980s:

> Within the private sector, this interest in health promotion has led to the extensive development and implementation of health promotion programs in the worksite, increases in the marketing of "healthy" foods, and increased societal interest in fitness. In the public sector this interest has led to national campaigns to control hypertension and cholesterol, the establishment of the Office of Disease Prevention and Health Promotion within the Public Health Service and the Center for Health Promotion and Education within the Centers for Disease Control [and Prevention], the development and implementation of community-wide health promotion programs by both governmental agencies and private foundations, and the establishment and monitoring of the 1990 Objectives for the Nation in health promotion. (p. 352)

Emphasis on health promotion was evident in publication of the *Lalonde Report* in Canada, John Knowles's "The Responsibility of the Individual," the Surgeon General's report on *Health Promotion/Disease Prevention in the United States*, and *Health Promotion: A Discussion Document on the Concept and Principles* in Europe. New journals were devoted exclusively to articles on health promotion programs and activities while existing journals both within and outside of traditional public health disciplines had theme issues on health promotion topics. International conferences on health promotion were held and health education training programs begun (McLeroy et al., 1988).

The emphasis on health promotion, however, increasingly emphasized public health initiatives at the individual behavior level, rather than the environmental level. Programs to help people stop smoking, lose weight, increase exercise, eat healthier foods, and so forth proliferated, and these programs were predominantly aimed at educating and motivating individuals to change unhealthy behaviors. These initiatives were in contrast to historic interventions such as sewage disposal or food inspection, which emphasized changing the environment, as we will explore in the Chapter 2.

PRECEDE–PROCEED and Health Promotion

By and large, health promotion programs used the now well-known model for conceptualizing community health promotion and planning: Green and Kreuter's (1991, 1999) **PRECEDE–PROCEED** model. The PRECEDE–PROCEED model was developed in the 1970s and has been applied since then with a few modifications in the 1990s, which we discuss shortly. PRECEDE stands for *Pre*disposing, *R*einforcing, and *E*nabling *C*onstructs in *E*ducational *D*iagnosis and *E*valuation. Green and Kreuter (1991) define predisposing factors as:

> . . . a person's or population's knowledge, attitudes, beliefs, values, and perceptions that facilitate or hinder motivation for change. Enabling factors are those skills, resources, or barriers that can help or hinder the desired behavioral changes as well as environmental changes. . . . Reinforcing factors, the rewards received, and the feedback the learner receives from others following adoption of the behavior, may encourage or discourage continuation of the behavior. (pp. 28–29)

PROCEED stands for *P*olicy, *R*egulatory, and *O*rganizational *C*onstructs in *E*ducational and *E*nvironmental *D*evelopment.

As the acronym PRECEDE denotes, the model is oriented toward improving health by changing individuals' behaviors through education, and not toward intervening at the environmental level to change conditions or structures. The question structured by the PRECEDE–PROCEED model is, "Why do people behave badly, that is, engage in unhealthy behaviors?" In addition, the first part of the two-part answer to this question, which is emphasized by PRECEDE–PROCEED, is lack of knowledge. Thus, education about the risks of certain behaviors and the benefits of others is a primary component of health promotion initiatives. These include initiatives to modify unfavorable dietary habits, sedentary lifestyle, substance abuse, smoking, and unsafe practices such as failure to use seat belts or follow safety precautions at work.

The second part of the answer structured by the PRECEDE–PROCEED model is related to attributes of the individual that hinder behavior change, including motivation to change, appraisal of threat, self-efficacy, response efficacy, and so forth. That is, once the knowledge about health behaviors is conveyed, the challenge is to motivate individuals to change their behavior from risky to healthy. Knowledge alone is not sufficient to bring about change in health behaviors.

Thus, a major tool of health promotion is the application of psychological theories to understand why people engage in unhealthy behaviors and how to stimulate them to modify these behaviors. A number of the most influential theories applied to health behavior include the Health Belief Model developed by Becker (1974); the Theory of Reasoned Action (Ajzen & Fishbein, 1980); the Protection Motivation Theory (Rogers, 1983); Bandura's (1986) Social Cognitive Theory, which emphasizes self-efficacy; and the Social Learning Theory (Rosenstock et al., 1988). These theories underlie the methods used in health promotion initiatives to motivate health behavior change.

The original PRECEDE–PROCEED model was described by Green in 1974. That version visualizes the assumed causal chain, which shows that behavioral problems produce health problems, which then, in turn, produce social problems, such as illegitimacy, unemployment, absenteeism, hostility, alienation, discrimination, riots, and crime. The effect of the environment on individual behavior is assumed under enabling factors such as availability of resources, accessibility, and referrals and reinforcing factors such as attitudes of program personnel. However, note that this is a very restricted environment, which is limited to the immediate setting of the health education program. There is also a nonbehavioral factors box in the model's algorithm, which contributes to health problems and could contain larger environmental factors, but is not the main focus of the model and is not seen as contributing to behavior problems.

Box 1.3. PRECEDE–PROCEED Applied to Safety in the Workplace

As an example of the use of the PRECEDE–PROCEED model, DeJoy (1996) describes how the model would be applied to workplace safety:

In the PRECEDE model, three sets of factors drive the prevention strategies.
Predisposing factors are the characteristics of the individual (beliefs, attitudes, values, etc.) and are conceptualized as providing the motivation for safety-related behavior—either safe or unsafe behavior. Threat-related beliefs and efficacy expectancies would be included here.
Enabling factors refer to objective aspects of the environment or system that block or promote safe or unsafe behaviors in the workplace. The skill and knowledge necessary to engage safely in the workplace would be included here, as would the availability and accessibility of protective equipment and other resources. Most barriers or costs would be classified as enabling factors.
Reinforcing factors involve any reward or punishment that follows or is anticipated as a consequence of the behavior. Performance feedback and the social approval/disapproval received from coworkers, supervisors, and managers would qualify as reinforcing factors in workplace settings.

(continued)

Clearly, the target for intervention in this example is the worker and their motivation to avoid workplace injuries. This orientation is apparent, when the author describes the predisposing factors as "providing the motivation for behavior," and also includes the worker's psychological factors such as beliefs about threat and efficacy. Enabling factors "allow motivation or aspiration to be realized" and include the worker's skill and knowledge. It is plain that the intervention strategy is to induce the practice of safety through education that enables the worker; application of psychological theories that address the worker's predisposing attitudes, beliefs, and values related to safety practices; and rewards or punishments that reinforce the worker's safety-related behavior.

Importantly, the environment—in this case, the physical workplace and the people who manage it—is seen as reinforcing and enabling the worker to engage in safety habits, but not as the target of the intervention. Rather, improving workplace safety is focused on motivating the individual worker to practice safety habits, not motivating the employer or the larger society to modify the workplace. The individual worker's motivation to practice workplace safety is the subject of the intervention, and the worker is viewed as the accountable party.

Also, note that the environment is quite proscribed. Its bounds are the specific workplace itself. The environment, in this example, does not include larger political and economic factors that may affect what occurs within the workplace. For instance, the political and economic factors that impact the availability of protective equipment and other resources required for safety are not considered. Regulations governing safety in the workplace are not considered, nor are the enforcement of regulations. This example is typical of health promotion programs, particularly through the 1990s. The larger environment could certainly be incorporated into the model, but it usually was not.

Why Health Promotion?

The health promotion trend, whereby the target of public health interventions was individuals' behavior instead of the environment, was, in part, because of the view that the distal causes of poor health—physical and social environmental factors including cultural, economic, and political factors—were too difficult to change.

Also, health promotion was tied to the desire for health care cost containment. Educating individuals about health was seen as a way to make people more self-sufficient in health, engage in self-care, and become better-informed consumers of health services. Because of concern about spiraling health care costs in the 1960s and onward, health promotion was presented as a means to control costs through the demand side (Green, 1999). This can be seen in the proliferation of research studies undertaken to improve health care utilization and decrease unhealthy behaviors through educational interventions for patients/consumers. Practitioners and funders of health services and public health research saw this effort as a "magic bullet" solution for behavioral problems presented to medical care and public health. Highly controlled randomized trials and fine-grained behavioral research resulted, testing ways to improve patient compliance.

They included ways to reduce broken appointments, make seeking medical care more appropriate, improve smoking cessation, and so forth. "The targets of the magic bullet interventions were as much those behaviors thought to account for some of the unnecessary and inappropriate uses of health services as those accounting for leading causes of death or disability" (p. 75).

It was also apparent that individual behaviors such as smoking, sedentary lifestyle, and poor dietary habits were highly related to the onset and progression of chronic diseases such as heart disease, pulmonary disease, and diabetes. If risky health behaviors could be changed, it was argued, the incidence of chronic diseases would be reduced. Of course, this is true.

KEY IDEA

The question, however, is whether trying to motivate individuals to change their behavior—through education, incentives, and disincentives—is the most effective and just means of accomplishing this goal. Is placing accountability for behavior change onto the individual, without changing the environment in which that behavior occurs, realistic and fair?

Criticisms of Health Promotion

Placing the locus of accountability for poor health on the individual is one of the major criticisms of the health promotion movement. Viewing the individual's behavior as the problem to be "fixed," rather than the context in which that behavior occurs, is seen as "blaming the victim." Under this view, the context of people's lives structures their health behaviors to a large degree, and so blaming individuals for having poor health behaviors is ineffective and unfair. For example, poor people and those of minority groups often live in neighborhoods with supermarkets that carry limited amounts of healthy foods, especially fruits and vegetables. Their shelves predominate, instead, with high-fat, high-sodium snack foods that have little nutritional value (Moore & Roux, 2006). Does the fairer and more effective public health intervention, aimed at improving the diet of people in such neighborhoods, target the residents themselves or the supermarkets? These are the kinds of questions that arise from the debate over the PRECEDE–PROCEED model.

Not surprisingly, beginning in the 1980s, the pendulum began to swing back to a focus on environmentally targeted interventions and an interest in understanding the interaction between individuals and their environment. Because of the "blaming-the-victim" argument, as well as the recognition that health education was not as effective as it had once been thought to be, interest in alternatives to the health promotion approach intensified. As Green himself noted in 1999, "The dominant emphasis has shifted from psychological and behavioral factors, which lend themselves to precise measure, to more difficult to measure and control factors, such as social, cultural, and political ones" (Green & Kreuter, 1999, p. 8). Further:

> In 1986, the First International Conference on Health Promotion produced the Ottawa Charter, which helped reorient policy, programs, and practices away from these proximal risk factors. The shift that followed was to the more distal risk factors in time, space, or scope, which we shall call risk conditions. These also influence health, either through the risk factors or by operating directly on human biology over time, but they are less likely than risk factors to be under the control of the individual at risk. (Green & Kreuter, 1999, p. 10)

Consistent with the pendulum swing, Green and Kreuter revised the PRECEDE–PROCEED model in 1991 to place more emphasis on the context of behavior. With respect to incorporating environmental influences, the model now contains a box in the model's algorithm labeled *environment*, which notably both influences and is influenced by behavior and lifestyle. This change in the PRECEDE–PROCEED model makes it in keeping with the general ecological model, which assumes that individuals are affected by their environment. In addition, the model now includes a policy regulation organization factor, which impacts the enabling factors and, through these, the environment. The main features and causal assumptions of the 1974 PRECEDE–PROCEED model remain the same—predisposing, reinforcing, and enabling factors affect behavior and lifestyle, which, in turn, impact health.

In 1999, Green and Kreuter made minor modifications to the PRECEDE–PROCEED model, and enlarged the role of the environment in their description of the factors influencing behavior. The risk factors and risk conditions—together with factors predisposing, enabling, and reinforcing them—are referred to in the PRECEDE–PROCEED model collectively as the determinants of health.

> These include adequate housing; secure income; healthful and safe community and work environment; enforcement of policies and regulations controlling the manufacture, marketing, labeling, and sale of potentially harmful products; and the use of these products (such as alcohol and tobacco) where they can harm others. (p. 10)

The PRECEDE–PROCEED model was once again revised in 2022 with improvements to conceptualizing the evaluation of programs. See **Figure 1.4**.

Although the revised models place more emphasis on the environment, the focus was still on providing a blueprint for changing the individual's behavior through education and relying on psychological theories for understanding how to motivate behavioral change. The context is identified in the models as necessary to achieve individual behavioral changes. However, in practice, changes to the context within health promotion programs are usually still limited and proscribed to the immediate setting. They do not aim to change underlying social structures or other larger environmental factors. See, for example, Lieberman et al. (2013) for a discussion.

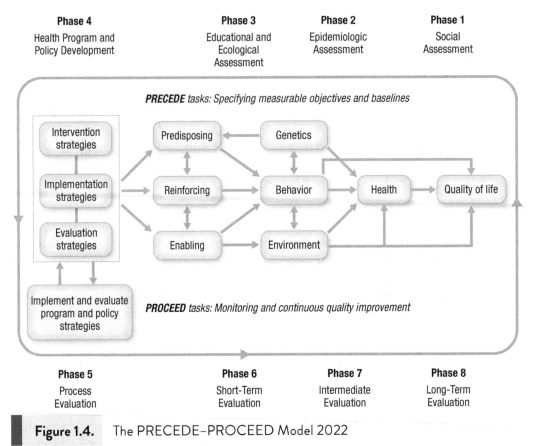

Figure 1.4. The PRECEDE–PROCEED Model 2022

Source: Green, L. W. (2022). *The PRECEDE-PROCEED model 2022 edition.* https://www.lgreen.net/precede -proceed-2022-edition

Population Health and Reemphasis of the Social Environment in Public Health Models

At the same time that health promotion was coming under attack, the population health approach was introduced and began to gain followers in the field of public health. Stirred by antipathy toward the emphasis on interventions that used education and psychologically based strategies to motivate individuals to change their behavior rather than changing the context or structure in which behavior occurs, this approach to public health focused on the distal social environment—power, wealth, and status—as the root cause of health problems. The evidence supporting this approach is the large body of research on disparities or inequalities in health status between the rich and the poor, the powerful and powerless, and those of high social status and those of low status. Incontrovertible findings that an individual's social status, wealth, and power have a profound influence on their chances of being healthy underwrite the population health approach to public health. The Whitehall study was one of the first to demonstrate what has become a consistent finding—people who are structurally disadvantaged are far more likely than the advantaged to have poor health.

Studies have asked, "Why do some people exercise and others do not?" "Why do some people eat nutritious foods and others do not?" "Why do some people lead sedentary lives and others do not?" "Why do some communities have support groups for behavior change and others do not?" "Why do some communities have opportunities for exercise and relaxation and others do not?" "Why are some communities free from toxic substances in the environment and others are not?" The answers are in the unequal distribution of power, wealth, and status that give the advantaged the opportunities and resources to live in healthier environments, engage in healthier behaviors, and have access to better health care.

As Marmot (2005) states:

> The gross inequalities in health that we see within and between countries present a challenge to the world. That there should be a spread of life expectancy of 48 years among countries and 20 years or more within countries is not inevitable. A burgeoning volume of research identifies social factors (i.e., wealth, power, and status) at the root of much of these inequalities in health. Social determinants are relevant to communicable and non-communicable disease alike. (p. 1099)

The population health approach has led to studies such as the research by Pickard et al. (2009) that offers explanations for undesirable health behaviors in terms of the social context of the individual. That is, the social context is viewed as having a causal impact on health behaviors.

The population health perspective is leading to more complex public health models that integrate distal and proximal social factors, physical environmental factors, and behavioral factors to predict disease, disability, and premature death. Health behaviors are viewed as patterned by the social environment, not "free-standing" (Chan et al., 2008; Purslow et al., 2008). For example, a recent study of the original Whitehall participants who have been followed for 24 years (Stringhini et al., 2010) investigated the role of health behaviors in the relationship between socioeconomic position and mortality. The behaviors studied included smoking, alcohol consumption, diet, and physical activity. The authors found that "there was an association between socioeconomic position and mortality that was substantially accounted for by adjustment for health behaviors, particularly when the behaviors were assessed repeatedly" (p. 1159).

Among champions of population health, the commitment to social justice is at the heart of public health's promise:

> Health disparities/inequalities include differences between the most advantaged group in a given category—e.g., the wealthiest, the most powerful racial/ethnic group—and all others, not only between the best and worst-off groups. Pursuing health equity means pursuing the elimination of such health disparities/inequalities. (Braveman, 2006, p. 167)

Everyone, not only the rich, the powerful, or those with social standing, is entitled to the conditions that produce health. It is in the tradition of public health to advocate for those who have unequal access to opportunities and resources in society as well as those with advantages, following in the footsteps of the public health engineering era, when people in all stations of life were provided with clean water, sewage and garbage disposal, and a clean food supply in the cities of industrializing nations.

Behavioral Versus Environmental Causes of Health Problems

Over the last 50 years, the emphasis of public health initiatives on behavior, rather than on environment, became widespread. Even though the ecological approach of public health views the individual as embedded in a physical and social environment and affected by it, the health promotion orientation led to an emphasis on behavior and a de-emphasis on the environment—both physical and social.

The President's Cancer Panel report (2010) provides an example of the divergence in orientation that has occurred and still exists. The report, *Reducing Environmental Cancer Risk: What We Can Do Now*, is unlike previous presidents' reports, which focused on individual behaviors, diagnosis, and treatment rather than the risk of environmental exposures. The 2010 report found that "a growing body of research documents myriad established and suspected environmental factors linked to genetic, immune, and endocrine dysfunction that can lead to cancer and other diseases." The panel advised that the "true burden of environmentally induced cancers has been grossly underestimated," and that the current estimates of 2% of all cancers caused by environmental toxins and 4% by occupational exposures is outdated.

DID YOU KNOW?

Of the more than 80,000 chemicals used in the United States today, only a few hundred have been tested for health effects. Environmental contaminants come from industrial and manufacturing processes, agriculture, household products, medical technologies, military practices, and the natural environment.

Reducing Environmental Cancer Risk: What We Can Do Now argues that the problem has not been addressed adequately by the National Cancer Program, which has focused on individual behaviors, screening, diagnosis, and treatment. It finds the current regulatory approach reactionary rather than precautionary—a substance's danger must be demonstrated incontrovertibly before action is taken to reduce exposure to it. Therefore, the "public bears the burden of proving that a given environmental exposure is harmful" (President's Cancer Panel, 2010, p. ii).

The still-existing tension between those who emphasize behavioral and those who emphasize environmental causes is demonstrated in the reaction to the 2010 President's Report. The panel urged the president to act on its findings, but reaction to the report was critical from Michael Thun, Vice President of Epidemiology and Surveillance Research at the American Cancer Society, who tried to bring the focus back to behavior. As reported in *The New York Times* (Grady, 2010), Dr. Thun stated that the report was "unbalanced by its implication that pollution is the major cause of cancer." Further:

> . . . Suggesting that the risk is much higher, when there is no proof, may divert attention from things that are much bigger causes of cancer, like smoking. If we could get rid of tobacco, we could get rid of 30 percent of cancer deaths, he said, adding that poor nutrition, obesity, and lack of exercise are also greater contributors to cancer risk than pollution. (Grady, 2010, para. 7–9)

This discussion exemplifies some of the complexities of taking a primary prevention approach to health, that is, to prevent health problems from beginning. There are many choices made when determining how to improve or maintain health, and one is the choice between an individual- or environmental-level intervention. Given the premise of the ecological model—that individuals are embedded in an environment, which they both influence and are influenced by—both components of the model are relevant.

Within the ecological model, both the individual and the context are potential sites of public health interventions, and both have been employed throughout the history of public health. For example, in the early part of the 20th century, there were interventions that focused on the individual level—teaching and encouraging individuals in immigrant communities to engage in certain health behaviors, such as handwashing, that prevent infectious diseases—and those that focused on the environmental level, notably the environmental engineering interventions that brought clean water, safe food supply, and sanitary disposal of waste to these communities and also prevented the spread of infectious diseases.

The emphasis on environmental over individual-level interventions changes over time, as we have seen in the discussion of public health models since 1960. Neither approach is ever entirely abandoned, but in different eras one may be emphasized over the other. Indeed, a study of tuberculosis control in the 19th and 20th centuries led Fairchild and Oppenheimer (1998) to argue for a more nuanced approach to public health practice in which strategies that address both individual and environmental causes of disease with broad and targeted interventions are employed.

KEY IDEA

"If the relative contribution of different interventions and factors is to be sorted out, pursuit of monocausal explanations for the retreat of TB, like monotypic intervention, is insufficient." (Fairchild & Oppenheimer, 1998, p. 1113)

These and other decisions about how to promote and maintain health in populations go to the heart of public health practice. Public health, as a field, plans and initiates prevention activities—primary, secondary, and tertiary. However, many important choices about these activities translate the public health mission into public health practice. Several choices are central to the actuality of public health:

- What health problems are addressed?
- Where interventions are targeted—environmental, individual, or multilevel?
- If targeted at the environmental level, are interventions focused on distal or proximal factors?
- Are methods voluntary or coercive?
- Are activities public or private enterprises?
- If private, are activities nonprofit or profit-making?

To clarify these choices and how they impact practice, we can examine the provision of clean water in the United States. Although water treatment has been practiced throughout human history as far back as 2000 BCE in ancient Greece and India, before the mid-1850s the motivation to treat water, usually with some form of filtering, was to improve taste and reduce turbidity. In the mid-1800s, the need to treat water to prevent infectious disease outbreaks was beginning to be understood, even before we knew that water could contain microorganisms that caused these diseases. How water became associated with specific diseases is the story of one of the most famous public health achievements—John Snow's identification, through application of epidemiologic principles, of the Broad Street pump as the source of the 1853 cholera epidemic in London. His work refused the belief that cholera was spread by "miasma in the atmosphere." The fascinating story is told at the end of the chapter in Appendix 1.1.

Knowledge about disease-causing microorganisms increased dramatically during the remainder of the 19th century because of advances in the microscope and other instruments. Cholera, typhoid, hepatitis, and other infectious diseases were understood to be waterborne and controllable through water treatment. Because of the tremendous death toll from such diseases, by the advent of the 20th century, water purification was considered an important public health issue, and methods to provide clean water were underway. The filtration systems of the past had been somewhat, but not entirely, effective against waterborne diseases. The first widely used method to eliminate waterborne disease organisms was chlorination. In 1970, public health concerns shifted from waterborne illnesses caused by microorganisms, to water pollution from pesticide residues, industrial waste, and organic chemicals. Regulations and water treatment plants were developed to respond to this source of water contamination as well (Jesperson, 2004).

In the United States, as in many other countries, providing clean water was viewed as a public good or utility. As a result, government at every level invested in water purification systems, and water treatment became a staple public health service. Government regulations set standards for water used for human consumption, and clean water was provided throughout the country by public or publicly regulated organizations. The exceptions were for people who lived in remote areas and obtained their water from private wells.

With respect to public health choices about how to improve health, this approach to preventing waterborne infectious diseases may be viewed as an archetypical primary prevention; purifying water supplies is intended to prevent infectious diseases such as cholera, typhoid, and hepatitis from occurring at all. As for the strategy chosen to prevent waterborne infectious diseases, water treatment systems such as those in the United States are environmental-level interventions. Our systems of preventing exposure to unclean water do not depend on individual behaviors such as boiling water or adding chlorine to water for individual use. Under the environmental-level approach that we have followed, clean water is delivered to individuals through a system that is planned, installed, monitored, and maintained by an organization, irrespective of an individual user's actions. Using and/or creating clean water is not the responsibility of the individual. In addition, the water treatment organization in the United States is generally a public utility, not a private enterprise.

Health Impact Pyramid

The **health impact pyramid** developed by Frieden (2010) provides a very useful framework for integrating behavioral and environmental approaches to public health practice (see **Figure 1.5**).

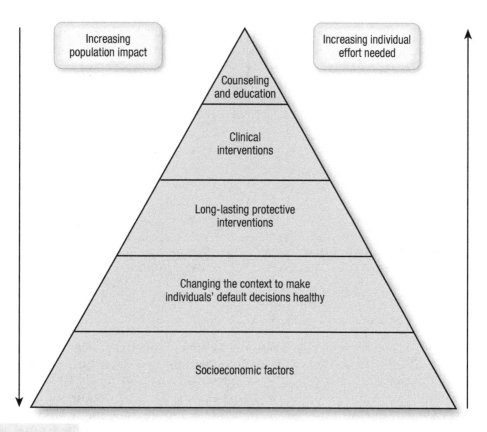

Figure 1.5. The Health Impact Pyramid

Source: Frieden, T. R. (2010). A framework for public health action: The health impact pyramid. *American Journal of Public Health, 100,* 591. https://doi.org/10.2105/AJPH.2009.185652

> A 5-tier pyramid best describes the impact of different types of public health interventions and provides a framework to improve health. At the base of this pyramid, indicating interventions with the greatest potential impact, are efforts to address socio-economic determinants of health. In ascending order are interventions that change the context to make individuals' default decisions healthy, clinical interventions that require limited contact but confer long-term protection, and ongoing direct clinical care, and health education and counseling. (Frieden, 2010, p. 590)

Note that the author accepts the population health perspective that structural inequality embodied in socioeconomic factors is the level with the most potential to improve health—a primary prevention strategy. Also note that the second level—changing the context—is a primary prevention strategy, which includes provision of clean water and safe food, as well as passage of laws that prevent injuries and exposure to disease-producing agents. Interventions at the top tiers are a mix of primary, secondary, and tertiary prevention "designed to help individuals, rather than entire populations, but they could theoretically have a large population impact if universally and effectively applied. In practice, however, even the best programs at the pyramid's higher levels achieve limited public health impact, largely because of their dependence on long-term individual behavior change" (Frieden, 2010, p. 591).

Since its publication in 2010, the health impact pyramid has begun to be used as a tool for describing different types of public health interventions. For example, an American Heart Association (AHA) publication states, "The improvement in socioeconomic status (first level) is a worthy goal for any society and the AHA Community Guide fully recognizes the critical importance of the social determinants of CVD [cardiovascular disease]" (Pearson et al., 2013). The report further argues that a combination of policies and programs at all five tiers will be the best way to improve health outcomes in populations.

GOING FORWARD

The purpose of this book is to open the field of public health to those new to it. Many complexities are not discussed in this attempt to make the overall values, goals, and practices of the field accessible to those unfamiliar with public health. With broad strokes, we hope to develop in the reader an appreciation of public health and an interest in learning more about the challenges and complications of "providing conditions in which people can be healthy."

So far, we have discussed public health in the ideal. However, the actual practice of public health does not always attain the ideal. In the next set of chapters, we discuss the public health system as it is currently practiced in the United States and its historical origins. This involves discussing the components of the public health system, including organization, financing, management, and performance, as well as the health problems that are addressed by public health. We will also outline the public health response to the COVID-19 pandemic and its impact in a case study (Chapter 9). In this brief review, we will see how public health practice today in the United States compares to the ideal of "assuring conditions in which people can be healthy." In the final chapter of the book, we discuss the prospects for public health in the United States.

DISCUSSION QUESTIONS

Q: What is the most important difference between the fields of medicine and public health?

Q: What do we mean by the determinants of health?

Q: What does research indicate is the impact of each determinant on human health?

Q: What are the major differences among the epidemiologic triangle, the PRECEDE–PROCEED model, and the health impact pyramid?

Q: What types of public health interventions are considered to be most effective?

DATA SOURCES

The authors encourage readers to investigate public health issues more fully than an introductory text such as this allows. By exploring the many, many sources of public health data available in the United States and in the world, readers can develop answers to their own questions and deepen their understanding of the field. To help in this regard, we provide at least one exercise for each chapter that requires using an existing, online source of data.

For Chapter 1, the following sources of data provide access to information related to the determinants of health:

- Physical environment such as housing and workplace safety
- Social environment such as socioeconomic status and social support
- Health behaviors such as exercise, nutrition, and smoking
- Behavioral Risk Factor Surveillance System (BRFSS): The BRFSS is the nation's premier source of information about health-related risk behaviors, chronic health conditions, and use of preventive health services. Begun in 1984, BRFSS now collects data in all 50 states as well as the District of Columbia and three U.S. territories. With about 400,000 completed telephone interviews with adults each year, it is the largest continuously conducted health survey in the world. Begin exploring here: https://www.cdc.gov/brfss/index.html
- National Health Interview Survey (NHIS): The NHIS has monitored the health of the nation since 1957. NHIS collects data on a wide range of health topics through personal household interviews. Survey results provide data

to track health status, health care access, and progress toward achieving national health objectives. Start your exploration here: https://www.cdc .gov/nchs/nhis/index.htm

- National Health and Nutrition Examination Survey (NHANES): NHANES is a program of studies designed to assess the health and nutritional status of adults and children in the United States. The survey is unique in that it combines interviews and physical examinations. Start here: https://www .cdc.gov/nchs/nhanes/index.htm

- Of course, the U.S. Census Bureau is a rich source of information that touches on nearly every public health issue in the United States including population numbers, trends, and characteristics and business and government statistics. Some of the Census Bureau's most relevant surveys are the American Community Survey (ACS), Current Population Survey (CPS), Economic Census, Annual Business Survey, and American Housing Survey. Start here to begin exploring: *https://www.census.gov/*

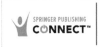 A robust set of instructor resources designed to supplement this text is located at **http://connect.springerpub.com/content/book/978-0-8261-8615-7.** Qualifying instructors may request access by emailing **textbook@springerpub.com.**

REFERENCES

Ajzen, I., & Fishbein, M. (1980). *Understanding attitudes and predicting social behavior.* Prentice-Hall.

Bandura, A. (1986). *Social foundations of thought and action: A social cognitive theory.* Prentice-Hall.

Becker, M. H. (1974). *The health belief model and personal health behavior.* C. B. Slack.

Berkman, L. F., & Glass, T. (2000). Social integration, social networks, social support, and health. In L. F. Berkman & I. Kawachi (Eds.), *Social epidemiology* (pp. 137–173). Oxford University Press.

Best, A. F., Haozous, E. A., de Gonzalez, A. B., Chernyavskiy, P., Freedman, N. D., Hartge, P., Thomas, D., Rosenberg, P. S., & Shiels, M. S. (2018). Premature death rates in the United States: Projections through 2030. *Lancet Public Health, 3*(8), e374–e384. https:// doi.org/10.1016/S2468-2667(18)30114-2.

Braveman, P. (2006). Health disparities and health equity: Concepts and measurement. *Annual Review of Public Health, 27,* 167–194. https://doi.org/10.1146/annurev .publhealth.27.021405.102103

Centers for Disease Control and Prevention. (2003). *Environmental public health indicators.* National Center for Environmental Health, Division of Environmental Hazards and Health Effects.

Centers for Disease Control and Prevention. (2010a). *Multistate outbreak of E. coli O157: H7 infections associated with beef from National Steak and Poultry.* http://www.cdc.gov/ecoli/2010/index.html

Centers for Disease Control and Prevention. (2011). *Health disparities and inequalities report.* http://www.cdc.gov/minorityhealth/CHDIReport.html

Centers for Disease Control and Prevention. (2020). *Health disparities.* https://www.cdc.gov/healthyyouth/disparities/

Centers for Disease Control and Prevention. (2022). *Picture of American: Prevention.* https://www.cdc.gov/pictureofamerica/pdfs/picture_of_america_prevention.pdf

Centers for Disease Control and Prevention. (2023). *Racism and health.* https://www.cdc.gov/minorityhealth/racism-disparities/index.html

Chan, R. H., Gordon, N. F., Chong, A., Alter, D. A., & Socioeconomic and Acute Myocardial Infarction Investigators. (2008). Influence of socioeconomic status on lifestyle behavior modifications among survivors of acute myocardial infarction. *American Journal of Cardiology, 102*(12), 1583–1588. https://doi.org/10.1016/j.amjcard.2008.08.022

Cohen, S. (2004). Social relationships and health. *American Psychologist, 59*, 676–684. https://doi.org/10.1037/0003-066X.59.8.676

DeJoy, D. (1996). Theoretical models of health behavior and workplace self-protective behavior. *Journal of Safety Research, 27*(2), 61–72. https://doi.org/10.1016/0022-4375(96)00007-2

Dooley, D., Fielding J., & Levi, L. (1996). Health and unemployment. *Annual Review of Public Health, 17*, 449–465. https://doi.org/10.1146/annurev.pu.17.050196.002313

Dubos, R. (1959). *Mirage of health: Utopias, progress, and biological change.* Harper & Brothers.

Evans, R. G., & Stoddart, G. L. (1994). Producing health, consuming health care. In R. G. Evans, M. L. Barer, & T. R. Marmor (Eds.), *Why are some people healthy and others not?* Aldine de Gruyter.

Fairchild, A. L., & Oppenheimer, G. M. (1998). Public health nihilism vs pragmatism: History, politics, and the control of tuberculosis. *American Journal of Public Health, 88*(7), 1105–1117. https://doi.org/10.2105/ajph.88.7.1105

Fos, P. J., & Fine, D. J. (2000). *Designing health care for populations: Applied epidemiology in health care administration.* Jossey-Bass.

Frieden, T. R. (2010). A framework for public health action: The health impact pyramid. *American Journal of Public Health, 100*(4), 590–595. https://doi.org/10.2105/AJPH.2009.185652

Friis, R. H., & Sellers, T. A. (1996). *Epidemiology for public health practice.* Aspen.

Grady, D. (2010). U.S. panel criticized as overstating cancer risks. *The New York Times.*

Green, L. W. (1974). Toward cost-benefit evaluations of health education: Some concepts, methods, and examples. *Health Education Monographs, 2*(Suppl. 1), 34–64. https://doi.org/10.1177/10901981740020S106

Green, L. W. (1999). Health education's contributions to public health in the twentieth century: A glimpse through health promotion's rear-view mirror. *Annual Review of Public Health, 20,* 67–88. https://doi.org/10.1146/ANNUREV.PUBLHEALTH.20.1.67

Green, L. W., & Kreuter, M. W. (1991). *Health promotion planning* (2nd ed.). Mayfield.

Green, L. W., & Kreuter, M. W. (1999). *Health promotion planning: An educational and ecological approach* (3rd ed.). Mayfield.

Heron, M. (2021). Deaths: Leading causes for 2019. *National Vital Statistics Reports, 70*(9). https://doi.org/10.15620/cdc:107021

Institute of Medicine. (1988). *The future of public health.* National Academy Press.

Institute of Medicine. (1999). *Toward environmental justice: Research, education, and health policy needs.* National Academies Press.

Jesperson, K. (2004). *Search for clean water continues.* National Evironmental Services Center. http://web.archive.org/web/20090520170248/http://www.nesc.wvu.edu/old_website/ndwc/ndwc_DWH_1.html

Kaplan, B. H., Cassel, J. C., & Gore, S. (1977). Social support and health. *Medical Care, 15*(Suppl. 5), 47–58. https://doi.org/10.1097/00005650-197705001-00006

Karasek, R., Baker, D., Marxer, F., Ahlbom, A., & Theorell, T. (1981). Job decision latitude, job demands, and cardiovascular disease: A prospective study of Swedish men. *American Journal of Public Health, 71*(7), 694–705. https://doi.org/10.2105/ajph.71.7.694

Karasek, R., Brisson, C., Kawakami, N., Houtman, I., Bongers, P., & Amick, B. (1998). The job content questionnaire: An instrument for internationally comparative assessments of psychosocial job characteristics. *Journal of Occupational Health Psychology, 3*(4), 322–355. https://doi.org/10.1037//1076-8998.3.4.322

Kasl, S. V., & Jones, B. A. (2000). The impact of job loss and retirement on health. In L. F. Berkman & I. Kawachi (Eds.), *Social epidemiology* (pp. 118–136). Oxford University Press.

Kasl, S. V., Rodriguez, E., & Lasch, K. E. (1998). The impact of unemployment on health and well-being. In B. P. Dohrenwend (Ed.), *Adversity, stress, and psychopathology* (pp. 111–131). Oxford University Press.

Krieger, N. (2000). Discrimination and health. In L. F. Berkman & I. Kawachi (Eds.), *Social epidemiology* (pp. 36–75). Oxford University Press.

Krieger, N., & Birn, A. E. (1998). A vision of social justice as the foundation of public health: Commemorating 150 years of the spirit of 1848. *American Journal of Public Health, 88*(11), 1603–1606. https://doi.org/10.2105/ajph.88.11.1603

Lasagna, L. (1962). *The doctor's dilemma.* Harper & Row.

Lieberman, L., Golden, S., & Earp, J. A. (2013). Structural approaches to health promotion: What do we need to know about policy and environmental change? *Health Education & Behavior, 40*(5), 520–525. https://doi.org/10.1177/1090198113503342

Lynch, J. W., Smith, G. D., Kaplan, G. A., & House, J. S. (2000). Income inequality and mortality: Importance to health of individual income, psychosocial environment, or material conditions. *British Medical Journal, 320,* 1200–1204. https://doi.org/10.1136/bmj.320.7243.1200

Marmot, M. (2005). Social determinants of health inequalities. *Lancet, 365*(9464), 1099–1104.

Marmot, M., Bobak, M., & Smith, G. D. (1995). Explanations for social inequalities in health. In B. C. Amick III, S. Levine, A. R. Tarlov, & D. C. Walsh (Eds.), *Society and health*. Oxford University Press.

Mays, V. M., Cochran, S. D., & Barnes, N. W. (2007). Race, race-based discrimination, and health outcomes among African Americans. *Annual Review of Psychology, 58*, 201–225. https://doi.org/10.1146/annurev.psych.57.102904.190212

McGinnis, J. M., & Foege, W. H. (1993). Actual causes of death in the United States. *Journal of the American Medical Association, 270*, 2207–2212. https://doi.org/10.1001/jama.1993.03510180077038

McGinnis, J. M., Williams-Russo, P., & Knickman, J. R. (2002). The case for more active policy attention to health promotion. *Health Affairs, 21*, 78–93. https://doi.org/10.1377/hlthaff.21.2.78

McLeroy, K. R., Bibeau, D., Steckler, A., & Glanz, K. (1988). An ecological perspective on health promotion programs. *Health Education Quarterly, 15*(4), 351–377. https://doi.org/10.1177/109019818801500401

Moore, L. V., & Roux, A. V. D. (2006). Associations of neighborhood characteristics with the location and type of food stores. *American Journal of Public Health, 96*(2), 325–331. https://doi.org/10.2105/AJPH.2004.058040

Myers, J. R. (2001). *Injuries among farm workers in the United States, 1995*. U.S. Department of Health & Human Services, Centers for Disease Control and Prevention, National Institute for Occupational Safety and Health.

National Human Genome Research Institute. (2018a). *Genetic disorders*. https://www.genome.gov/For-Patients-and-Families/Genetic-Disorders

National Human Genome Research Institute. (2018b). *Genomics and medicine*. https://www.genome.gov/health/Genomics-and-Medicine

National Institute of Occupational Safety and Health. (2018). *Agricultural safety: Farm safety survey*. https://www.cdc.gov/niosh/topics/aginjury/fss/default.html

Pearson, T., Palaniappan, L., Artinian, N., Carnethon, M., Criqui, M., Daniels, S., Fonarow, G. C., Fortmann, S. P., Franklin, B. A., Galloway, J. M., Goff Jr, D. C., Heath, G. W., Holland Frank, A. T., Kris-Etherton, P. M., Labarthe, D. R., Murabito, J. M., Sacco, R. L., Sasson, C., Turner, M. B., & American Heart Association Council on Epidemiology and Prevention (2013). American Heart Association guide for improving cardiovascular health at the community level, 2013 update: A scientific statement for public health practitioners, healthcare providers, and health policy makers. *Circulation, 127*, 1730–1753. https://doi.org/10.1161/CIR.0b013e31828f8a94

Pencheon, D., Guest, C., Melzer, D., & Gray, J. A. M. (Eds.). (2001). *Oxford handbook of public health practice*. Oxford University Press.

Peterson, R. K. D. (1995). Insects, disease, and military history: The Napoleonic campaigns and historical perception. *American Entomologist, 41*, 147–160. https://doi.org/10.1093/ae/41.3.147

Pickard, R. B., Miller, A. N., & Kirkpatrick, F. (2009). *A decade on the mean streets: A new typology for understanding health choices of those living in poverty's grasp.* American Public Health Association Annual Meeting.

President's Cancer Panel & National Cancer Institute. (2010). *Reducing environmental cancer risk: What we can do now.* U.S. Department of Health & Human Services, National Institutes of Health.

Purslow, L. R., Young, E. H., Wareham, N. J., Forouhi, N., Brunner, E. J., Luben, R. N., Welch, A. A., Khaw, K.-T., Bingham, S. A., & Sandhu, M. S. (2008). Socioeconomic position and risk of short-term weight gain: Prospective study of 14,619 middle-aged men and women. *BMC Public Health, 8,* 112. https://doi.org/10.1186/1471-2458-8-112

Rogers, R. W. (1983). Cognitive and psychological processes in fear appeals and attitude change: A revised theory of protection motivation. In J. T. Cacioppo & R. E. Petty (Eds.), *Social psychophysiology: A sourcebook* (pp. 153–176). Guilford Press.

Rosenstock, I. M., Strecher, V. J., & Becker, M. H. (1988). Social learning theory and the health belief model. *Health Education Quarterly, 15*(2), 175–183. https://doi.org/10.1177/109019818801500203

Samet, J. M., Marbury, M. C., & Spengler, J. D. (1987). Health effects and sources of indoor air pollution. Part 1. *American Review of Respiratory Diseases, 136,* 1486–1508. https://doi.org/10.1164/ajrccm/136.6.1486

Smedley, B. D., Stith, A. Y., & Nelson, A. R. (Eds.). (2003). *Unequal treatment: Confronting racial and ethnic disparities in health care.* National Academies Press.

Smith, R. (2008, July 8). The end of disease and the beginning of health. *thebmjopinion.* https://blogs.bmj.com/bmj/2008/07/08/richard-smith-the-end-of-disease-and-the-beginning-of-health/

Stokes, J. III, Noren, J. J., & Shindell, S. (1982). Definitions of terms and concepts applicable to clinical preventive medicine. *Journal of Community Health, 8*(1), 33–41. https://doi.org/10.1007/BF01324395

Stokols, D. (1996). Translating social ecological theory into guidelines for community health promotion. *American Journal of Health Promotion, 10*(4), 282–298. https://doi.org/10.4278/0890-1171-10.4.282

Stringhini, S., Sabia, S., Shipley, M., Brunner, E., Nabi, H., Kivimaki, M., & Singh-Manoux, A. (2010). Association of socioeconomic position with health behaviors and mortality. *Journal of the American Medical Association, 303*(12), 1159–1166. https://doi.org/10.1001/jama.2010.297

Summers, J. (1989). *Soho: A history of London's most colourful neighborhood.* Bloomsbury.

Theorell, T. (2000). Working conditions and health. In L. F. Berkman & I. Kawachi (Eds.), *Social epidemiology* (pp. 95–117). Oxford University Press.

Thoits, P. A. (1982). Life stress, social support, and psychological vulnerability: Epidemiological considerations. *Journal of Community Psychology, 10*(4), 341–362. https://doi.org/10.1002/1520-6629(198210)10:43.0.co;2-j

U.S. Department of Health & Human Services, & Health Resources & Services Administration. (2022). *MUA find.* https://data.hrsa.gov/tools/shortage-area/mua-find

U.S. Environmental Protection Agency. (2006). *Indoor air quality in large buildings.* www.epa.gov/iaq/largebldgs

World Health Organization. (2022a). *Constitution.* https://www.who.int/about/governance/constitution

World Health Organization. (2022b). *Determinants of health.* https://www.who.int/news-room/questions-and-answers/item/determinants-of-health

Young, T. K. (1998). *Population health: Concepts and methods.* Oxford University Press.

Appendix 1.1. John Snow, the Broad Street Pump, and the Demise of Cholera in 19th-Century London

"When a wave of Asiatic cholera first hit England in late 1831, it was thought to be spread by "miasma in the atmosphere." By the time of the Soho outbreak 23 years later, medical knowledge about the disease had barely changed, though one man, Dr. John Snow, a surgeon (actually an anesthesiologist) and pioneer of the science of epidemiology, had recently published a report speculating that it was spread by contaminated water—an idea with which neither the authorities nor the rest of the medical profession had much truck. Whenever cholera broke out—which it did four times between 1831 and 1854—nothing whatsoever was done to contain it, and it rampaged through the industrial cities, leaving tens of thousands dead in its wake. The year 1853 saw outbreaks in Newcastle and Gateshead as well as in London, where a total of 10,675 people died of the disease. In the 1854 London epidemic the worst-hit areas at first were Southwark and Lambeth. Soho suffered only a few, seemingly isolated, cases in late August. Then, on the night of the 31st, what Dr. Snow later called "the most terrible outbreak of cholera which ever occurred in the kingdom" broke out.

It was as violent as it was sudden. During the next three days, 127 people living in or around Broad Street died. Few families, rich or poor, were spared the loss of at least one member. Within a week, three-quarters of the residents had fled from their homes, leaving their shops shuttered, their houses locked and the streets deserted. Only those who could not afford to leave remained there. It was like the Great Plague all over again.

By 10 September, the number of fatal attacks had reached 500 and the death rate of the St Anne's, Berwick Street and Golden Square subdivisions of the parish had risen to 12.8%—more than double that for the rest of London. That it did not rise even higher was thanks only to Dr. John Snow.

Snow lived in Frith Street, so his local contacts made him ideally placed to monitor the epidemic which had broken out on his doorstep. His previous researches had convinced him that cholera, which, as he had noted, "always commences with disturbances of the functions of the alimentary canal," was spread by a poison passed from victim to victim through sewage-tainted water; and he had traced a recent outbreak in South London to contaminated water supplied by the Vauxhall Water Company—a theory that the authorities and the water company itself were, not surprisingly, reluctant to believe. Now he saw his chance to prove his theories once and for all, by linking the Soho outbreak to a single source of polluted water.

From day one he patrolled the district, interviewing the families of the victims. His research led him to a pump on the corner of Broad Street and Cambridge Street, at the epicenter of the epidemic. "I found," he wrote afterwards, "that

(continued)

nearly all the deaths had taken place within a short distance of the pump." In fact, in houses much nearer another pump, there had only been 10 deaths—and of those, five victims had always drunk the water from the Broad Street pump, and three were schoolchildren, who had probably drunk from the pump on their way to school.

Dr. Snow took a sample of water from the pump, and, on examining it under a microscope, found that it contained "white, flocculent particles." By 7 September, he was convinced that these were the source of infection, and he took his findings to the Board of Guardians of St James's Parish, in whose parish the pump fell.

Though they were reluctant to believe him, they agreed to remove the pump handle as an experiment. When they did so, the spread of cholera dramatically stopped. [Actually the outbreak had already lessened for several days.]" (Summers, 1989, pp. 113–117)

2 Origins of Public Health

How is public health practiced in the United States today? To examine this issue, we will first discuss the origins of public health in the Industrial Revolution of the 18th and 19th centuries. Early industrialization, and the human misery that was its consequence, set the stage for public health as a professional field—its sense of identity, organization, goals, methods, and "sensibility." In previous eras, societies have practiced "public health" in that they may have provided healthful conditions for their people. The Romans built the great aqueducts, for instance, to bring clean water to the city. The Venetians during the 17th and 18th centuries controlled plague through public measures, including surveillance and control of travel:

> During the 17th and 18th centuries, measures were taken by the Venetian administration to combat plague on the Ionian Islands. At that time, although the scientific basis of plague was unknown, the Venetians recognized its infectious nature and successfully decreased its spread by implementing an information network. Additionally, by activating a system of inspection that involved establishing garrisons

along the coasts, the Venetians were able to control all local movements in plague-infested areas, which were immediately isolated. In contrast, the neighboring coast of mainland Greece, which was under Ottoman rule, was a plague-endemic area during the same period. . . . even in the absence of scientific knowledge, close observation and social and political measures can effectively restrain infectious outbreaks to the point of disappearance. (Konstantinidou et al., 2009, p. 39)

However, modern public health aims are, in addition to the prevention and control of disease and injury in populations—a goal in evidence throughout human history—the aspiration for social justice. This public health "sensibility" is intolerant of disparities in health between those who have wealth, power, and status, and those who do not (Krieger & Birn, 1998). This "sensibility" was clearly apparent in the early period of the Industrial Revolution and led to the great achievements that we ascribe to public health in the 19th and 20th centuries and strive to emulate today.

CLASSIFICATION OF HEALTH PROBLEMS

Before considering the origins of modern public health, we need a classification scheme for health problems. We can consider health problems to be of two broad types: diseases and injuries. Diseases can be classified as infectious or noninfectious, with **infectious diseases** caused by pathogenic microorganisms—bacteria, viruses, fungi, multicellular parasites, and prions—that can be transmitted from person to person or from other species to persons. The term "communicable disease" is used interchangeably with infectious disease as a result. Examples of infectious diseases are tuberculosis, plague, cholera, influenza, and human immunodeficiency virus (HIV). **Noninfectious diseases** are those that are not caused by a pathogenic microbe, but by factors that are not communicable or contagious such as environmental exposures to toxins, nutritional deficiencies, health behaviors, and genetic inheritance. They include dietary and autoimmune conditions, diabetes, cardiovascular disease, as well as hereditary diseases such as hemophilia. Mental health conditions such as depression, anxiety, and others are noninfectious. Noninfectious diseases are sometimes referred to as chronic diseases. However, the concept of chronic and acute may be applied to either infectious or noninfectious diseases. For example, HIV infection has become a chronic condition, at least in developed countries such as the United States, and nutritional deficiency diseases, once diagnosed, can be acute; that is, curable without lingering or permanent effects.

Injuries are the other broad category of health problems. Useful classifications of injuries for public health practice are identifying them as intentional and unintentional. **Intentional injuries** are self-inflicted, such as suicide, or inflicted by a person or persons on others, such as homicide. Intentional injuries may result in death or morbidity. Domestic violence, child abuse, and elder abuse are intentional injuries. **Unintentional or accidental injuries**, again, can be self-inflicted or inflicted by others and result in mortality or morbidity. The most common unintentional injuries result from motor vehicle crashes, but the home and work-place are sites of a great many unintentional injuries as well, including burns, falls, drownings, poisonings, and lacerations.

Distinguishing between diseases and injuries, infectious and noninfectious diseases, and intentional and unintentional injuries facilitates an understanding of the causes of health problems, and, therefore, strategies to prevent them.

ORIGINS OF MODERN PUBLIC HEALTH

The history of modern public health in the United States and elsewhere has its roots in the Industrial Revolution. The exemplar is Britain. During industrialization, cities grew rapidly as factories replaced the domestic system of production, beginning with textiles. The poor living and working conditions in the burgeoning industrial cities, where infectious diseases were prevalent and frequently epidemic, are well documented. Housing was crowded, sanitation was grossly inadequate, clean water was scarce, and a healthful diet was beyond the means of most people. Work consisted of long days in unsafe and poorly ventilated factories, often exposed to toxic substances (Pike, 1966; Thompson, 1964; Toynbee, 1957). Following are descriptions of housing and factory conditions in Britain, where industrialization first took root and had a profound effect on public health everywhere, including the United States, particularly in the development of the public health "sensibility."

Life During the Industrial Revolution

Living Conditions

In the 1800s, London was an unsavory place to live for most people. The smells of raw sewage, horse and cattle manure, slaughter houses, unwashed bodies, and coal fires filled the air. Fog from the smoke of these fires made breathing difficult. Housing was cramped, often airless, and without a clean water supply or sanitary disposal of garbage and sewage. Diet was poor. On housing in London, Dr. Vinen, a medical officer of health, reported in 1856 on the living conditions typical of the day:

> In one small miserably dirty dilapidated room, occupied by a man, his wife and four children, in which they live day and night, was a child in its coffin that had died of measles eleven days before and, although decomposition was going on, it had not even been fastened down. The excuse made for its not having been buried before was that burials by the parish did not take place unless there were more than one to convey away at a time . . . In another miserable apartment scarce seven feet wide lived five persons and in which there was not one atom of furniture of any kind; the room contained nothing but a heap of filthy rags on the floor . . . The front door is never closed day or night and in consequence the staircase and landing form a nightly resort for thieves and prostitutes, where every kind of nuisance is committed . . . There are two yards

at the back of this house, in each of which is an open privy; one of them is so abominably filthy and emitted a smell so foul that I was almost overpowered. (Spartacus Educational, 2010f, Dr. Vinen, para. 1)

Factory Life

Factories of the period were grim places to work. Many interviews with adult and child laborers testify to the conditions that often led to injury, permanent disability, and disease. Long hours, little rest, poor ventilation, exposure to dangerous equipment and chemicals, and harsh enforcement of workplace rules were the norm. There is no substitute for the words of those who experienced the conditions themselves.

John Birley, a worker in a 19th-century mill, was interviewed by *The Ashton Chronicle* in 1849 about his life in Cressbrook Mill, where he began working when he was about 7 years old (Spartacus Educational, 2010e):

> Our regular time was from five in the morning till nine or ten at night; and on Saturday, till eleven, and often twelve o'clock at night, and then we were sent to clean the machinery on the Sunday. No time was allowed for breakfast and no sitting for dinner and no time for tea. We went to the mill at five o'clock and worked till about eight or nine when they brought us our breakfast, which consisted of water-porridge, with oatcake in it and onions to flavour it. Dinner consisted of Derbyshire oatcakes cut into four pieces, and ranged into two stacks. One was buttered and the other treacled. By the side of the oatcake were cans of milk. We drank the milk and with the oatcake in our hand, we went back to work without sitting down. (John Birley, para. 1)

A child who was interviewed by Michael Sadler's Parliamentary Committee in 1832 gave the following account of how factory hours were kept (Spartacus Educational, 2010i):

> I worked at Mr. Braid's Mill at Duntruin. We worked as long as we could see. I could not say at what hour we stopped. There was no clock in the mill. There was nobody but the master and the master's son [who] had a watch and so we did not know the time. The operatives were not permitted to have a watch. There was one man who had a watch but it was taken from him because he told the men the time. (James Patterson, para. 1)

Factory accidents were a major safety problem.

> Unguarded machinery was a major problem for children working in factories. One hospital reported that every year it treated nearly a thousand people for wounds and mutilations caused by machines in factories. A report commissioned by the House of Commons in 1832 said that: "there are factories, no means few in number, nor confined to the smaller mills, in which serious accidents are continually occurring, and

in which, notwithstanding, dangerous parts of the machinery are allowed to remain unfenced." The report added that the workers were often "abandoned from the moment that an accident occurs; their wages are stopped, no medical attendance is provided, and whatever the extent of the injury, no compensation is afforded." In 1842 a German visitor noted that he had seen so many people in the streets of Manchester without arms and legs that it was like "living in the midst of the army just returned from a campaign." (Spartacus Educational, 2010c, paras. 1–3)

Poorly ventilated factory buildings were another serious problem (Spartacus Educational, 2010d).

A report published in July 1833 stated that most factories were "dirty; low-roofed; ill-ventilated; ill-drained; no conveniences for washing or dressing; no contrivance for carrying off dust and other effluvia." Sir Anthony Carlisle, a doctor at Westminster Hospital, visited some textile mills in 1832. He later gave evidence to the House of Commons on the dangers that factory pollution was causing for the young people working in factories: "labour is undergone in an atmosphere heated to a temperature of 70 to 80 and upwards." He pointed out that going from a "very hot room into damp cold air will inevitably produce inflammations of the lungs."

Doctors were also concerned about the "dust from flax and the flue from cotton" in the air that the young workers were breathing in. Dr. Charles Aston Key told Michael Sadler that this "impure air breathed for a great length of time must be productive of disease, or exceedingly weaken the body." Dr. Thomas Young, who studied textile workers in Bolton, reported that factory pollution was causing major health problems.

> Most young workers complained of feeling sick during their first few weeks of working in a factory. Robert Blincoe said he felt that the dust and flue was suffocating him. This initial reaction to factory pollution became known as *mill fever*. Symptoms included sickness and headaches. The dust and floating cotton fibre in the atmosphere was a major factor in the high incidence of tuberculosis, bronchitis, asthma, and byssinosis[1] amongst cotton workers. (paras. 1–5)

Child Labor

Child labor in textile factories and coal mines was perhaps the most appalling fact of the early period of industrialization. Following are interviews with two children about their experiences in the textile factories of London. The interviews were conducted for government investigations into the working conditions of children (Spartacus Educational, 2010b). Again, there is no substitute for the words of those who experienced these conditions themselves.

Charles Aberdeen was interviewed by Michael Sadler and his House of Commons Committee on 23rd July, 1832.

Question: *How young have you known children go into silk mills?*

Answer: I have known three at 6 [years of age]; but very few at that age.

Question: *What were your hours of labor?*

Answer: From six in the morning till seven at night.

Question: *Was it found necessary to beat children to keep them up to their employment?*

Answer: Certainly.

Question: *Did the beating increase towards evening?*

Answer: Their strength relaxes more towards the evening; they get tired, and they twist themselves about on their legs, and stand on the sides of their feet.

Question: *As an overlooker did you stimulate them to labor by severity?*

Answer: Certainly, my employer always considered this indispensable.

Question: *Did you not find it very irksome to your feelings, to have to take those means of urging the children to the work?*

Answer: Extremely so; I have been compelled to urge them on to work when I knew they could not bear it; but I was obliged to make them strain every nerve to do the work, and I can say I have been disgusted with myself and with my situation; I felt myself degraded and reduced to the level of a slave driver in such cases.

Question: *Is not tying the broken ends, or piecing, an employment that requires great activity?*

Answer: Yes.

Question: *Does not the material often cut the hands of those poor children?*

Answer: Frequently; but some more than others. I have seen them stand at their work, with their hands cut, till the blood has been running down to the ends of their fingers.

Question: *Is there more work required of the children than there used to be when you first knew the business?*

Answer: Yes; on account of the competition [that] exists between masters. One undersells the other; consequently the master endeavors to get an equal quantity of work done for less money. (Spartacus Educational, 2010b, Factory Workers section, William Rastrick)

Eliza Marshall was born in Doncaster in 1815. At the age of 9 her family moved to Leeds, where she found work at a local textile factory. Eliza was interviewed by Michael Sadler and his House of Commons Committee on 26th May, 1832.

Question: *What [were] your hours of work?*

Answer: When I first went to the mill we worked [from] six in the morning till seven in the evening. After a time we began at five in the morning, and worked till ten at night.

Question: *Were you very much fatigued by that length of labor?*

Answer: Yes.

Question: *Did they beat you?*

Answer: When I was younger they used to do it often.

Question: *Did the labor affect your limbs?*

Answer: Yes, when we worked over-hours I was worse by a great deal; I had stuff to rub my knees; and I used to rub my joints a quarter of an hour, and sometimes an hour or two.

Question: *Were you straight before that?*

Answer: Yes, I was; my master knows that well enough; and when I have asked for my wages, he said that I could not run about as I had been used to do.

Question: *Are you crooked now?*

Answer: Yes, I have an iron on my leg; my knee is contracted.

Question: *Have the surgeons in the Infirmary told you by what your deformity was occasioned?*

Answer: Yes, one of them said it was by standing; the marrow is dried out of the bone, so that there is no natural strength in it.

Question: *You were quite straight till you had to labor so long in those mills?*

Answer: Yes, I was as straight as anyone. (Spartacus Educational, 2010b, Factory Workers section, Eliza Marshall, para. 2)

Following is an interview with a man who became a piecer in a mill as a child (Spartacus Educational, 2010h):

When I achieved the manly age of 10 I obtained half-time employment at Dowry Mill as a "little piecer." . . . The noise was what impressed me most. Clatter, rattle, bang, the swish of thrusting levers and the crowding of hundreds of men, women and children at their work. Long rows of huge spinning frames, with thousands of whirling spindles, slid forward several feet, paused and then slid smoothly back again, continuing the process unceasingly hour after hour while cotton became yarn and yarn changed to weaving material. Often the threads on the spindles broke as they were stretched and twisted and spun. These broken ends had to be instantly repaired; the piecer ran forward and joined them swiftly, with a deft touch that is an art of its own.

I remember no golden summers, no triumphs at games and sports, no tramps through dark woods or over shadow-racing hills. Only meals at which there never seemed to be enough food, dreary journeys through smoke-fouled streets, in mornings when I nodded with tiredness and in evenings when my legs trembled under me from exhaustion. (J. R. Clynes, paras. 1–4)

Finally, here is another account of childhood spent in a mill from a young man interviewed by William Dodd in 1842 (Spartacus Educational, 2010a):

I am about twenty-five years old. I have been a piecer at Mr. Cousen's worsted mill; I have worked nowhere else. I commenced working in a worsted mill at nine years of age. Our hours of labour were from six in the morning to seven and eight at night, with thirty minutes off at noon for dinner. We had no time for breakfast or drinking. The children conceive it to be a very great mischief; to be kept so long in labour; and I believe their parents would be very glad if it was not so. I found it very hard and laborious employment. I had 2s. per week at first. We had to stoop, to bend our bodies and our legs.

I was a healthy and strong boy, when I first went to the mill. When I was about eight years old, I could walk from Leeds to Bradford (ten miles) without any pain or difficulty, and with a little fatigue; now I cannot stand without crutches! I cannot walk at all! Perhaps I might creep up stairs. I go up stairs backwards every night! I found my limbs begin to fail, after I had been working about a year. It came on with great pain in my legs and knees. I am very much fatigued towards the end of the day. I cannot work in the mill now.

The overlooker beat me up to my work! I have been beaten till I was black and blue and I have had my ears torn! Once I was very ill with it. He beat me then, because I mixed a few empty bobbins, not having any place to put them in separate. We were beaten most at the latter end of the day, when we grew tired and fatigued. The highest wages I ever had in the factory, were 5s. 6d. per week.

My mother is dead; my father was obliged to send me to the mill, in order to keep me. I had to attend at the mill after my limbs began to fail. I could not then do as well as I could before. I had one shilling a week taken off my wages. I had lost several inches in height. I [frequently] had to stand thirteen and fourteen hours a day, and to be continually engaged. I was perfectly straight before I entered on this labour.

Other boys were deformed in the same way. A good many boys suffered in their health, in consequence of the severity of their work. I am sure this pain, and grievous deformity, came from my long hours of labour. My father, and my friends, believe so too. It is the opinion of all the medical men who have seen me. (Benjamin Gomersal, paras. 1–5)

Health Problems of the Times

The squalid and unsafe living and working conditions in industrialized cities of 19th-century Britain led to infectious disease outbreaks and epidemics, especially among the poor. Children were at most risk of death from infectious disease. The appalling working and living conditions of the poor and working classes during the industrialization of Europe, the United States, and similar countries also had a profound impact on the risk of injuries and noninfectious diseases. Lack of attention to safety in the workplace was a major cause of injuries and disabilities. In addition, the wages that families received for necessities were often insufficient to pay for healthful foods, and as a result, nutritional deficiency diseases were common.

Emergence of the Public Health Sensibility

The living and working conditions for the ordinary person during this period provoked a progressive outcry for change. Child labor was especially galvanizing. Work in the factories and coal mines was long, hard, and dirty for all laborers. However, protection of children and women became a cause for many progressive leaders of the time. The following excerpt from a poem written in 1836 by Caroline Sheridan Norton (anonymous at the time) is an example of the sentiments held by many persons about child labor practices in Britain at the time (Norton, 1836). Prefacing the poem, which was meant to be presented in Parliament, the author stated the following:

> The abuses even, of such a business, must be cautiously dealt with; lest, in eradicating them, we shake or disorder the whole fabric. We admit, however, that the case of CHILDREN employed in the Cotton Factories is one of those that call fairly for legislative regulation (para. 1):
>> These then are his Companions: he, too young
>> To share their base and saddening merriment,
>> Sits by: his little head in silence hung;
>> His limbs cramped up; his body weakly bent;
>> Toiling obedient, till long hours so spent
>> Produce Exhaustion's slumber, dull and deep.
>> The Watcher's stroke–bold–sudden–violent–
>> Urges him from that lethargy of sleep,
>> And bids him wake to Life–to labour and to weep!
>> But the day hath its End. Forth then he hies
>> With jaded, faltering step, and brow of pain;
>> Creeps to that shed–his HOME–where happy lies
>> The sleeping babe that cannot toil for Gain;
>> Where his remorseful Mother tempts in vain
>> With the best portion of their frugal fare:
>> Too sick to eat–too weary to complain–
>> He turns him idly from the untasted share,
>> Slumbering sinks down unfed, and mocks her useless care. (Norton,
> 1836, A Voice from the Factories, paras. 48–49)

The author added about the poem:

> I will only add, that I have in *no* instance overcharged or exaggerated, by poetical fictions, the picture drawn by the Commissioners appointed to inquire into this subject. I have strictly adhered to the printed Reports; to that which I believe to be the melancholy truth; and that which I have, in some instances, myself had an opportunity of witnessing.
>
> I earnestly hope I shall live to see this evil abolished. There will be delay—there will be opposition: such has ever been the case with all questions involving interests, and more especially where the preponderating interest has been on the side of the existing abuse. Yet, as the noble-hearted and compassionate Howard became immortally connected with the removal of the abuses which for centuries disgraced our prison discipline; as the perseverance of Wilberforce created the dawn of the long-delayed emancipation of the negroes; so, my Lord, I trust to see *your* name enrolled with the names of these great and good men, as the Liberator and Defender of those helpless beings, on whom are inflicted many of the evils both of slavery and imprisonment, without the odium of either. (Norton, 1836, Dedicated to the Right Honourable Lord Ashley, paras. 7–8)

Another famous speech, given by Lord Byron before the House of Lords in 1812, defended the Luddites who had engaged in violence provoked by the loss of employment due to the industrialization of textile manufacture:

> During the short time I recently passed in Nottingham, not twelve hours elapsed without some fresh act of violence; and on that day I left the county I was informed that forty Frames had been broken the preceding evening, as usual, without resistance and without detection.
>
> Such was the state of that county, and such I have reason to believe it to be at this moment. But whilst these outrages must be admitted to exist to an alarming extent, it cannot be denied that they have arisen from circumstances of the most unparalleled distress: the perseverance of these miserable men in their proceedings, tends to prove that nothing but absolute want could have driven a large, and once honest and industrious, body of the people, into the commission of excesses so hazardous to themselves, their families, and the community.
>
> They were not ashamed to beg, but there was none to relieve them: their own means of subsistence were cut off, all other employment preoccupied; and their excesses, however to be deplored and condemned, can hardly be subject to surprise.
>
> As the sword is the worst argument that can be used, so should it be the last. In this instance it has been the first; but providentially as yet only in the scabbard. The present measure will, indeed, pluck it from the sheath; yet had proper meetings been held in the earlier stages of these riots, had the grievances of these men and their masters (for they also had their grievances) been fairly weighed and justly examined,

I do think that means might have been devised to restore these workmen to their avocations, and tranquillity [*sic*] to the country. (Spartacus Educational, 2010g, Lord Byron, paras. 1–4)

KEY IDEA

In the public outcry over the working and living conditions in England during this period, especially for children, we see the emergence of the public health sensibility—the belief in the importance of equity, fairness, and human dignity. These attributes are at the heart of public health purpose. All people deserve equity and fairness and dignity, regardless of their power or wealth.

EMERGENCE OF MODERN PUBLIC HEALTH PRACTICES

Infectious Disease Outbreaks and the Response

The high rate of infectious diseases in the industrializing British cities, including the cholera outbreaks of 1817, 1849, and 1854 in London, brought about a public health response. The 1854 outbreak was the one for which John Snow identified the Broad Street pump as the cause, and although it was not known that the bacteria *Vibrio cholera* was present in the water gathered at the pump, it was evident from Snow's epidemiologic investigation that it was the source of the disease outbreak.

The method used to address the problem of infectious diseases in Britain and other industrializing countries during the 1800s was environmental engineering—the archetypical primary prevention strategy—which modified the environment for all persons at risk. Although the microbial agents of infectious diseases were unknown at the time, public health engineering programs in the 1800s provided clean water and removal of sewage and garbage to reduce the problem of infectious disease outbreaks.

> By the 1800s, people began to understand that unsanitary living conditions and water contamination contributed to disease epidemics. This new awareness prompted major cities to take measures to control waste and garbage. In the mid-1850s, Chicago built the first major sewage system in the United States to treat wastewater. Soon, many other U.S. cities followed Chicago's lead. (National Oceanic and Atmospheric Administration, 2010, para. 2)

Later in the century, the scientific discoveries that led to vaccines and antimicrobial therapies, such as penicillin, resulted in further reduction in the threat of infectious diseases. These avenues of discovery and responses to infectious diseases became a template for future public health activity to control infectious disease.

Injuries and Noninfectious Diseases and Response

The working conditions that led to injury and disability during the Industrial Revolution in Britain also produced a public response in the form of health policies. Many people wished to see an end to the abuse of workers under the factory system. With respect to child labor, the public response was an investigation of conditions by officials in the government and eventual passage of legislation. In 1831, the Sadler Committee, chaired by Michael Thomas Sadler, was charged with investigating conditions of child labor in cotton and linen factories. In 1833, a parliamentary commission was appointed to investigate working conditions in other textile industries. In 1842, a committee chaired by Lord Ashley investigated conditions in coal mines. Following is a summary of the laws enacted in Britain from 1819 to 1891 to protect workers, particularly children:

> 1819—Cotton Mills Act: Limits working days for children in cotton mills to 16 hours for those under 16 years. Children younger than the age of 9 should not be employed, but magistrates did not enforce this.
>
> 1833—Factory Act: Improves conditions for children working in cotton and woolen factories. Young children were working very long hours in workplaces where conditions were often terrible. The basic act was as follows:
>
> 1. There should be no child workers younger than 9 years of age.
> 2. Employers must have a medical or age certificate for child workers.
> 3. Children between the ages of 9 and 13 to work no more than 8 hours a day.
> 4. Children between the ages of 13 and 18 to work no more than 12 hours a day.
> 5. Children are not to work at night.
> 6. There should be two hours [of] schooling each day for children under 13 years.
> 7. Four factory inspectors must be appointed to enforce the law throughout the whole of the country.

However, the passing of this Act did not mean that the mistreatment of children stopped overnight.

> 1842—Mines and Collieries Act: Women and girls, and boys younger than the age of 10, are not allowed to work underground. Boys younger than the age of 15 are not allowed to work on machinery.
>
> 1844—Factory Act: Children younger than 13 years to work no more than 6.5 hours a day. Women and children aged 13 to 18 to work no more than 12 hours a day.
>
> 1847—Factory Act: Women and children younger than 18 years are limited to a 10 hour work day.
>
> 1860—Coal Mines Regulation Act: Boys younger than 12 years are not allowed underground unless they can read and write.
>
> 1867—Factory Act Extension: Extended existing legislation to all factories with 50 or more people employed. Specific industries included

some with even less than 50 employees. These were blast furnaces, iron and steel mills, glass, paper making, tobacco, printing and bookbinding.

1875—Chimney Sweep Act: Requires that all chimney sweeps be licensed. Licenses were issued only to sweeps not using climbing boys.

1878—Factory and Workshops Act: Employment of children younger than 10 years is banned. Regulations of control safety, ventilation, and meals.

1891—Factory Act: This made the requirements for fencing machinery more stringent. Under the heading "Conditions of Employment," two considerable additions were included to previous legislation. The first is the prohibition on employers to employ women within 4 weeks after confinement; the second is the raising of minimum age at which a child can be set to work from 10 to 11 years old. (United Kingdom Parliament, 2014)

Public response to the health problems brought about by the Industrial Revolution—both infectious diseases and injuries—laid the foundation for public health as a professional field in Britain and other industrializing countries in Europe and the Americas. From the cauldron, which was the industrializing cities of the 19th century, came what have become permanent public health commitments to workplace safety, child and maternal health, safe and healthful housing conditions, sanitary disposal of waste, and a safe and nutritious food supply. Concern for "vulnerable" populations and the desire to reduce health disparities and increase health equity are at the heart of many, if not most, public health goals and activities today. This "public health sensibility," it also can be argued, arose among progressive elites in response to the inequities and hardships of the poor and working people during the Industrial Revolution.

With the justification and emerging methods to improve health in place, public health needed evidence to evaluate these methods and to demonstrate their success. Epidemiology was to fulfill this need, and the *International Classification of Diseases* (ICD) was one of epidemiology's first and most essential tools, providing the data for scientific studies of disease causation, treatment, and prevention.

THE *INTERNATIONAL CLASSIFICATION OF DISEASES* AND THE RISE OF EPIDEMIOLOGY

KEY IDEA

If the broad mission of public health is to "fulfill society's interest in assuring conditions in which people can be healthy," it is epidemiology that underlies this endeavor with the systematic study of conditions that undermine human health.

Formally, **epidemiology** "is the study of the distribution and determinants of health-related states or events in specified populations, and the application of this study to the control of health problems" (Public Health Science and Surveillance, 2012, para. 2). Generally considered an integral or foundational component of public health practice, epidemiology aims to shape policy decisions and support evidence-based practice by identifying risk factors for disease and targets for intervention (Department of Epidemiology, 2020; Public Health Science and Surveillance, 2012). The *ICD* is an essential tool in the epidemiologists' toolbox.

DID YOU KNOW?

Dr. John Snow (1813–1858) is often referred to as the father of epidemiology. He was an obstetrician and anesthesiologist practicing in London during the first half of the 19th century. At that time, cholera was a leading cause of death throughout the world. There were frequent, large-scale cholera outbreaks in European cities, which were thought to be the result of "bad air." Dr. Snow's 1854 epidemiologic investigation of a cholera epidemic in London's Soho district linked the outbreak to the now famous Broad Street pump. Through careful observation, he noted that residents using water from the Broad Street pump, which was located near an outlet for sewage, were affected at much higher rates than those using uncontaminated water. While the parish's Board of Guardians was skeptical, they agreed to remove the Broad Street pump handle as an experiment, and the spread of cholera in the district was halted.

Public health requires facts about death in order to develop and evaluate practices that prevent premature death. For example, the United States, like many other industrialized countries, has the capability to report a 90% reduction in infant mortality and 99% reduction in maternal mortality between 1900 and 1999 (Centers for Disease Control and Prevention [CDC], 1999). This kind of information is used to evaluate what is effective and what is not in public health and health care practices. In order to obtain information for these purposes, we need to know and systematically record the causes of death.

The earliest efforts to systematically track deaths and their causes are believed to have begun in the mid-15th century Italian cities (in response to the Black Death). However, the earliest statistical analysis of death records (instead of individual trajectories) is attributed to John Graunt in his analysis of the deaths reported in the *London Bills of Mortality* (also established in response to the Black Death) circa 1662 (Moriyama et al., 2011). The first question he attempted to answer was the proportion of liveborn children who died before reaching the age of 6 years, and his estimate of 36% is considered accurate (World Health Organization [WHO], 2021, January 1).

> However, it was William Farr who asked and answered the question, "can lifetime be prolonged by a knowledge of the causes that cut it short?" Appointed in 1837 to the post of Compiler of Abstracts at the General Register Office of England and Wales, which registered births, marriages, and deaths, he not only compiled statistics on death and disease across the regions, he used his access to the data to identify public health concerns. For example, Farr published a report in 1864 showing a disproportionately high number of deaths among miners in

Cornwall and concluded that pulmonary diseases due to labor conditions inside the mines were the chief cause of their high mortality rate. (Granados, 2022)

Perhaps most significant was Farr's collaboration with Florence Nightingale. As the nursing administrator of the British Army's hospital network during the Crimean War, Nightingale was determined to change a system that saw thousands of soldiers live long enough to suffer through the limited supplies and filthy, overcrowded facilities of their own army. Historically, government leaders accepted the loss of common soldiers as inevitable and that communicable diseases were unavoidable. Working systematically upon her return in 1855 to prove otherwise, she addressed inconsistently collected data and perhaps more significantly developed compelling data visualizations and comparisons. For example, she showed peacetime soldiers living in army barracks died at higher rates than civilian men of similar ages. The result was new data-collection operations considered the best in Europe that also proved the success of the reforms they motivated. By 1863, mortality from preventable disease among soldiers was less than the comparable civilian population. Similar efforts in the name of civilian public health resulted in the British Public Health Act of 1875, which established requirements for well-built sewers, clean running water and regulated building codes (Andrews, 2022).

Underlying these analyses are the systematic, comprehensive collection of incidences of death with a common classification of disease that allows comparison over time and between populations (Moriyama et al., 2011). As Farr, whose early nomenclatures were a basis for the initial international standards, noted:

> The advantages of a uniform statistical nomenclature, however imperfect, are so obvious, that it is surprising no attention has been paid to its enforcement in Bills of Mortality. Each disease has, in many instances, been denoted by three or four terms, and each term has been applied to as many different diseases: vague, inconvenient names have been employed, or complications have been registered instead of primary diseases. The nomenclature is of as much importance in this department of inquiry as weights and measures in the physical sciences, and should be settled without delay. (WHO, 2021, p. 1)

The **International Classification of Diseases (ICD)** is the current "platform" for this and which allows for analysis of the causes of mortality and morbidity in different countries or regions of the world over time. As authors Kiran Rabheru, Julie E. Byles, and Alexandre Kalaches note in their summary of discussions about a particular category of codes:

> Embedded within the *ICD* are diagnostic categories that are very influential in the operation of global health-care systems. Clinically, the diagnostic categories form the basis for recording and tracking statistics about illnesses; health data pertaining to primary, secondary, and tertiary care; and causes of death on death certificates. Diagnostic

codes are also embedded within the *ICD* and are used as tools for decision support, resource allocation, and financial reimbursement for health-care services and delivery. Large-scale use of data based on *ICD* diagnostic codes includes adjudication of insurance coverage, other payment systems for health-care services, planning and administration of patient quality and safety, and large-scale research. (Rabheru et al., 2022, p. E457)

As of January 1, 2022, the *ICD* is on its 11th revision (designated *ICD-11*) and has been a long time in the making. Whether traced to French physician and botanist Dr. Francois Bossier de Sauvages de Lacroix's initial categorization of 10 distinct classes of diseases in 1763, or the system Farr presented to the International Statistical Congress in 1855 (the general arrangement of which survived as the basis of the International List of Causes of Death adopted by the International Statistical Institute in 1893), the system in use today is the result of tremendous effort, consideration and refinement over many decades (Hirsch et al., 2016; Moriyama et al., 2011; WHO, 2021).

The initial charter for the *ICD* called for revisions every 10 years and this pattern was mostly followed through the 9th revision of the *ICD*. However, the limitations of this approach were becoming apparent with too much time between revisions to capture new needs and not enough time to allow for more significant restructuring of the coding system itself especially as the system was expanded to support hospital statistics and billing uses. While *ICD-9* was adopted in 1976 sharing the same format and even as many codes as *ICD-8* (adopted 1966), *ICD-10* with its new structure was not adopted until 1990. *ICD-11* was adopted in 2019 as another major update designed "to serve semantic interoperability of individual data, reusability of recorded data, for use cases other than health statistics, including decision support, resource allocation, reimbursement, guidelines and more" (WHO, 2021, 2022a, 2022b).

Beyond technical changes, these revisions also capture an evolving understanding of disease and their causes as well as new diseases (Moriyama et al., 2011). It was possible, in 17- and 18-century England, to die of Bleach, Blasted or be Devoured by Lice. One of the forerunners of the *ICD*, had categories such as "deaths from congenital debility, malformations or monstrosity" and "deaths from ill-defined diseases." More recent versions capture world or at least U.S. priorities of the time—proposed additions for 2001 included extra codes for anthrax while 2013 saw codes for gluten sensitivity (Gee, 2015; Schulz, 2014; WHO, 2020). In early 2020, extra codes were added to the *ICD-10* on an emergency basis to track COVID-19 diagnoses and identification of SARS-CoV-2 virus distinct from other coronavirus. *ICD-11* includes a code for burnout (WHO, 2019).

It should be understood that the inclusion and exclusion of codes—and therefore the ability to provide statistical summaries (as well as other use cases)—is a "consideration of the past, current, and future potential for improvement" from interventions based on distinguishing a condition or situation through a new code (Rabheru et al., 2022). In order for a code to be introduced for a condition, the

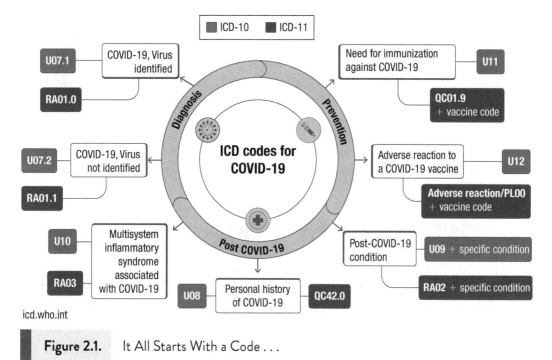

icd.who.int

Figure 2.1. It All Starts With a Code . . .

Source: World Health Organization. (n.d.). *It all starts with a code . . .* https://www.who.int/standards/classifications/classification-of-diseases/emergency-use-icd-codes-for-covid-19-disease-outbreak

condition must be sufficiently understood and identifiable through the process to record qualifying events. Old records will not contain direct references to diseases more recently discovered or better understood. For example, retrospective analysis of old blood samples found SARS-CoV-2 was present in the United States as far back as December 2019 but specific codes for COVID-19 were introduced on an emergency basis only in March of 2020 (CDC, 2020; NIH, 2021). See **Figure 2.1**.

Additionally, the availability or lack of codes and categories can frame how diseases are treated, as authors Kiran Rabheru, Julie E. Byles, and Alexandre Kalaches summarize from their discussions with WHO on the ultimately rejected proposals to add codes for "Old Age" to *ICD-11*:

> *ICD*'s diagnostic categories substantially affect patient care, health care management, and resource allocation. In the context of highly prevalent and ubiquitous societal ageism, erroneous and arbitrary use of the "old age" code, based on chronological age alone, would compromise safety and quality of health care for older people. Furthermore, clinical decision making based on ageism would lead to failure in identifying modifiable risk factors and treatment options, resulting in poorer health care and quality of life outcomes. Opportunities for primary, secondary, and tertiary prevention, symptom management, and social and environmental supports could be overlooked. (Rabheru et al., 2022, p. E459)

Finally, it should be noted that:

> On death certificates, the causes we identify are constrained in one specific way: to the immediate physical breakdown that triggered the events that killed you. "If someone dies of a heart attack," Harvey Fineberg, the president of the Institute of Medicine, says, "you don't say he died of high cholesterol, sedentary life style, and a forty-pack-year history of smoking." For that matter, he notes, we no longer say that "you died of despair, you died of poverty, you died of heartbreak. But certainly those are all pretty clear risks for premature death." (Schulz, 2014, para. 37)

DID YOU KNOW?

Information about the causes of death is obtained from death certificates and how they are coded and compiled:

> For the purpose of national mortality statistics, every death is attributed to one underlying condition, based on information reported on the death certificate and using the international rules for selecting the underlying cause of death from the conditions stated on the certificate. The underlying cause is defined by the World Health Organization (WHO) as "the disease or injury that initiated the train of events leading directly to death, or the circumstances of the accident or violence that produced the fatal injury." Generally, more medical information is reported on death certificates than is directly reflected in the underlying cause of death. Conditions that are not selected as underlying causes of death constitute the nonunderlying causes of death, also known as multiple cause of death. . . . Selected causes of death of public health and medical importance are compiled into tabulation lists and are ranked according to the number of deaths assigned to these causes. The top-ranking causes determine the leading causes of death. (National Center for Health Statistics [NCHS], 2010, p. 502)

Fundamental to modern public health is the availability of valid and reliable data about deaths—their number and causes, as well as the circumstances surrounding them. From such data, patterns can be detected that continually expand our knowledge about the effectiveness of interventions to prevent premature death and improve life. By standardizing the causes of death, the *ICD* is essential to this endeavor. Death certificates, which record the *ICD* code for each death, have become the indispensable tool of epidemiology.

SUCCESS OF PUBLIC HEALTH (AND SETBACKS)

Infectious diseases were the major cause of morbidity and mortality in Britain, as well as the rest of the world, through the end of the 19th century. Common infectious diseases included smallpox, chicken pox, cholera, malaria, diphtheria, and scarlet fever. Some diseases were not fatal, but others were responsible for most of the deaths at the turn of the century. Some, such as smallpox, could be disfiguring for life.

Environmental engineering projects that were begun in the 1800s resulted in improved control of infectious diseases and some of the greatest successes of public health. Later, advancements in the microscope and microbiology led to effective treatments for infectious diseases that in the past were death sentences. They also led to the development of vaccines to prevent infectious diseases from occurring.

> Control of infectious diseases has resulted from clean water and improved sanitation. Infections such as typhoid and cholera transmitted by contaminated water, a major cause of illness and death early in the 20th century, have been reduced dramatically by improved sanitation. In addition, the discovery of antimicrobial therapy has been critical to successful public health efforts to control infections such as tuberculosis and sexually transmitted diseases (STDs). (CDC, 1999, p. 242)

Success Reflected in Cause of Death

These developments—primary prevention through sanitary engineering and vaccines, and secondary prevention through antibiotics and other antimicrobial drugs—changed dramatically the causes of death for people in the 20th century, as well as their age of death. Thus, the success of public health efforts with regard to many infectious diseases—through primary and secondary prevention— was evident in changes in the leading causes of death and in life expectancy after the 19th century.

The United States is a good example of how the causes of death changed after 1900. The leading causes of death in 1900 in the United States (see Table 2.1) reflect the significance of infectious diseases. Deaths from infectious diseases were continuing to decline in 1900, but were still major health threats. At the turn of the century, the first three causes of death were infectious diseases—pneumonia and influenza; tuberculosis; diarrhea and enteritis; and ulceration of the intestines. These, along with diphtheria, accounted for 34% of all deaths at that time.

By 2006, infectious diseases were far less prevalent causes of death than noninfectious diseases. Heart, cerebrovascular, and respiratory diseases, cancer, and diabetes topped the list (see Table 2.2). The only infectious diseases among the 10 leading causes of death—influenza and pneumonia, and septicemia—accounted for only 4% of all deaths. Further, most pneumonia and septicemia deaths occurred during hospitalizations at the end of life, not among the young.

Success Reflected in Life Expectancy

Life expectancy also reflects success in controlling infectious disease.

> Life expectancy is a measure often used to gauge the overall health of a population. As a summary measure of mortality, life expectancy represents the average number of years of life that could be expected if current death rates were to remain constant. Shifts in life expectancy

Table 2.1. Leading Causes of Death: United States, 1900

Cause of Death	Number of Deaths	% of All Deaths
All causes	343,217	100
Pneumonia (all forms) and influenza	40,362	11.76
Tuberculosis (all forms)	38,820	11.31
Diarrhea, enteritis, and ulceration of the intestines	28,491	8.30
Diseases of the heart	27,427	7.99
Intracranial lesions of vascular origin (stroke)	21,353	6.22
Nephritis (all forms)	17,699	5.16
All accidents	14,429	4.20
Cancer and other malignant tumors	12,769	3.72
Senility	10,015	2.92
Diphtheria	8,056	2.35

Source: National Center for Health Statistics. (2010). *Leading causes of death, 1900–1998.* http://cdc.gov/nchs/data/dvs/lead1900_98.pdf

Table 2.2. Leading Causes of Death: United States, 2006

Cause of Death	Number of Deaths	% of All Deaths
All causes	2,426,264	100
Diseases of the heart	631,636	26.03
Malignant neoplasm	559,888	23.08
Cerebrovascular diseases	137,119	5.65
Chronic lower respiratory diseases	124,583	5.13
Unintentional injury	121,599	5.01
Diabetes mellitus	72,449	2.99
Alzheimer disease	72,432	2.99
Influenza and pneumonia	56,326	2.32
Nephritis, nephritic syndrome, and nephrosis	45,344	1.87
Septicemia	34,234	1.41

Source: National Center for Health Statistics. (2010). *Health United States 2009 with special feature on medical technology.* Author.

are often used to describe trends in mortality. Life expectancy at birth is strongly influenced by infant and child mortality. Life expectancy later in life reflects death rates at or above a given age and is independent of the effect of mortality at younger ages. (National Center for Health Statistics [NCHS], 2010, p. 44)

The control of infectious diseases, which began with the sanitary and housing improvements in the 1800s and ended with microbial treatments and vaccines in the late 19th and 20th centuries, was a major cause of increased life expectancy in the first half of the 20th century. This is particularly true for young people who were most at risk for death from diseases such as cholera, typhoid, diphtheria, and other infections. As an example, Table 2.3 contains the life expectancies for all people from 1900 through 2006 in the United States (Arias, 2010).[2] Between 1900 and 2006, children at birth and at the age of 1 year experienced a 58% and 40% increase in life expectancy, respectively, largely in the first half of the century. About 65% and 62%, respectively, of the overall increase for these ages came prior to 1951.

Table 2.3. Life Expectancy by Age: Death Registration States, 1900–1902 to 1909–1911, and United States, 1929–1931 to 2006

Age and race	Average Number of Years of Life Remaining						
	1900–1902	1909–1911	1929–1931	1949–1951	1969–1971	1989–1991	2006
All races							
0	49.24	51.49	59.20	68.07	70.75	75.37	77.7
1	55.20	57.11	61.94	69.16	71.19	75.08	77.2
5	54.98	56.21	59.29	65.54	67.43	71.22	73.3
10	51.14	52.15	54.84	60.74	62.57	66.29	68.4
20	42.79	43.53	45.94	51.20	53.00	56.63	58.6
30	35.51	35.70	37.75	41.91	43.71	47.23	49.2
40	28.34	28.20	29.67	32.81	34.52	37.98	39.7
50	21.26	20.98	22.06	24.40	25.93	29.03	30.7
60	14.76	14.42	15.24	17.04	18.34	20.90	22.4
70	9.30	9.11	9.58	10.92	12.00	13.96	14.9
80	5.30	5.25	5.50	6.34	7.10	8.40	8.7

Source: Arias, E. (2010). United States life tables, 2006. *National Vital Statistics Reports, 58*(21), 1–40. https://pubmed.ncbi.nlm.nih.gov/21043319/#:~:text=It%20increased%20for%20males%20

In contrast, life expectancy for adults 60 years and older increased further after 1951. People 60, 70, and 80 years old experienced an increase in life expectancy between 1900 and 2006 of 52%, 60%, and 64%, respectively. However, only about 28% of this increase for each age group occurred prior to 1951. In the age of the great infectious disease epidemics, the control measures had only small effects on those who survived childhood.

Setbacks Reflected in Cause of Death and Life Expectancy

Infectious diseases are still a problem and an increasing one. The COVID-19 pandemic, which emerged late in 2019, is the most recent and deadly. It was the third leading cause of death in 2021 with 416,893 deaths, exceeded only by heart disease and cancer. It is also having an impact on life expectancy (see Chapter 9).

Even before COVID-19, new infectious diseases were emerging. For example, HIV, an infectious disease that appeared in the 1980s and had no antidote, has affected on mortality among young people. Old infectious diseases have become resistant to standard treatments. For example, methicillin-resistant *Staphylococcus aureus* (MRSA), both community- and hospital-acquired, is a great concern. As the Centers for Disease Control and Prevention [CDC] reports: "MRSA can be fatal. In 1974, MRSA infections accounted for 2% of the total number of staph infections; in 1995 it was 22%; in 2004 it was 63%. CDC estimated that 94,360 invasive MRSA infections occurred in the United States in 2005; 18,650 of these were associated with death" (CDC, 2010).

10 Great Achievements of Public Health Since 1900

Public health has had many accomplishments since its successes in infectious disease control in the 19th and early 20th centuries. The CDC (1999) has developed a list of the 10 greatest public health achievements in the United States since 1900. The average life span has increased by more than 30 years in the United States, and the CDC attributes 25 years of this gain to public health measures. The 10 achievements selected by the CDC were "based on the opportunity for prevention and the impact on death, illness, and disability" (p. 241). They are listed as follows.

Ten Great Public Health Achievements—United States, 1900 to 1999

1. *Vaccination.* Vaccination has resulted in eradication of smallpox; elimination of poliomyelitis in the Americas; and control of measles, rubella, tetanus, diphtheria, *Haemophilus influenza* type b, and other infectious diseases in the United States and other parts of the world.

2. *Motor vehicle safety.* Improvements in motor vehicle safety have resulted from engineering efforts to make both vehicles and highways safer, and from successful efforts to change personal behavior (e.g., increased use of safety belts, child safety seats, and motorcycle helmets, and decreased drinking and driving). These efforts have contributed to large reductions in motor vehicle-related deaths.

3. *Safer workplaces.* Work-related health problems such as coal workers' pneumoconiosis (black lung) and silicosis—common at the beginning of the century—have come under better control. Severe injuries and deaths

related to mining, manufacturing, construction, and transportation have also decreased; since 1980, safer workplaces have resulted in a reduction of approximately 40% in the rate of fatal occupational injuries.

4. *Control of infectious diseases.* Control of infectious diseases has resulted from clean water and improved sanitation. Infections such as typhoid and cholera transmitted by contaminated water, a major cause of illness and death early in the 20th century, have been reduced dramatically by improved sanitation. In addition, the discovery of antimicrobial therapy has been critical to successful public health efforts to control infections such as tuberculosis and sexually transmitted diseases (STDs).

5. *Decline in deaths from coronary heart disease and stroke.* Decline in deaths from coronary heart disease and stroke have resulted from risk-factor modification such as smoking cessation and blood pressure control, coupled with improved access to early detection and better treatment. Since 1972, death rates for coronary heart disease have decreased 51%.

6. *Safer and healthier foods.* Since 1900, safer and healthier foods have resulted from decreases in microbial contamination and increases in nutritional content. Identifying essential micronutrients and establishing food-fortification programs have almost eliminated major nutritional deficiency diseases such as rickets, goiter, and pellagra in the United States.

7. *Healthier mothers and babies.* Healthier mothers and babies have resulted from better hygiene and nutrition, availability of antibiotics, greater access to health care, and technologic advances in maternal and neonatal medicine. Since 1900, infant mortality has decreased 90%, and maternal mortality has decreased 99%.

8. *Family planning.* Access to family planning and contraceptive services has altered social and economic roles of women. Family planning has provided health benefits such as smaller family size and longer intervals between the birth of children; increased opportunities for preconceptional counseling and screening; fewer infant, child, and maternal deaths; and the use of barrier contraceptives to prevent pregnancy and transmission of HIV and other STDs.

9. *Fluoridation of drinking water.* Fluoridation of drinking water began in 1945, and in 1999 reached an estimated 144 million persons in the United States. Fluoridation safely and inexpensively benefits both children and adults by effectively preventing tooth decay, regardless of socioeconomic status or access to care. Fluoridation has played an important role in the reductions in tooth decay (40%–70% in children) and of tooth loss in adults (40%–60%).

10. *Recognition of tobacco use as a health hazard.* Recognition of tobacco use as a health hazard and subsequent public health antismoking campaigns have resulted in changes in social norms to prevent initiation of tobacco use, promote cessation of use, and reduce exposure to environmental tobacco smoke. Since the 1964 Surgeon General's report on the health risks of smoking, the prevalence of smoking among adults has decreased, and millions of smoking-related deaths have been prevented. (CDC, 1999, pp. 242–243)

The list of greatest public health achievements was updated in 2011 by the CDC, Domestic Public Health Achievements Team. The updated list expanded descriptions of the public health impact on control of infectious diseases, as well as occupational safety. In addition, the following achievements were added:

Cancer Prevention

Evidence-based screening recommendations were established to reduce mortality from colorectal cancer and female breast and cervical cancer. Several interventions inspired by these recommendations resulted in improved cancer screening rates.

Childhood Lead Poisoning Prevention

Efforts to prevent childhood lead poisoning succeeded. From 1976–1980 to 2003–2008, findings from the National Health and Nutrition Examination Surveys found a steep decline, from 88.2% to 0.9%, in the percentage of children aged 1 to 5 years with blood lead levels ≥10 mcg/dL. The risks for elevated blood lead levels based on socioeconomic status and race also were reduced significantly.

Public Health Preparedness and Response

After the international and domestic terrorist actions of 2001 highlighted gaps in the nation's public health preparedness, improvements were made to expand the capacity of the public health system to respond including improving the laboratory, epidemiology, surveillance, and response capabilities of the public health system. (CDC, 2011, p. 621)

CHAPTER SUMMARY

Through the 19th century and into the 20th century, public health in the United States organized principally as a government effort and expanded its impact on the important health issues of the time. Public health practice continued to be influenced by the health and safety problems—infectious diseases and injuries—that predominated in the industrializing cities of Britain, the United States, and elsewhere during the Industrial Revolution, and the prevention measures that had been successful then. These included provisions of clean water, sanitary removal of sewage and garbage, safe housing, clean food supply, and safe workplaces.

Development and provision of vaccines to prevent infectious diseases became an essential component of the public health toolkit. Public health also added initiatives in response to changing health needs, particularly the increase in noninfectious diseases such as heart, vascular, and respiratory diseases; diabetes; and cancer. Reducing health behaviors related to noninfectious disease risk including smoking, poor diet, and sedentary lifestyle became an integral part of public health practice.

As medical care became more effective, ensuring availability of hospital and physician services for those whose access was limited by poverty, geography, and health status became an important focus of public health efforts. The development of automobiles and the influence of motor vehicle–related accidents on morbidity and mortality put this issue on the public health agenda as well. Emerging infectious diseases, particularly HIV and the antibiotic-resistant strains of old infectious diseases have become important to public health. Threaded throughout the expanded public health agenda remains the drive to ensure that persons with the least power, influence, and resources have the opportunity to lead safe and healthy lives, just as the plight of child factory workers in the early 1800s moved British reformers to action on their behalf. The emphasis today on ending health disparities is testament to this enduring public health goal and the "public health sensibility" motivating it. This is not to say that public health has been entirely effective. Much has been done, but much remains to be done, as discussed in the last chapter.

DISCUSSION QUESTIONS

Q: How do the 10 greatest achievements of public health relate to the health impact pyramid?

Q: How do the 10 greatest achievements of public health relate to the PRECEDE–PROCEED model?

Q: Who were the champions of reform during the Industrial Revolution?

Q: How were public health reforms achieved during the Industrial Revolution?

Q: What is the relationship of child labor to public health achievements during the Industrial Revolution?

Q: Why is the *ICD* important to the development of public health practice?

NOTES

1. Byssinosis is a lung disease caused by breathing cotton dust or dusts from other fibers such as flax, hemp, or sisal.
2. Alaska and Hawaii were included beginning in 1959. For decennial periods prior to 1929–1931, data are for groups of registration states as follows: 1900–1902 and 1909–1911, 10 states and the District of Columbia (DC); 1919–1921, 34 states and DC Beginning 1970, excludes deaths of nonresidents of the United States.

A robust set of instructor resources designed to supplement this text is located at http://connect.springerpub.com/content/book/978-0-8261-8615-7. Qualifying instructors may request access by emailing textbook@springerpub.com.

REFERENCES

Andrews, R. J. (2022). Florence Nightingale's data revolution. *Scientific American, 327*(2), 78–85. https://doi.org/10.1038/scientificamerican0822-78

Arias, E. (2010). United States life tables, 2006. *National Vital Statistics Reports, 58*(21), 1–40. https://pubmed.ncbi.nlm.nih.gov/21043319/#:~:text=It%20increased%20for%20males%20

Centers for Disease Control and Prevention. (1999). Achievements in public health, 1900-1999: Healthier mothers and babies. *Morbidity and Mortality Weekly Review, 48*(38), 849–858. https://www.cdc.gov/mmwr/preview/mmwrhtml/mm4838a2.htm

Centers for Disease Control and Prevention. (1999). Ten great public health achievements—United States, 1900–1999. *Morbidity and Mortality Weekly Report, 48*(12), 241–243. https://pubmed.ncbi.nlm.nih.gov/10220250/

Centers for Disease Control and Prevention. (2007). *CDC estimates 94,000 invasive drug-resistant staph infections occurred in the U.S. in 2005.* https://www.cdc.gov/media/pressrel/2007/r071016.htm

Centers for Disease Control and Prevention. (2011). Ten great public health achievements—United States, 2001—2010. *Morbidity and Mortality Weekly Report (MMWR), 60*(19), 619–623. https://pubmed.ncbi.nlm.nih.gov/21597455/

Centers for Disease Control and Prevention. (2020). *New ICD-10-CM code for the 2019 novel coronavirus (COVID-19), April 1, 2020.* https://www.cdc.gov/nchs/data/icd/Announcement-New-ICD-code-for-coronavirus-3-18-2020.pdf

Department of Epidemiology, Columbia University. (2020). *What is epidemiology?* https://www.publichealth.columbia.edu/public-health-now/news/what-epidemiology

Gee, A. (2015). Death by flaming water ski, and other misfortunes. *The New Yorker.* https://www.newyorker.com/tech/annals-of-technology/death-by-flaming-water-ski-and-other-misfortunes-in-the-international-classification-of-diseases

Granados, J. A. T. (2022). William Farr: British physician. *Encyclopaedia Britannica.* https://www.britannica.com/biography/William-Farr

Hirsch, J. A., Nicola, G., McGinty, G., Liu, R. W., Barr, R. M., Chittle, M. D., & Manchikanti, L. (2016). *ICD-10*: History and context. *American Journal of Neuroradiology, 37*, 596–99. https://doi.org/10.3174/ajnr.A4696

Konstantinidou, K., Mantadakis, E., Falagas, M. E., Sardi, T., & Samonis, G. (2009). Venetian rule and control of plague epidemics on the Ionian Islands during 17th and 18th centuries. *Emerging Infectious Diseases, 15*(1), 39–43. https://doi.org/10.3201/eid1501.071545

Krieger, N., & Birn, A. E. (1998). A vision of social justice as the foundation of public health: Commemorating 150 years of the spirit of 1848. *American Journal of Public Health, 88*(11), 1603–1606. https://doi.org/10.2105/ajph.88.11.1603

Moriyama, I. M., Loy, R. M., & Robb-Smith, A. H. T. (2011). *History of the statistical classification of diseases and causes of death.* National Center for Health Statistics. https://www.cdc.gov/nchs/data/misc/classification_diseases2011.pdf

National Center for Health Statistics. (2010). *Health United States 2009 with special feature on medical technology*. Author.

National Institutes of Health. (2021). *NIH study offers new evidence of early SARS-CoV-2 infections in U.S.* https://www.nih.gov/news-events/news-releases/nih-study-offers-new-evidence-early-sars-cov-2-infections-us

National Oceanic and Atmospheric Administration. (2010). *Nonpoint source pollution: A brief history of pollution*. https://oceanservice.noaa.gov/education/tutorial_pollution/02history.html

Norton, C. S. (1836). *A voice from the factories*. John Murray. http://digital.library.upenn.edu/women/norton/avftf/avftf.html

Pike, E. R. (1966). *Hard times: Human documents of the industrial revolution*. Praeger.

Public Health Science and Surveillance, & Centers for Disease Control and Prevention. (2012). *Introduction to epidemiology: Definition of epidemiology*. https://www.cdc.gov/csels/dsepd/ss1978/lesson1/section1.html

Rabheru, K., Byles, J. E., & Kalache, A. (2022). How 'old age' was withdrawn as a diagnosis from ICD-11. *The Lancet, 3*(7), E457–E459. https://doi.org/10.1016/S2666-7568(22)00102-7

Schulz, K. (2014). Final forms: What death certificates can tell us, and what they can't. *The New Yorker*. https://www.newyorker.com/magazine/2014/04/07/final-forms

Spartacus Educational. (2010a). *Benjamin Gomersal*. https://spartacus-educational.com/IRgomersal.htm

Spartacus Educational. (2010b). *William Rastrick*. https://spartacus-educational.com/IRrastrick.htm

Spartacus Educational. (2010c). *Factory accidents*. https://spartacus-educational.com/IRaccidents.htm

Spartacus Educational. (2010d). *Factory pollution*. https://spartacus-educational.com/IRpollution.htm

Spartacus Educational. (2010e). *John Birley*. https://spartacus-educational.com/IRbirley.htm

Spartacus Educational. (2010f). *London*. https://spartacus-educational.com/ITlondon.htm

Spartacus Educational. (2010g). *Lord Byron*. https://spartacus-educational.com/PRbyron.htm

Spartacus Educational. (2010h). *Piecers in the textile industry*. https://spartacus-educational.com/IRpiecers.htm

Spartacus Educational. (2010i). *Working hours*. https://spartacus-educational.com/IRtime.htm

Thompson, E. P. (1964). *The making of the English working class*. Pantheon Books.

Toynbee, A. (1957). *The industrial revolution*. Beacon Press.

United Kingdom Parliament. (2014). *Living heritage: Reforming parliament in the 19th century.* http://www.parliament.uk/about/living-heritage/transformingsociety/livinglearning/19thcentury/overview/

World Health Organization. (2019). *Burn-out an 'occupational phenomenon': International classification of diseases.* https://www.who.int/news/item/28-05-2019-burn-out-an-occupational-phenomenon-international-classification-of-diseases

World Health Organization. (2020). *It all starts with a code . . . .* https://www.who.int/standards/classifications/classification-of-diseases/emergency-use-icd-codes-for-covid-19-disease-outbreak

World Health Organization. (2021). *History of the development of the ICD.* https://www.who.int/publications/m/item/history-of-the-development-of-the-icd

World Health Organization. (2022a). *International statistical classification of diseases and related health problems (ICD).* https://www.who.int/standards/classifications/classification-of-diseases

World Health Organization. (2022b). ICD-11 *reference guide: An introduction to* ICD-11. https://icdcdn.who.int/icd11referenceguide/en/html/index.html#part-1-an-introduction-to-icd11

3 | Organization and Financing of Public Health

LEARNING OBJECTIVES

Students will learn . . .

1. The legal basis for public health practice at the federal, state, and local levels.

2. The organization of public health services at the federal, state, and local levels.

3. The three core functions and the 10 essential services and who performs them.

4. The major public health agencies at the federal level and their roles.

5. The source and amount of public health funding.

The 2003 Institute of Medicine (IOM) report, *The Future of the Public's Health in the 21st Century*, emphasizes that public health extends beyond government and encompasses, "the efforts, science, art, and approaches used by all sectors of society (public, private, and civil society) to assure, maintain, protect, promote, and improve the health of the people" (Committee on Assuring the Health of the Public in the 21st Century, 2002, p. 20). The report defines six critical "actors" who are in a position to greatly affect health: communities, the health care delivery system, employers and business, the media, academia, and government.

Public health systems are commonly defined as "all public, private, and voluntary entities that contribute to the delivery of essential public health services within a jurisdiction." This concept ensures that all entities' contributions to the health and well-being of the community or state are recognized in assessing the provision of public health services. The public health system includes:

- Public health agencies at state and local levels
- Healthcare providers
- Public safety agencies
- Human service and charity organizations
- Education and youth development organizations
- Recreation and arts-related organizations

- Economic and philanthropic organizations
- Environmental agencies and organizations (CDC, 2023, para. 1)

Other definitions of public health also emphasize the collaboration between the public and private sectors in the organization and activities of public health. Van Wave et al. (2010) assert that:

> The public health system is defined as the collective resources, infrastructure, and effort of all public, private, and voluntary entities and their respective roles, relationships, and interactions that contribute to the delivery of essential public health services to the population within a jurisdiction. (p. 284)

The CDC states: "The governmental public health agency—both at the state and local levels—is a major contributor and leader in the public health system, but these governmental agencies cannot provide the full spectrum of Essential Services alone" (CDC, 2007, p. 6). The IOM (1988, p. 41) defines the public health system as the "activities undertaken within the formal structure of government and the associated efforts of private and voluntary organizations and individuals." Further, the IOM (2003) finds that a public health system is a complex network of individuals and organizations that have the potential to play critical roles in creating the conditions of health. They can act for health individually, but when they work together toward a health goal, they act as a system—a public health system (p. 28).

Although there is much to recommend this broader understanding of the public health system, it is also too extensive for an introduction. In this chapter, we will focus on the governmental public health system, with some attention to the private actors who frequently collaborate with it (e.g., academia, nonprofit health organizations, and professional associations). The decision to focus on government is, in part, practical: Taking an especially broad view of the public health "system," which encompasses a multitude of actors in all areas of society—largely without any formalized organization, relationships, or roles—renders it largely resistant to generalization, and, as we will see, the governmental system is itself sufficiently complex all on its own. The decision is also, however, substantive:

> Governmental public health agencies constitute the backbone of the public health system and bear primary, legally mandated responsibility for assuring the delivery of essential public health services. Therefore, the role of government in assuring the nation's health is one that must be continued and sustained. (IOM, 2003, p. 27)

Government has a unique and special responsibility to promote public health. Governments also have the resources and legal authority to implement public health policies and focus public health missions that private actors generally lack. Accordingly, the focus of the discussion of the U.S. public health system will be on the government agencies; we should not lose sight of the fact that government frequently partners with other actors—academia, nongovernmental organizations (NGOs), professional associations, philanthropic organizations, the private health care delivery system, as well as business and media—in developing and delivering public health services.

The integrating force for the public health system—the "glue"—is the official public health agency infrastructure. Only government has jurisdiction, the power to create and enforce laws, and the mandate to secure our fundamental rights. In the United States, such duties rest within the governments of the fifty states and five territories, each of which has an organized public health unit that oversees the conduct of the government's public health programs and fulfills the roles that "cannot be properly delegated." (Tilson & Berkowitz, 2006, p. 904)

Government is also key because "public health" functions, at least in large part, are to provide for people who are not suitably or effectively provided for by the private sector.

ORGANIZATION OF THE PUBLIC HEALTH SYSTEM

The governmental public health system in the United States is comprised of several departments and agencies within the federal government, at least one state-level agency for every state and territory in the country, and approximately 2,800 local health agencies. Hundreds of thousands of public health workers staff these agencies (Association of State and Territorial Health Officials [ASTHO], 2020; National Association of County and City Health Officials [NACCHO], 2020a; U.S. Department of Health and Human Services [DHHS], 2022a). Given our cognitive preference to find order in systems and our predispositions about the structure of organizations, it may be tempting to imagine from this rudimentary description that the U.S. public health system is a centralized, cohesive, hierarchically arranged organization in which the federal government sets policy and marshals resources, which it then distributes to the states, which in turn establish the infrastructure for implementation of those polices and provision of public health services to the population through local health departments (LHDs), which then deliver them.

In truth, however, the governmental public health system in the United States is highly decentralized. The federal government has little direct control over state public health matters. States are generally responsible for their own public health systems, and in most circumstances, states delegate at least some of that authority to local political units—cities, towns, counties, and so forth—that set and implement their own public health policies. Rather than exercising *authority* over health matters in the United States, the federal government's role is primarily one of *influence*. This influence is broadly either of the "persuasive" variety, whereby research and recommendations conducted at the federal level inform the decisions of more local public health policymakers and actors, or of the "financial" variety, whereby the federal government provides financial support to state and local public health agencies, frequently on the condition that the funds be used in a particular manner. The limited authority the federal government does have is generally restricted to those issues that have been recognized as affecting commercial or business conditions across state lines. Thus, the U.S. government public health system is a highly complex system of discrete, often independent, decentralized, and varied agencies.

The decentralized and largely local character of the public health system is, in substantial part, a consequence of the legal, political, and historical context in which the public health system developed and operates. Largely, the organization of the public health system and the delivery of public health services can be traced to the principles of federalism governing the broader political and governmental organization of the United States (Turnock & Atchison, 2002). Under the U.S. federal system, sovereign power is shared between the federal government and the states, with certain powers delegated to the federal government exclusively, certain powers retained by the states exclusively, and some powers held by both the federal and state governments (subject to the limitations of federal supremacy). The 10th Amendment provides that any power not specifically delegated to the federal government in the Constitution be retained by the states. Among the powers the Constitution provides to the federal government is the power to tax and spend and to regulate interstate commerce. As will be discussed further, the activities of the federal government in support of public health generally derive from these powers. One power not specified in the Constitution, however, is the "police power"—the power to regulate and coerce persons for the benefit and welfare of society. Because it is not specified, it is among the plenary powers remaining with the states. It has long been recognized that the authority to regulate in the interest of public health derives from the police power ("The states of this Union may, in the exercise of their police powers, pass quarantine and health laws." *Passenger Cases*, [1849] Wayne, J., concurring). States, therefore, have primary authority for public health in the United States.

Consistent with federalism's placement of value on local self-determination, states often further pass on the police power, at least to some extent, to smaller and more local units of government (counties, cities, towns, etc.). This is true in the area of public health. Many states have delegated public health responsibilities to local governments or boards of health. Further, "home rule" statutes in 48 states authorize local governments, depending on factors including their size and class, to address public health issues directly through local laws (McCarty et al., 2009). That public health concerns are considered under the federal system to be principally matters of local focus is consistent with the historic emergence of public health practice and regulation in the United States. "Public health in the United States did not begin as a systematic, rational, centrally directed activity following a coherent plan but rather as a fitful, episodic, and necessity-driven response to immediate local threats" (Fee & Brown, 2002). Public health concerns—and health matters in general, for that matter—did not historically emerge as national issues, but as local ones, and the allocation of government responsibility—with state and the local government having primary responsibility for implementing public health regulations and delivery of public health services—reflects this.

That governmental public health authority and delivery in the United States is decentralized is not necessarily problematic. Consistent with principles of federalism, theories of political economy suggest that superior public services may flow from decentralized governmental authority, because the more local the government, the closer it is to the population it serves, making it more informed of and responsive to the needs of its population (Mays et al., 2006, 2007). However, in the last half century, the ability of the U.S. public health system to deliver the services required of it has come under scrutiny. The IOM's 1988 landmark report, *The Future of Public Health*, which is a frequent reference point for analysis and evaluation of the U.S. public health system, stimulated interest in assessment and improvement of the public health enterprise (Tilson & Berkowitz, 2006; Turnock ·& Atchison, 2002). The report noted that "[i]n recent years, there has been a growing sense that public health, as a profession, as a governmental activity, and as a commitment of society is neither clearly defined, adequately supported, nor fully understood" (IOM, 1988, p. v). It concluded that the nation, in overlooking the public health system, was unable to achieve public health goals (IOM, 1988).

The legal and constitutional framework in which public health activities are conducted contributes to the "disarray" and fractured system of public health identified by the IOM. A consequence of limited scope of federal government's authority in regulating health is that there is no central public health authority with nationwide reach; no entity or agency has comprehensive authority for the operation of the public health system. Instead, as the IOM observed, because public health regulations and services are implemented primarily at the state and local levels, public health goals emerge within different political units and communities, each with their own health problems and concerns, political systems, resource availability, organizations, and values (IOM, 1988). Therefore, public health systems vary widely from community to community, with each prioritizing different problems and offering different responses and solutions to public health issues. While this characteristic may enhance local control, appropriateness, and flexibility of local agencies to meet the needs of a particular population, it also leads to fragmentation and uneven distribution in the type and quality of services provided (Baker et al., 2005). Further, with responsibility for health dispersed across federal, state, and local agencies and governments, coordination in response to health problems or in pursuit of health goals is often frustrated by fragmented system organization. The division of authority has led to inconsistency, poor resource allocation, and lack of clarity about the agencies' respective responsibilities (Baker & Koplan, 2002). In light of this, the IOM concluded that "viewed from a national perspective, the national public health system is a scene of tremendous variety and disarray as different communities work out different solutions to public health problems" (IOM, 1988, p. 74).

The IOM did not conclude that the structure of the U.S. public health system was inherently flawed. Rather, it acknowledged that states have primary authority over public health matters, that LHDs provide the "front" line in the delivery of public health services, and that the federal government has the resources to facilitate improvement of the public health infrastructure. It emphasized that no community should be without the protections of a public health system and concluded that this was possible only through the local components of an organized nationwide system of state-level agencies (IOM, 1988; Tilson & Berkowitz, 2006). Rather than propose a reorganization of the public health system, the IOM concentrated on the enterprise of public health, and identified three core functions that should be conducted by public health agencies at all levels of government:

1. Assessment—activities concerning community diagnosis such as surveillance and epidemiology;
2. Policy development—determination and prioritization of problems, goals, solutions, and resource allocation; and
3. Assurance—guaranteeing that necessary public health services are provided.

The IOM acknowledges that implementation of the core functions would vary from place to place. "The specific actions appropriate to strengthen public health will vary from area to area and must blend professional knowledge with community values" (IOM, 1988, p. 18).

10 Essential Services

In 1994, the DHHS convened a committee with representatives from all major public health constituencies, including the American Public Health Association (APHA), the Association of Schools of Public Health (ASPH), the ASTHO, the Environmental Council of the States (ECS), the NACCHO, the National Association of State Alcohol and Drug Abuse Directors, the National Association of State Mental Health Program Directors, the Public Health Foundation (PHF), and the divisions of DHHS constituting the U.S. Public Health Service. The Public Health Functions Steering Committee released a consensus statement titled *Public Health in America*, which stated the vision, mission, purposes, and essential functions of public health in the United States (DHHS et al., 1994). According to the statement, public health:

- Prevents epidemics and the spread of disease,
- Protects against environmental hazards,
- Prevents injuries,
- Promotes and encourages healthy behaviors,
- Responds to disasters and assists communities in recovery, and
- Ensures the quality and accessibility of health services.

The committee also identified 10 essential services of public health, which were revised in 2020 by the Public Health National Center for Innovations and the de Beaumont Foundation. The revision was intended to "bring the framework in line with current and future public health practice" (CDC, 2021a). The essential public health services (revised) are:

1. Assess and monitor population health status, factors that influence health, and community needs and assets;
2. Investigate, diagnose, and address health problems and hazards affecting the population;
3. Communicate effectively to inform and educate people about health, factors that influence it, and how to improve it;
4. Strengthen, support, and mobilize communities and partnerships to improve health;

5. Create, champion, and implement policies, plans, and laws that impact health;

6. Utilize legal and regulatory actions designed to improve and protect the public's health;

7. Ensure an effective system that enables equitable access to the individual services and care needed to be healthy;

8. Build and support a diverse and skilled public health workforce;

9. Improve and innovate public health functions through ongoing evaluation, research, and continuous quality improvement; and

10. Build and maintain a strong organizational infrastructure for public health.

The list of 10 essential services translates the three core functions identified by the IOM into a more specific set of activities. "These embody the protections and services that every citizen has the right to expect, and every government has the obligation to assure. No matter what the unique features of any single community, the concept of the 10 essential services recognizes that every community needs a robust and reliable agency infrastructure" (Tilson & Berkowitz, 2006, p. 905). The 10 essential services provide the foundation for the nation's public health strategy, including the *Healthy People* objectives, which are discussed in Chapter 6, and the development of the National Public Health Performance Standards (CDC, 2022a; DHHS and Office of Disease Prevention and Health Promotion, 2022). See **Figure 3.1.**

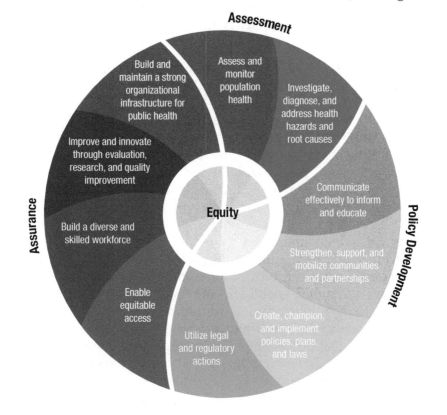

Figure 3.1.   The 10 Essential Public Health Services

Source: Centers for Disease Control and Prevention, Public Health Professionals Gateway. (2023). *10 essential public health services.* https://www.cdc.gov/publichealthgateway/publichealthservices/essentialhealthservices.html

The 10 Essential Public Health Services provide a framework for public health to protect and promote the health of all people in all communities. To achieve equity, the Essential Public Health Services actively promote policies, systems, and overall community conditions that enable optimal health for all and seek to remove systemic and structural barriers that have resulted in health inequities. Such barriers include poverty, racism, gender discrimination, ableism, and other forms of oppression. Everyone should have a fair and just opportunity to achieve optimal health and well-being. (CDC, 2021a, para. 3)

FEDERAL PUBLIC HEALTH

Despite the constitutional restrictions on the federal government's role in regulating public health, it nevertheless plays a very large role in the U.S. public health system. The two powers constitutionally delegated to the federal government mentioned before—the power to tax and spend for the general welfare and the power to regulate interstate commerce—provide the basis for most federal activity in the public health arena. The federal government's key activities can generally be categorized as falling under at least one of four groups: (a) allocation and distribution of resources to public health actors; (b) information generation and distribution; (c) health care access assurance; and (d) regulation and enforcement. In many cases, an activity may be characterized as falling under more than one category.

The power to tax and spend is exactly what it sounds like: The federal government is authorized to collect and distribute funds to promote the welfare of the nation. "Spending" may be either the funding of projects and programs carried out by the government itself, financing contracts with external parties, or making direct contributions of funds (e.g., through grants). Most of the federal government's public health activities are based on its power to tax and spend. For example, pursuant to this power, the federal government conducts extensive health monitoring, surveillance, and epidemiologic studies; it conducts and funds health and biomedical research; it surveys the nation's health status and health needs; it develops policies, guidelines, and standards for public health practice; it provides direct and indirect funding to state and local public health agencies, as well as private organizations such as community health centers; it supports public information and education campaigns on health-related matters; it conducts and funds public health education and research; it provides education and training to the public health workforce; and it funds or provides access to personal health services through such programs as community health centers, Medicaid, Medicare, State Children's Health Insurance Program (SCHIP), and health care for veterans. The taxing power is also used to encourage or discourage certain behaviors. For example, the federal government may encourage private business to provide health insurance to employees through tax credits, and it may discourage the consumption of tobacco products or alcohol through the imposition of excise or "sin" taxes.

The federal government's health-related regulatory authority is generally de-rived from the Commerce Clause—the constitutional provision permitting the federal government to regulate interstate commerce. Although generally more limited in scope than its activities financing public health research and services or providing access to health care, the federal government does impose and en-force regulations and laws in several public health areas affecting the country generally. For example, federal agencies enforce regulations concerning drug, food, and occupational safety, as well as environmental protection. The federal government's regulatory activities in each of these arenas are based in its author-ity under the Commerce Clause. If there were political will, federal control could be imposed. The same reasoning could be applied to communicable disease monitoring—disease affects business and does not respect political boundaries.

Department of Health and Human Services

The central, though not the only, federal agency responsible for public health and health care in the United States is the **DHHS**. Its mission is "to enhance the health and well-being of all Americans, by providing for effective health and human services and by fostering sound, sustained advances in the sciences underlying medicine, public health, and social services" (DHHS, 2022a, para. 1). Through 12 operating divisions, the DHHS administers more than 100 health-related pro-grams in a wide range of areas, including health and biomedical research, ep-idemiology and surveillance, disease prevention and immunization, food and drug safety, providing access to primary health care for certain populations, and bioterrorism response preparedness. These programs "protect the health of all Americans and provide essential human services, especially for those who are least able to help themselves" (DHHS, 2022b, para. 1).

In 2022, the DHHS directly employed approximately 84,000 people and had a budget with $1.7 trillion in outlays. About 80% of the budget funded the Medic-aid and Medicare programs. Many of the other mandatory programs concerned children and family well-being (DHHS, 2022c). See **Table 3.1**.

Discretionary programs accounted for 10% of the budget (DHHS, 2022c). See **Figure 3.2**.

Of the 12 operating divisions within the DHHS, nine are components of the U.S. Public Health Service. There are two staff offices within the Office of the Secre-tary, which are also designated components of the U.S. Public Health Service and which operate to coordinate the agency's public health activities. They are the Office of Global Affairs (OGA) and the Office of the Assistant Secretary for Preparedness and Response. These operating divisions and staff offices them-selves each contain many subagencies and offices, administering hundreds of programs within the DHHS. **Table 3.2** lists the DHHS operating divisions and their respective missions and budgets.

As **Table 3.2** indicates, the scope of activities and services undertaken by the DHHS is vast, and indeed, many of the identified subagencies and offices have

Table 3.1. Composition of the DHHS Budget: Mandatory Programs (in Millions of Dollars)

Mandatory Programs (Outlays)[a]	2020	2021	2022	2022 ± 2021
Medicare	768,618	720,312	767,325	+47,013
Medicaid	458,468	521,127	570,687	+49,560
Temporary assistance for needy families[b]	17,182	17,278	17,878	+S00
Foster care and adoption assistance	8,836	10,764	10,241	−523
Children's health insurance program[c]	16,880	17,220	17,142	−78
Child support enforcement	4,424	4,388	4,157	−231
Child care entitlement	2.979	3,187	13,973	+10,786
Social services block grant	1,727	1,583	1,640	+57
Other mandatory programs[d]	14.93E	65,913	90,460	+24,547
Offsetting collections	−1,219	−1,169	−597	+572
Subtotal, Mandatory outlays	**1,292,833**	**1,360,603**	**1,492,906**	**+132,303**
Total, DHHS Outlays	**1,504,270**	**1,547,463**	**1,662,293**	**+114,830**

[a]Totals may not add due to rounding.
[b]Includes outlays for the Temporary Assistance for Needy Families (TANF) and the TANF Contingency Fund.
[c]Includes outlays for the Child Enrollment Contingency Fund.
[d]Includes outlays for No Surprises Implementation Fund, Defense Production Act Medical Supplies Enhancement, Prepare Americans for Future Pandemics, Invest in Maternal Health, the Public Health Resilience, and all other remaining mandatory outlays not broken out in the Mandatory Programs table.

DHHS, Department of Health and Human Services; TANF, Temporary Assistance for Needy Families.

Source: Department of Health and Human Services. (2023). *Fiscal year 2022: Budget in brief*. https://www.hhs.gov/sites/default/files/fy-2022-budget-in-brief.pdf

their own branches and divisions, each with its own mission and program responsibilities. A comprehensive discussion of the activities and programs of the DHHS agencies is far beyond what can be accomplished here. Furthermore, reorganization at the federal level is occurring rapidly, particularly in response to the COVID-19 pandemic. What follows should not, by any means, be considered an exhaustive or complete description of the agencies discussed, but is rather intended to give an idea of some of the key programs and activities of the DHHS agencies, and how the federal government supports the 10 essential public health services.

Our discussion of the 12 DHHS operating divisions begins with the CDC, the preeminent public health organization in the United States.

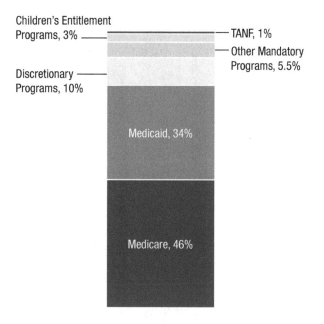

Figure 3.2.   The FY 2022 DHSS Budget—$1.7 Trillion in Outlays

DHHS, Department of Health and Human Services; FY, fiscal year; TANF, Temporary Assistance for Needy Families.

Source: U.S. Department of Health and Human Services. (2022c). *Fiscal year 2022: Budget in brief.* https://www.hhs.gov/sites/default/files/fy-2022-budget-in-brief.pdf

Centers for Disease Control and Prevention

Established in 1946 as the Communicable Disease Center, the CDC is the foremost epidemiologic, surveillance, and disease prevention agency in the federal government. Among its key functions is to monitor and report on the nation's health, detect health problems and disease outbreaks, research and implement disease prevention strategies, develop and advocate sound public health policies, promote healthy behaviors, and provide public health leadership and training. The CDC is the nation's go-to agency for public health. It is the voice of public health for the nation. The CDC houses some of the best epidemiologists; biomedical, behavioral, and social scientists; prevention researchers; health policy analysts; and health economists in the world. Many know the CDC for its outstanding work related to infectious diseases. Its staff travels to sites worldwide when infectious disease outbreaks occur. The CDC publishes the essential *Morbidity and Mortality Weekly Report* (*MMWR*), which contains the latest information on reportable diseases, new hazards, and other emerging health conditions. The CDC has also been a leader in bioterrorism threats research and practice. The CDC has become actively involved in noninfectious disease prevention, as well as the area of chronic diseases and injury control. The CDC has been called "the nation's premier and largest public health organization" (Hartsaw, 2009, p. 141).

At the time of writing, the CDC was undergoing reorganization, particularly as a result of the COVID-19 pandemic response (see Chapter 9). Data improvement and data analytics are important foci of reorganization.

Table 3.2. Department of Health and Human Services (DHHS) Operating Divisions, 2022

Operating Division[a]	Mission and Budget[b]
Administration for Children and Families (ACF)	*Mission:* to foster health and well-being by providing federal leadership, partnership, and resources for the compassionate and effective delivery of human services. *FY2022 Budget Outlays:* $98,367
Administration for Community Living (ACL)	*Mission:* to maximize the independence, well-being, and health of older adults, people with disabilities across the lifespan, and their families and caregivers. *FY2022 Budget Outlays:* $5,005
Administration for Strategic Preparedness and Response (ASPR)[c]	*Mission:* (a) to lead the nation's medical and public health preparedness for, response to, and recovery from disasters and public health emergencies. (b) to collaborate with hospitals; health care coalitions; biotech firms; community members; state, local, tribal, and territorial governments; and other partners across the country to improve readiness and response capabilities. *FY2022 Budget Outlays:* (through Public Health and Social Services Emergency Fund and others)
Agency for Healthcare Research and Quality (AHRQ)[c]	*Mission:* to produce evidence to make health care safer, higher quality, more accessible, equitable, and affordable, and to work within the U.S. Department of Health and Human Services and with other partners to make sure that the evidence is understood and used. *FY2022 Budget Outlays:* $344
Agency for Toxic Substances and Disease Registry (ATSDR)[c]	*Mission:* to protect communities from harmful health effects related to exposure to natural and man-made hazardous substances by responding to environmental health emergencies; investigating emerging environmental health threats; conducting research on the health impacts of hazardous waste sites; and building capabilities of and providing actionable guidance to state and local health partners. *FY2022 Budget Outlays:* (included in CDC budget)
Centers for Disease Control and Prevention (CDC)[c]	*Mission:* to protect America from health, safety, and security threats, both foreign and in the United States. Whether diseases start at home or abroad, are chronic or acute, curable or preventable, human error or deliberate attack, the CDC fights disease and supports communities and citizens to do the same. *FY2022 Budget Outlays:* $16,108

Centers for Medicare & Medicaid Services (CMS)	Mission: CMS OMH will lead the advancement and integration of health equity in the development, evaluation, and implementation of CMS's policies, programs, and partnerships. FY2022 Budget Outlays: $1,379,251
Food and Drug Administration (FDA)[c]	Mission: (a) to protect the public health by ensuring the safety, efficacy, and security of human and veterinary drugs, biological products, and medical devices; and by ensuring the safety of our nation's food supply, cosmetics, and products that emit radiation. (b) to regulate the manufacturing, marketing, and distribution of tobacco products to protect the public health and to reduce tobacco use by minors. (c) to expand the knowledge base in medical and associated sciences in order to enhance the nation's economic well-being and ensure a continued high return on the public investment in research; and (d) to exemplify and promote the highest level of scientific integrity; public accountability, and social responsibility in the conduct of science. FY2022 Budget Outlays: $3,857
Health Resources and Services Administration (HRSA)[c]	Mission: to improve health outcomes and achieve health equity through access to quality services, a skilled health workforce, and innovative, high-value programs. FY2022 Budget Outlays: $17,628
Indian Health Services (IHS)[c]	Mission: to raise the physical, mental, social, and spiritual health of American Indians and Alaska Natives to the highest level. FY2022 Budget Outlays: $10,951
National Institutes of Health (NIH)[c]	Mission: to seek fundamental knowledge about the nature and behavior of living systems and the application of that knowledge to enhance health, lengthen life, and reduce illness and disability. FY2022 Budget Outlays: $45,213
Substance Abuse and Mental Health Services Administration (SAMHSA)[c]	Mission: SAMHSA's mission is to reduce the impact of substance use and mental illness on America's communities. FY2022 Budget Outlays: $9,651

[a] Alphabetical.
[b] Budget outlays in millions of dollars.
[c] U.S. Public Health Service.

FY, fiscal year; OMH, Office of Minority Health.

Source: U.S. Department of Health and Human Services. (2022a). *About HHS.* https://www.hhs.gov/about/index.html; U.S. Department of Health and Human Services. (2022c). *Budget in brief: Fiscal year 2022.* https://www.hhs.gov/sites/default/files/fy-2022-budget-in-brief.pdf

KEY IDEA

Overall, every CDC division and program is being affected by an increased focus on data improvement and better application of data to meet its mission.

The **Public Health Data Modernization Initiative** is "at the heart of a national effort to improve the data that can improve health. This cross-cutting strategy will move us from tracking threats to anticipating them" (CDC, 2022b, para. 1). The initiative focuses on:

- Accelerating health-related data modernization capabilities across private and public entities,
- Improving the skills of the public health workforce in data science and informatics, and
- Innovating in areas of modeling and predictive analysis, artificial intelligence, and machine-learning approaches to improving health.

In fiscal year (FY) 2021, under the CARES (Coronavirus Aid, Relief, and Economic Security) Act, additional funds were provided for data surveillance and analytical infrastructure:

- "Leverage data for surveillance, detection, and improving jurisdictions' situational awareness to allow localized, targeted responses and decision making using more real-time data to respond to outbreaks like COVID-19.
- Expand the electronic exchange and integration of information between public health and health care, including electronic health records, which is essential for timely, accurate, and accessible disease surveillance.
- Support for public health's data science, informatics, and IT workforce; expanding core data, informatics, and IT capacity; advancing interoperable systems and tools; strengthening and expanding collaboration" (CDC, 2022b, para. 4).

The Data Modernization Initiative's Strategic Plan summarizes the CDC's vision for enhanced data utilization:

> CDC's Data Modernization Initiative (DMI) is how our nation will move from siloed and brittle public health data systems to connected, resilient, adaptable, and sustainable "response-ready" systems that can help us solve problems before they happen and reduce the harm caused by the problems that do happen. (CDC, 2021b, para. 1)

The scope of the CDC's activities is too great to be presented comprehensively here, but a few examples follow. See **Figure 3.3**, for all of the centers and offices within the CDC and their organizational structure as of March 2021 (CDC, 2021a).

Infectious Diseases

At present, the CDC has three centers to prevent, control, and detect communicable diseases: the National Center for Immunization and Respiratory Diseases

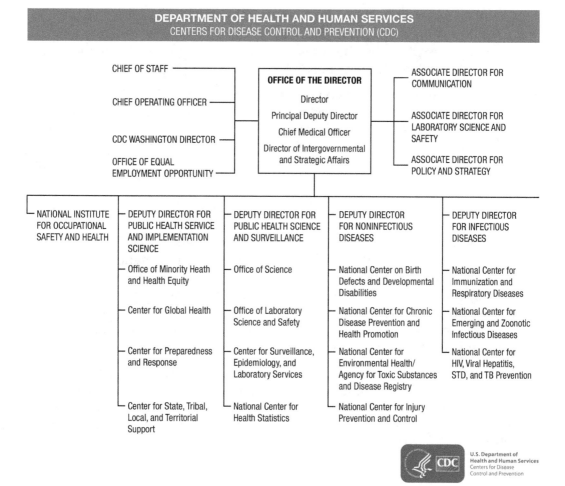

Figure 3.3.   Organizational Chart: Centers for Disease Control and Prevention, 2021

STD, sexually transmitted disease; TB, tuberculosis.

Source: From https://www.cdc.gov/about/pdf/organization/cdc-org-chart.pdf

(NCIRD); National Center for Emerging and Zoonotic Infectious Diseases (NCEZD); and National Center for HIV/AIDS, Viral Hepatitis, Sexually Transmitted Infection, and Tuberculosis Prevention (NCHHSTP).

The *NCIRD* has four divisions:

- Bacterial diseases,
- Influenza,
- Viral diseases, and
- Immunization services (NCIRD, 2023).

The priorities of the Division of Bacterial Diseases are to accelerate development, introduction, and evaluation of vaccines for bacterial respiratory diseases including pneumonia, meningitis and neonatal sepsis; to identify, assess, and implement improved and innovative methods for laboratory, statistical, and epidemiologic sciences that impact bacterial disease; to strengthen surveillance and early detection of bacterial diseases; and communicate effectively with the public about these diseases. This division works globally, as well as in the United States, as do the other divisions in NCIRD.

The focus of the Influenza Division is improving influenza detection and control, vaccine effectiveness, and risk assessment and readiness for influenza epidemics and pandemics. The Division of Viral Diseases seeks to optimize the use of vaccines to prevent viral diseases; identify new ways to prevent viral diseases; and respond effectively to viral disease outbreaks, particularly by improving local, state, and global response capacity.

The Immunization Services Division seeks to protect individuals and communities from vaccine-preventable diseases. The division administers the Vaccines for Children program and Section 317 immunization grants to state health departments. It provides technical support for immunization information systems and conducts research and evaluation of programs to improve vaccine uptake and delivery of vaccines. The Division provides financial support for immunization programs and provider and public education about vaccination. Program effectiveness is monitored through the National Immunization Surveys administered by the National Center for Health Statistics (NCHS).

The *NCEZD* "works to protect people at home and around the world from emerging and zoonotic infections ranging from A to Z—anthrax to Zika. We are living in an interconnected world where an outbreak of infectious disease is just a plane ride away" (NCEZD, 2023, August 1, para. 1). The work of the NCEZD reflects this broad mandate and encompasses:

- Foodborne and waterborne illnesses;
- Infections that spread in hospitals;
- Infections that are resistant to antibiotics;
- Deadly diseases like Ebola and anthrax;
- Illnesses that affect immigrants, migrants, refugees, and travelers;
- Diseases caused by contact with animals; and
- Diseases spread by mosquitoes, ticks, and fleas.

Within the several divisions comprising the office, the CDC conducts extensive disease epidemiology, laboratory programs, and basic and applied research relating to infectious disease, and plans for and coordinates prevention and outbreak response. With a $678 million budget in the fiscal year (FY) 2022 (DHHS, 2022c), investments are being made to modernize the CDC's technology and methods to detect and track infectious diseases more effectively. The Advanced Molecular Detection and Response to Infectious Disease Outbreaks initiative represents a fundamental change and modernization in the CDC's current public health microbiology and bioinformatics capabilities. It supports investments in bioinformatics, database development, data warehousing, and analytics to make use of recent technologic advances and allows the CDC to derive information from increasingly complex data sets.

Two initiatives within the NCEZID facilitate partnerships and a holistic approach to disease prevention:

- System for Enteric Disease Response, Investigation, and Coordination (SEDRIC), and
- One Health.

SEDRIC is a web-based platform developed by the CDC and Palantir Technologies. It facilitates collaborative, multistate outbreak investigations of foodborne and animal contact diseases (enteric; NCEZID, 2022b). "One Health is a collaborative, multisectoral, and transdisciplinary approach—working at the local, regional, national, and global levels—with the goal of achieving optimal health outcomes recognizing the interconnection between people, animals, plants, and their shared environment" (NCEZID, 2022a, para. 1). The CDC's One Health office serves as the head of the World Organisation for Animal Health (WOAH) Collaborating Center for Emerging and Reemerging Zoonotic Diseases. One Health office staff also serve as agency liaisons to the Food and Agriculture Organization of the United Nations (FAO; https://www.fao.org/home/en/) and WOAH. SEDRIC and One Health are critical to allowing the CDC to continue as the nation's premier public health agency in the area of infectious disease control and prevention (NCEZID, 2022a).

The *NCHHSTP* is responsible for public health surveillance, prevention research, and programs to prevent and control HIV and AIDS, sexually transmitted diseases (STDs), viral hepatitis, and tuberculosis (TB). The center works in collaboration with governmental and nongovernmental partners at community, state, and national levels on research, surveillance, technical assistance, evaluation, and development of prevention programs. In FY 2022, the center's budget was $1,421 million, an increase of $107 million over the FY 2021 budget (DHHS, 2022c). NCHHSTP is particularly interested in engaging young people. These related activities include:

- Advancing school-based health and disease prevention programs,
- Developing data and educational materials to support clinicians, and
- Developing communication materials to support disease prevention among highly affected groups (NCHHSTP, 2023).

Noninfectious Diseases and Injuries

Many units within the CDC focus on noninfectious diseases and injuries. They are:

- National Center on Birth Defects and Developmental Disabilities;
- National Center for Chronic Disease Prevention and Health Promotion;
- National Center for Environmental Health, including the Agency for Toxic Substances and Disease Registry;
- National Center for Injury Prevention and Control; and
- National Institute for Occupational Safety and Health (NIOSH).

The *National Center on Birth Defects and Developmental Disabilities (NCBDDD)* conducts research and supports extramural research designed to identify the causes of birth defects, developmental disabilities, and blood disorders and to promote the well-being of persons with disabilities. The center also funds prevention and education programs. The NCBDDD reports that one in 33 are born with a birth defect, 1 in 44 have autism spectrum disorder, and one in four adults has some kind of disability. "Birth defects are common, costly, and critical. Our unique state-based birth defects tracking and public health research provide a wealth of information that we use to identify causes of birth defects, find opportunities to prevent them, and improve the health of those living with birth defects" (NCBDDD, 2021, para. 2).

The *National Center for Chronic Disease Prevention and Health Promotion (NCCDPHP)* works to prevent and control chronic diseases, by reducing the risk factors for chronic diseases, particularly among groups affected by health disparities. With an FY 2022 budget (https://www.dcd.gov/chronicdisease/programs-impact/budget/index.htm) of more than $1.3 billion, the Center focuses on many of the leading causes of morbidity and mortality such as cancer, diabetes, heart disease and stroke, nutrition/obesity, and tobacco use. See **Figure 3.4**. The center provides funding and assistance to help state, tribal, and territorial health agencies to:

- Support data collection on disease risk factors, incidence, and death;
- Conduct research on disease risk and prevention strategies;
- Implement disease prevention programs; and
- Provide educational materials for health professionals, policymakers, and the public on issues pertaining to chronic disease prevention and control.

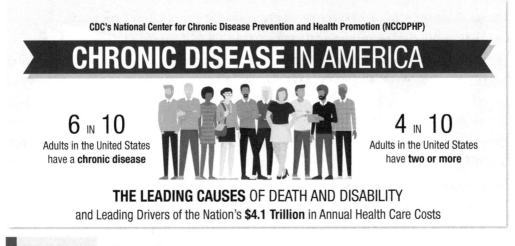

Figure 3.4.   Chronic Diseases in America

Source: From bottom of page: https://www.cdc.gov/chronicdisease/center/index.htm

Among the programs administered by the *National Center for Chronic Disease Prevention and Health Promotion* is the Preventive Health and Health Services (PHHS) Block Grant program, which provides noncategorical funding to states, territories, and tribes to support both public health agency capacity development and chronic disease prevention programs. The PHHS Block Grant Program gives recipients the latitude to fund any of 1,200+ national health objectives available in the nation's *Healthy People* 2020 health improvement plan.

Grants made under the $149 million annual program are designed to be flexible, providing states funding to fill gaps in programs that address the leading causes of death and disability in a manner determined by the grantees based on the particular needs of the population served. See **Figure** 3.5. The funds are frequently used to support clinical services, preventive screening, public education, workforce development, surveillance, and chronic disease prevention programs (NCCDPHP, 2022). The large infrastructure allotment is for people, systems, and communications resources that span multiple programs.

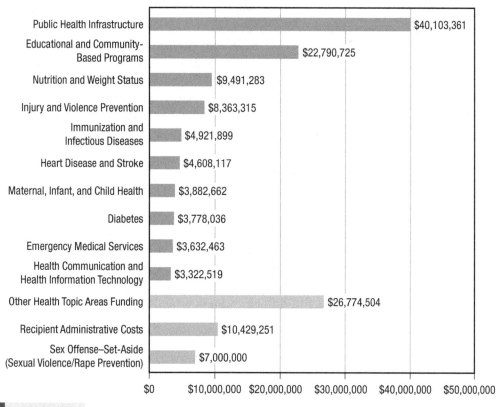

Total PHHS Block Grant Recipient Funding Allocation, FY 2020
$149,098,135

Public Health Infrastructure	$40,103,361
Educational and Community-Based Programs	$22,790,725
Nutrition and Weight Status	$9,491,283
Injury and Violence Prevention	$8,363,315
Immunization and Infectious Diseases	$4,921,899
Heart Disease and Stroke	$4,608,117
Maternal, Infant, and Child Health	$3,882,662
Diabetes	$3,778,036
Emergency Medical Services	$3,632,463
Health Communication and Health Information Technology	$3,322,519
Other Health Topic Areas Funding	$26,774,504
Recipient Administrative Costs	$10,429,251
Sex Offense–Set-Aside (Sexual Violence/Rape Prevention)	$7,000,000

Figure 3.5.   Total PHHS Block Grant Recipient Funding Allocation, FY 2020

PHHS, Preventive Health and Health Services.

Source: From https://www.cdc.gov/phhsblockgrant/funding/index.htm

The *National Center for Environmental Health (NCEH)* works to prevent illness, disability, and death resulting from human interaction with environmental toxins. The center conducts surveillance and applied research, supports educational campaigns, develops standards and guidelines, and offers training to state and local health agencies in environmental health prevention and response. It works in conjunction with the *Agency for Toxic Substances and Disease Registry (ATSDR)*, a congressionally mandated agency charged with conducting public health assessments of waste sites, conducting health surveillance and registries related to toxic substances, and providing information, education, and training concerning hazardous substances.

The *National Center for Injury Prevention and Control (NCIPC)* works to prevent injuries and violence, and to reduce their consequences. The Center conducts injury and violent death surveillance and supports research and injury prevention programs in such areas as domestic violence and firearm violence. The Center also funds extramural research on injury prevention, care, and rehabilitation, and supports Injury Control Research Centers at several academic institutions across the country.

The *National Institute for Occupational Safety and Health (NIOSH)* was created in conjunction with the U.S. Department of Labor's Occupational Safety and Health Administration (OSHA). Whereas OSHA has the responsibility of developing and enforcing workplace safety and health regulations, NIOSH was formed to provide the research in the field of occupational safety and health necessary to do so effectively. NIOSH conducts research, develops guidance and recommendations on workplace safety, disseminates information, and, upon request, conducts workplace health hazard evaluations. In addition to its own research, NIOSH sponsors research and training through extramural programs and enters cooperative agreements with state health departments, academia, unions, and nongovernmental organizations (NGOs) to participate in collaborative surveillance and research projects.

National Center for Health Statistics

The *NCHS* is the premier organization for the collection, processing, analysis, and dissemination of health data for the nation. The NCHS collects data from birth and death records, medical records, interview surveys, and through direct physical exams and laboratory testing. Some of NCHS's major ongoing surveys and data collection systems, from which information is drawn about the nation's health, health care, and the determinants of health, include the following (NCHS, 2023):

- National Health and Nutrition Examination Survey (NHANES)
- National Health Care Surveys (NHCS)
  - National Ambulatory Medical Care Survey (NAMCS)
  - National Hospital Ambulatory Medical Care Survey (NHAMCS)
  - National Hospital Care Survey
  - National Post-Acute and Long Term Care Survey

- National Health Interview Survey (NHIS)
- National Immunization Surveys (NIS)
- National Survey of Family Growth (NSFG)
- National Vital Statistics System (NVSS)
  - Birth Data
  - Mortality Data
  - Fetal Death Data
  - Linked Births/Infant Deaths

You can access the NCHS Summary of Current Surveys and Data Collection Systems here: https://www.cdc.gov/nchs/data/factsheets/factsheet-summary -current-surveys.pdf

Data from the NCHS surveys and systems are available to the public through the NCHS website (www.cdc.gov/nchs/) as public use files. The NCHS also produces innumerable standardized reports based on these data. The NCHS data are essential for developing, implementing, and evaluating public health policy in the United States. They allow:

- Documentation of population and subpopulation health status;
- Identification of health and health care disparities by race or ethnicity, socioeconomic status, region, and other population characteristics;
- Description of health care system experiences;
- Monitoring health status and health care delivery trends;
- Identification of health problems;
- Support of biomedical and health services research;
- Provision of information for policy; and
- Evaluation of health policies and programs impact (NCHS, 2022).

Other Centers for Disease Control and Prevention Offices and Centers

Other offices and centers include the Center of Surveillance, Epidemiology, and Laboratory Services; Center for Public Health Preparedness and Response; Center for State, Tribal, Local and Territorial Support; Center for Global Health; and Office of Minority Health and Health Equity.

The CDC's *Center for State, Tribal, Local and Territorial Support* aims to improve the capacity and performance of the public health system at all levels of organization by providing guidance on activities related to state, tribal and local, and public health agencies. The Center provides technical assistance and direct funding to state and local agencies to support the delivery of public health services and programs in accordance with CDC guidelines and standards in areas such as health promotion and disease prevention, public health policy, technology and communications infrastructure, and workforce development.

Through its *Center for Global Health*, the CDC works with international partners to prevent and control infectious and chronic diseases and to build sustainable global public health capacity through the development of epidemiologic and laboratory resources and the international public health workforce. Activities of the *Center for Global Health* include programs in global disease detection through which the CDC works with international public health actors such as ministries of health and the World Health Organization (WHO) to develop capacity for the rapid detection, identification, and containment of infectious diseases and bioterrorist threats internationally. The *Center for Global Health* also supports programs in AIDS prevention and treatment, and the prevention and control or eradication of polio, measles, influenza, and malaria. CDC staff work in more than 60 countries in support of the global health mission.

Administration for Children and Families

The *Administration for Children and Families (ACF)* works in partnership with states and communities to provide critical assistance to vulnerable families while helping families and children achieve a path to success. AFC programs work to find safe and supportive homes for abused children, counsel newly arrived refugees as they begin their new lives in America, and work to remove and provide opportunities to troubled teens who are homeless. In 2021, the AFC administered more than 60 programs. Its budget of more than $62 billion was the second largest in the DHHS. Examples of programs and the percentage of the FY 2022 budget allotted to each program under the AFC include Temporary Assistance for Needy Families (TANF), Head Start, Foster Care and Permanency, Child Care and Development, Child Support Enforcement, Low Income Home Energy Assistance Program (LIHEAP), Social Services Block Grant (SSBG), and Refugee and Entrant Assistance. See **Figure 3.6** (ACF, 2023).

Administration for Strategic Preparedness and Response

The *Administration for Strategic Preparedness and Response (ASPR)* is the lead government agency for medical and public health preparedness and response to disasters and public health emergencies. The ASPR collaborates widely with private and public sector organizations including hospitals; health care systems; biotechnology firms; communities; state, local, tribal, and territorial governments; and others to improve the country's readiness and response capabilities. The priorities are responding to the COVID-19 pandemic, restoring damages due to the pandemic, and preparing for future emergencies. ASPR seeks to contribute to an inclusive public health community that meets the challenges to the nation's health security (ASPR, 2022).

Health Resources and Services Administration

The activities of the *Health Resources and Services Administration (HRSA)* are principally to further the essential services related to workforce development and ensure access to health care services. Comprising seven bureaus and 11 offices and

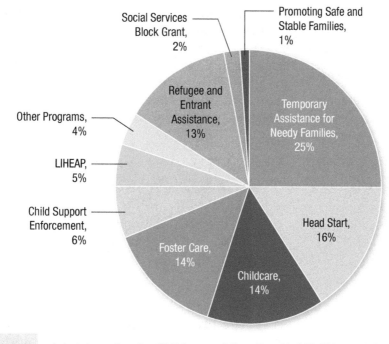

Figure 3.6.   Administration for Children and Families (ACF) FY 2022 Budget

LINEAP, Low Income Home Energy Assistance Program; TANF, Temporary Assistance for Needy Families.

Source: Administration for Children and Families. (2023). *FY 2023 budget.* https://www.acf.hhs.gov/about/budget.

with a staff of more than 1,800, HRSA is the primary federal agency for improving access to health care services for people who are uninsured, isolated, or particularly vulnerable. HRSA provides leadership and financial support to health care providers in every state and U.S. territory. Primarily a grant-giving and oversight agency, HRSA distributes most of its budget to community-based organizations, colleges and universities, hospitals, local and state governments, associations, and foundations.

The bureaus include:

- Bureau of Health Workforce,
- Bureau of Primary Health Care,
- Federal Office of Rural Health Policy,
- Health Systems Bureau,
- HIV/AIDS Bureau,
- Maternal and Child Health Bureau, and
- Provider Relief Bureau.

HRSA's *Bureau of Health Workforce* makes grants to health professions' training programs and funds scholarships and loan repayment programs for health professionals.

It also provides scholarship and educational loan repayment opportunities in exchange for clinicians' agreement to serve in communities with critical shortages of health care providers. The Bureau creates shortage designations, which identify an area, population, or facility experiencing a shortage of health care services. The shortage designations help distribute participants to places of most need. Other federal programs use shortage designations for their own resource distribution. There are several types of shortage designations:

- Health Professional Shortage Areas (HPSAs),
- Maternity Care Target Areas (MCTAs),
- Medically Underserved Areas (MUAs) and Medically Underserved Populations (MUPs),
- Exceptional Medically Underserved Population (Exceptional MUP), and
- Governor's-Designated Secretary-Certified Shortage Areas for Rural Health Clinics (HRSA, Bureau of Health Workforce, 2022).

HRSA's *HIV/AIDS Bureau* administers the Ryan White HIV/AIDS Program, which provides funding to grantees for HIV/AIDS outreach and AIDS Drug Assistance Programs (ADAPs). The program is designed to help those who do not have sufficient health care coverage or financial resources to cope with HIV and AIDS. The *Maternal and Child Health Bureau* administers the Maternal and Child Health Block Grant to states. The grants are designed to expand access to comprehensive prenatal and postnatal care for women; support health assessments, diagnostics, and treatment for children; and expand access to immunization and other preventive care for children. The *Federal Office of Rural Health Policy* supports many rural health programs including rural health networks, black lung clinics, telehealth, and veterans rural health access programs (HRSA, 2021b).

HRSA's *Bureau of Primary Health Care* provides funding for nonprofit, community-run health centers delivering comprehensive primary and preventive health care for people who otherwise lack access to health care. "Over the last 57 years, health centers have grown to become the cornerstone of community-based primary health care in the United States. By integrating medical, dental, behavioral, and other health care services, health centers provide patients the right care, at the right time, in the right place" (HRSA, 2022, para. 1). Populations served by community health centers include people with low incomes, the uninsured, those with limited English proficiency, migrant and seasonal farm workers, individuals and families who are homeless, and those living in public housing. Health centers provide care on a sliding fee scale and see patients without regard for their ability to pay. There are approximately 1,400 community health centers, delivering health care services at 13,500 sites. The centers serve approximately 29 million people, including migrant farm workers and homeless persons. One in 11 people in the United States receives medical care from a HRSA-funded health center (HRSA, 2021a).

Food and Drug Administration

The *Food and Drug Administration (FDA)* is the agency charged with regulating drugs and most food products in the United States. The FDA is "responsible for protecting the public health by ensuring the safety, efficacy, and security of human and veterinary drugs, biological products, and medical devices; and by ensuring the safety of our nation's food supply, cosmetics, and products that emit radiation" (FDA, 2018, para. 2).

The FDA is responsible for:

- Regulating the manufacturing, marketing, and distribution of tobacco products and to reduce tobacco use by minors;
- Speeding innovations to make medical products more effective, safer, and more affordable; and
- Helping the public get the accurate, science-based information needed to use medical products and foods (FDA, 2018).

Among the FDA's seven centers are the:

- Center for Biologics Evaluation and Research,
- Center for Drug Evaluation and Research,
- Center for Food Safety and Applied Nutrition,
- Center for Tobacco Products, and
- National Center for Toxicologic Research.

Over-the-counter and prescription drugs, including generic drugs, are regulated by the FDA's *Center for Drug Evaluation and Research*. The FDA evaluates drug safety and efficacy and ensures that the labeling and marketing of approved drugs are accurate. Vaccines, blood, and biologics are regulated by the FDA's *Center for Biologics Evaluation and Research*. The *Center for Food Safety and Applied Nutrition* works to ensure that the food supply is safe, sanitary, and honestly labeled. The *Center for Tobacco Products* was established to oversee the regulation of the marketing and promotion of tobacco products and set performance standards for tobacco products to protect public health. The FDA also operates the *National Center for Toxicological Research*, which conducts research to evaluate the biological effects of potentially toxic chemicals or microorganisms and to understand toxicological processes needed to inform the FDA's regulatory decisions (FDA, 2018).

Indian Health Service

The *Indian Health Service (IHS)* is responsible for providing federal health services to American Indians and Alaska Natives. The IHS provides a comprehensive health service delivery system for approximately 2 million American Indians and Alaskan Natives who belong to 574 federally recognized tribes in the United

States. It is the principal federal health care provider and health advocate for native people. The IHS operates or finances over 650 hospitals, clinics, and health stations on or near Indian reservations.

In addition to providing direct health care services, the IHS also undertakes broader health promotion activities. For example, the Office of Environmental Health and Engineering promotes the development of safe water and waste treatment programs. The IHS has also launched a Health Promotion and Disease Prevention (HP/DP) initiative that aims to develop and implement effective health promotion and chronic disease prevention programs, particularly in areas of concern for the native population, including increasing incidence of chronic diseases related to lifestyle issues such as obesity, physical inactivity, poor diet, substance abuse, and injuries (IHS, 2022).

Substance Abuse and Mental Health Services Administration

The *Substance Abuse and Mental Health Services Administration (SAMHSA)* works to improve the quality and availability of substance abuse prevention, addiction treatment, and mental health services. SAMHSA provides funding through block grants to state and local governments to support substance abuse and mental health services, including treatment for serious substance abuse problems or mental health problems; supports education programs for the general public and health care providers; improves substance abuse prevention and treatment services through the identification and dissemination of best practices; and conducts surveillance and monitoring of the prevalence and incidence of substance abuse.

Administration for Community Living

The *Administration for Community Living (ACL)* is focused on ensuring that older adults and people with disabilities are able to have the option to live at home and fully participate in their communities. Created in April 2012, the ACL brought together three previously separate entities within the DHHS: the Administration on Aging, the Office on Disability, and the Administration on Intellectual and Developmental Disabilities (AIDD).

National Institutes of Health

The *National Institutes of Health (NIH)* is the primary federal agency conducting and supporting biomedical research. Composed of 27 institutes and centers, the NIH conducts and funds research into the causes, treatment, cure, and prevention of a broad range of disease. Among the NIH institutes and centers are the National Cancer Institute; National Heart, Lung, and Blood Institute; National Institute on Aging; National Human Genome Research Institute; National Center for Complementary and Integrative Health; and National Center for Advancing Translational Sciences. An important resource for all public health and health care professionals in the United States and throughout the world is the National Library of Medicine, which collects, organizes, and makes available biomedical science information. Its web-based databases include PubMed/Medline and MedlinePlus.

The vast majority of the NIH's budget goes to support extramural research at universities and other research institutions. Included in its portfolio is a substantial body of disease prevention research. Research on disease prevention is an important part of the NIH mission. The institutes and centers have a broad portfolio of prevention research and training, as well as programs to disseminate the findings to scientists, health professionals, and the public. Ultimately, knowledge gained from NIH-supported prevention research enables the application of sound science in clinical practice, health policy, and community health programs, thereby improving the health of the public (NIH, 2022).

Centers for Medicare & Medicaid Services

The *Centers for Medicare & Medicaid Services (CMS)* administers the largest health insurance programs in the country, with a 2022 budget of approximately $1.4 trillion and 63.9 million Medicare enrollees and 6.8 million Medicaid enrollees in 2021 (DHHS, 2022c). The CMS administers Medicare, which provides publicly financed health insurance for elderly and disabled Americans, and Medicaid, a program administered jointly by the federal government and the states, which provides publicly financed health coverage for low-income persons and nursing home coverage for low-income elderly adults. Although primarily considered a health care insurance program for low-income people, Medicaid-reimbursed services may also include such public health activities as Early and Periodic Screening, Diagnostic and Treatment (EPSDT) services for children, family planning services, cancer screening, school health services, and adult immunizations. Further, Medicaid payments also support public health providers such as health centers, public hospitals, community mental health providers, and STD clinics, which are dependent on Medicaid revenues to sustain their operations (Perlino, 2006).

CMS also administers the *Children's Health Insurance Program (CHIP)*, which insures children from low-income families who earn too much to qualify for Medicaid. However, each state has its own rules about the family income that allows eligibility for CHIP. In addition, CMS administers the *Center for Consumer Information and Insurance Oversight (CCIIO)*, which contributes to implementing the Affordable Care Act, signed into law March 23, 2010. CCIIO oversees the provisions related to private health insurance. In particular, CCIIO is working with states to establish new Health Insurance Marketplaces (CMS, 2022). The CMS budget primarily funds Medicare and Medicaid. See **Figure 3.7** (DHHS, 2022c).

Agency for Healthcare Research and Quality

The *Agency for Healthcare Research and Quality (AHRQ)* is the lead federal agency charged with improving the quality, safety, efficiency, and effectiveness of health care for all Americans. It does not make policy, but rather, with a budget of approximately $455 million in FY 2022, AHRQ conducts and supports a broad range of health services research within research institutions, hospitals, and health care systems that informs and enhances decision-making, and improves

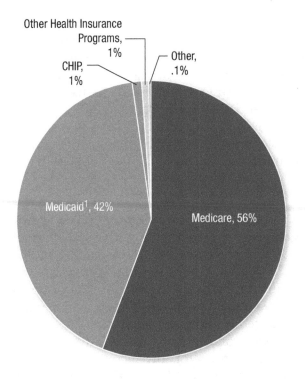

Figure 3.7. FY 2022 Net Federal Outlays Proposed Law—$1.4 Trillion

[1]Medicaid represents total federal spending only.

Source: U.S. Department of Health and Human Services. (2022c). *Budget in brief: Fiscal year 2022.* https://www
.hhs.gov/sites/default/files/fy-2022-budget-in-brief.pdf

health care services, organization, and financing. AHRQ's research, which is both conducted internally and through grants and contracts to universities, health care systems, hospitals, and physician practices, focuses on a set of broad issues relating to both clinical services and the system in which those services are provided, including comparative effectiveness, patient safety, health information technology, prevention and care management for chronic conditions, and value research.

Overall, AHRQ's priorities are:

- Investing in health systems research that generates evidence about how to deliver high-quality, safe, high-value healthcare.
- Creating tools and strategies for health systems and frontline clinicians to support practice improvement.
- Providing data and analytics to help decision-makers understand the healthcare system and identify opportunities for improvement. (AHRQ, 2022, para. 1)

Important data tools developed by AHRQ include the Healthcare Cost and Utilization Project (HCUP), the Consumer Assessment of Healthcare Providers and Systems, and the Medical Expenditure Panel Survey (MEPS).

Other Federal Agencies

Federal agencies other than those in the DHHS have important public health roles. These include the U.S. Department of Agriculture (USDA), Environmental Protection Agency (EPA), U.S. Department of Labor (DOL), Department of Veterans Affairs (VA), and Department of Defense (DOD).

U.S. Department of Agriculture

The *U.S. Department of Agriculture (USDA)* plays a vital regulatory role in the public health system through its Food Safety and Inspection Service—the public health agency responsible for the safety and labeling of the commercial supply of meat, poultry, and egg products. The USDA also plays a role in directly ensuring health through its Food and Nutrition Service, which oversees funding of food assistance programs such as the Supplemental Nutrition Assistance Program (SNAP, formerly the Food Stamp Program), which subsidizes food purchases for low-income people; the National School Lunch Program, which provides subsidies to schools for meals in exchange for serving lunches that meet federal nutritional requirements to students, and offers free or reduced price lunches to eligible children; and the Women Infants and Children (WIC) program, which provides federal grants to states for supplemental foods, health care referrals, and nutrition education for low-income pregnant, breastfeeding, and nonbreastfeeding postpartum women and to infants and children up to age 5 who are found to be at nutritional risk. In 2022, participation levels for these programs were estimated at 45.4 million per month for SNAP, 30 million per day for the National School Lunch Program, and 6.4 million per month for WIC. The 2022 budget increased funding to extend meal service flexibilities to schools and child care centers, ensuring that all children received healthy meals at no cost during the school year. It also expanded the Summer Electronic Benefit Transfer (EBT), which provides food for school-aged children during the summer and proposed lowering eligibility for the National School Lunch Program (Community Eligibility Provision [CEP]) so that more schools might be able to afford it (USDA, 2022).

U.S. Environmental Protection Agency

The mission of the *U.S. Environmental Protection Agency (EPA)* is to protect human health and the environment by regulating the release of pollutants in the air, land, and water and conducting or providing grants for environmental remediation. The EPA grant categories are air and radiation, water, drinking water, hazardous waste, and pesticides and toxics. Among the many laws administered, fully or partly, by the EPA are the Clean Air Act; the Clean Water Act; the Comprehensive Environmental Response, Compensation and Liability Act; the Safe Drinking Water Act; and the Toxic Substances Control Act. Nearly half of the EPA's budget is expended through grants to states, nonprofits, educational institutions, and others for various projects, from scientific studies to site cleanups (EPA, 2021, 2022).

U.S. Department of Labor

The *U.S. Department of Labor (DOL)*, through the *Occupational Safety and Health Administration (OSHA)*, regulates the health and safety of workplaces, either directly or through approval of state occupational safety programs that exceed federal requirements. OSHA regulations are based on *National Institute for Occupational Safety and Health (NIOSH)* research and regulate matters ranging from the permissible exposures limits for hazardous substances in the workplace to the use of portable power tools. Another vital program of the DOL is the *Bureau of Labor Statistics (BLS)*, which collects, analyses, and disseminates data that describe American's work experience including earnings by demographics, industry, and occupation; worker characteristics; employment by occupation; work experience over time; labor turnover; unemployment; and consumer expenditures (BLS, 2022; OSHA, 2022).

U.S. Department of Veterans Affairs and Department of Defense

The *Department of Veterans Affairs (VA)* and the *Department of Defense (DOD)* provide access to health care services to veterans and active military personnel. The VA operates the nation's largest integrated health care system, providing care at 1,298 health care facilities (https://www.va.gov/find-locations/?facilityType/ =health), including 171 medical centers and 1,113 outpatient sites of care of varying complexity (VA outpatient clinics). The VA health care system serves 9 million enrolled Veterans each year (VA, 2022).

Summary of Federal Public Health

The enormity and complexity of the federal public health system are daunting, resisting a pithy summary. The number of departments, agencies, offices, centers, and so forth, as well as the number of health problems addressed, and the size of the public health budgets challenge students' full understanding of the federal effort. A few key points are:

- The federal departments involved in some important aspect of public health include the DHHS, USDA, EPA, DOL, VA, and DOD.
- Each one participates in some aspect of the 10 Essential Public Health Services—Assurance, Policy Development, and Assessment—designed to promote equitable access to the conditions which promote health.
- The DHHS is the principal government public health agency.
- Within the DHHS, the CDC is the principal agency that produces evidence-based public health information and communicates it to the public and to public health and health care professionals.
- Other DHHS divisions of special importance to public health are the ACF, HRSA, CMS, FDA, and NIH.

STATE PUBLIC HEALTH

As described earlier, the primary legal authority for public health in the United States rests with the states. Although the federal government undertakes extensive public health activities, as we have seen, those programs are generally categorized under resource allocation and distribution, information generation and distribution, health care access assurance, and, to a more limited extent, regulation and enforcement in matters affecting the country broadly (e.g., drug and food safety). The states generally have responsibility, at least at first, for implementing public health programs and delivering public health services. So, while the federal government has, for example, established the National Electronic Disease Surveillance System whereby state and local health agencies may report incidences of reportable diseases, the decision whether or to what degree to participate in the system is left to the individual states. The ASTHO—citing considerable variation among states and local agencies—finds the public health system "comprehensive, yet inconsistent" (ASTHO, 2009, p. 8), a result of the states' legal authority for public health and their independent decision-making powers.

Organization and Governance

There is at least one state-level government authority with primary responsibility for public health in every state, and in state governments alone (ASTHO, 2017). State health departments are structured and organized in a multitude of ways, located in different parts of state government, and differ in the extent and nature of the authority granted to them.

> The structure of a state public health agency refers to the agency's placement within the larger departmental/organizational structure of the state. The location of the state health agency will affect how agencies operate in terms of budgeting, decision making, and programmatic responsibility. State public health agencies can either be freestanding/independent agencies or a unit of a larger combined health and human services organization, also referred to as an umbrella agency or super agency. State public health agencies located within a larger agency often reside in that agency with other programs such as Medicaid and Medicare, public assistance, and substance abuse and mental health services. (ASTHO, 2017, p. 18)

Most state health departments (55%) are freestanding, independent agencies, and 42% are a unit within a larger health and human services organization—an "umbrella" agency or "superagency" (ASTHO, 2017). The California Department of Public Health is one example of a public health department located within an umbrella agency, the California Health and Human Services Agency (CHHSA). CHHSA oversees 12 departments and five offices including the departments of Public Health, Aging, Child Support Services, Health Care Services (Medicaid and other public insurance administration), Community Services and

Development, Developmental Services, Emergency Medical Services Authority, Managed Health Care, State Hospitals, and Social Services (CHHS, 2022).

Each state health agency is led by a state health official (SHO)—called a state health secretary or commissioner of health. In 2016, 66% of SHOs were appointed by the governor, 14% were appointed by a parent agency secretary, 10% were appointed by a board or commission, and 10% were appointed by another entity. SHOs have a variety of backgrounds. In 2016, 64% held a medical degree, and 44% had an MPH degree. Once appointed, 74% require confirmation by the legislature, governor, or a board or commission. The median tenure for a SHO has been stable at 1.8 years since 2012 (ASTHO, 2017).

State public health agencies also vary in the authorities granted to them. Most state health departments (70%) are authorized to declare health emergencies and to collect key health data. Less than one half of state health departments, however, have the authority to adopt public health laws and regulations. Health departments have even less authority over budgetary and leadership issues. Overall funding and administrative decisions generally rest with the legislature or executive branch of state government. For example, less than 30% of state health agencies have budget authority, and almost none may select the agency head, establish taxes in support of public health, or place tax and levy measures on the ballot, those powers being reserved for the governor or legislature (ASTHO, 2017).

Twenty-seven states have boards or councils of health, which variously promulgate rules and advise elected officials on policy. A minority of state boards of health formulate public health policies, legislative agendas, or public health budgets for the state (Beitsch et al., 2006). Boards of health, typically comprised of citizens, consumers, members of the business community, and public health professionals, play a decreasingly important role in state public health activities (ASTHO, 2017; Beitsch et al., 2006).

The relationship between state health departments and local departments also exhibits considerable variation. See **Figure 3.8**. "Centralized/largely centralized" refers to a governance structure in which state employees primarily lead local health units and the state retains authority over most decisions related to the budget, issuing public health orders, and selecting the local health official. "Decentralized/largely decentralized" refers to a governance structure in which local government employees primarily lead local health units and the local governments retain authority over most key decisions (ASTHO, 2017).

The overwhelming majority of state health agencies report partnering with NGOs on various programs and activities. Most frequently, state agencies partner with universities and schools, community organizations, hospitals and other health care providers, insurers, and community health centers. More than half of state agencies also report partnering with businesses, the media, and environmental and conservation organizations.

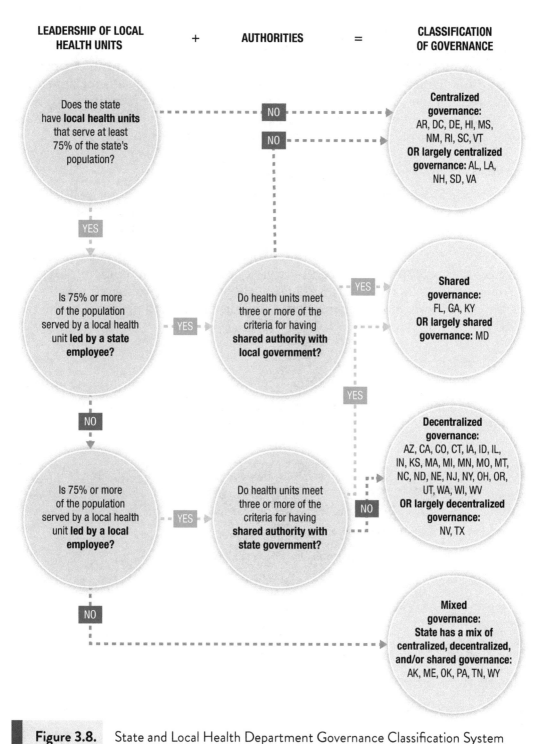

Figure 3.8.   State and Local Health Department Governance Classification System

*If the majority (75% or more) but not all of the state population meets the designation, then the state is largely centralized, decentralized, or shared.

Source: Association of State and Territorial Health Officials. (2017). *ASTHO profile of state and territorial public health* (Vol. 4). https://www.astho.org/globalassets/pdf/profile/profile-stph-vol-4.pdf

Other issues related to the organization of public health services at the state level concern the locus of responsibility. Is there a separate agency for environment and environmental health? Is public health responsible for mental health and substance abuse, or is there a separate agency? This would also be the case for aging and child health. If there are separate agencies, do they work and coordinate efforts in a positive way? These issues are answered differently in different states and have consequences for the coordination and provision of public health services.

Services and Activities

State public health departments engage in a wide range of public health activities. Federal initiatives are an important mandate for states, and Table 3.3 indicates that most state health departments are responsible for them.

The following is information about some of the major groupings of public health services and activities performed by states: surveillance and epidemiology; environmental health; maternal and child health; emergency preparedness; immunization services; regulation, inspection, and licensing; and personal health care (ASTHO, 2017).

Surveillance and Epidemiology

Every state public health department conducts some level of public health surveillance, monitoring, and epidemiologic activities. Almost all state public health departments collect data related to risk factors and disease incidence, including

Table 3.3. State Health Agency Responsibility for Federal Initiatives, 2016 ($N = 50$)

Federal Initiative	N	%
Maternal and child health/Title V program	49	98
Preventive Health and Health Services Block Grant (CDC)	49	98
CDC Public Health Emergency Preparedness (PHEP) cooperative agreement	48	96
Immunization funding, Section 317 program	48	96
Women, Infants, and Children program (USDA)	48	96
Hospital Preparedness Program (HPP) cooperative agreement (ASPR)	46	92
Vital statistics (NCHS)	45	90
Injury prevention (CDC)	44	88
HIV pharmacies (ADAP)	44	88
National Comprehensive Cancer Control Program grant (CDC)	41	82

Source: Association of State and Territorial Health Officials. (2017). *ASTHO profile of state and territorial public health* (Vol. 4). https://www.astho.org/globalassets/pdf/profile/profile-stph-vol-4.pdf

chronic and infectious diseases, exposures, and access to care. The most common data collection activities, with 96% of departments engaging in data collection, include behavioral risk factors, communicable and infectious diseases, reportable diseases, and vital statistics. Activities are not based on size of the population served, governance classification, or geographic region.

Environmental Health

The overwhelming majority of state health agencies (approximately 90%) oversee environmental health epidemiology and food safety education. Less frequently, but in most instances, the state health agency is involved in toxicology, as well as radiation, radon, poison, vector control, indoor air quality, and water supply safety.

Maternal and Child Health

Almost 80% of states offer services to children with special health care needs, and 57% states also administer the Women, Infants, and Children (WIC) nutrition program and provide family planning and prenatal care services. About half of all state health departments are involved in early intervention services for children, maternal and child health home visits, and family planning services.

Emergency Preparedness

All state health agencies have some responsibility to prepare for disaster response and emergencies. All state health departments have responsibility for responding to communicable disease outbreaks, nearly all have responsibilities for responding to bioterrorism events, and almost 90% have responsibility for responding to chemical, nuclear, and natural disasters.

Immunization Services

Over 90% of state health agencies are responsible for vaccine order management and inventory distribution of childhood and adult immunizations. Approximately 46% administer childhood immunization and about 42% administer adult immunizations. The number of individuals immunized by state health agencies is dependent on the agency's geographic location. Eighty-five percent of agencies in centralized states provide childhood and adult vaccine administration in comparison to those in decentralized states, which administer about 22% of childhood and adult vaccines. In decentralized states, vaccination services are often provided by primary health care providers or LHDs.

Regulation, Inspection, and Licensing

Most state health agencies have some involvement (along with other agencies at the federal, state, and/or local level) in the regulation and enforcement of laws that protect health and ensure safety. Activities include inspection or licensing of a variety of public health system partners such as entities that provide direct care, including hospitals (42 states), clinics (23 states), and hospice facilities (36 states). Other activities include regulation, inspection, and licensing of entities that process and serve food; recreational sites such as beaches, campgrounds, and public swimming pools; water sources; waste disposal sites and entities; and tobacco retailers. Most state public health departments, however, do not license health professionals. This is typically a function of another agency or department of state government. Fewer than 25% of state health agencies directly license nurses, physicians, physician assistants, or dentists. Vital and health statistics may start at the state or local government level. Marriage, births, and deaths are state or local functions. Notification of reportable diseases starts at the local level and is sent to the state.

Personal Health Care

Except for HIV/AIDS and STDs, state health agencies generally do not provide treatment for communicable and chronic diseases. Approximately 60% screen for tuberculosis and STDs, including HIV/AIDS. Over 70% of agencies provide newborn screening services. The frequency of screenings for breast, cervical, colon, and rectal cancers are dependent on the size of the population served. Agencies in centralized states provide these services more often than those in decentralized states. Most state health agencies provide or regulate at least some clinical services in oral health, emergency medical services, minority health, and rural health. A minority of states provide services for victims of sexual assault and violence, substance abuse prevention, or pharmacy services.

State Public Health Priorities

State health agency officials listed their top five priorities: (a) improving public health and public health infrastructure; (b) assurance of access to health care systems and services; (c) increasing the availability and use of data and evidence; (d) quality improvement, performance management, and accreditation-related services; and (e) implementation of effective health policies.

Quality improvement and improved effectiveness is a growing interest among state health departments in accreditation. The *Public Health Accreditation Board (PHAB)* accredits public health departments to strengthen public health infrastructure and transform governmental public health. This is a voluntary activity.

> Through public health accreditation and promotion of innovation, we support health departments in their work to promote and protect the health of the communities they serve. We believe both accreditation and innovation are critical to public health transformation; together they can ensure that health departments are continually improving in line with national public health standards while building health and equity. (PHAB, 2022, para. 2)

The three prerequisites for submitting an application for PHAB accreditation are:

- Conduct a state health assessment,
- Create a state health improvement plan, and
- Develop an agency-wide strategic plan.

In 2016, 94% of state health agencies reported completing a state health assessment. The percentage of state health agencies that had developed or begun a state health improvement plan increased from 23% in 2007 to 64% in 2016. As of 2016, 96% of state health departments had developed an agency-wide strategic plan. When the survey was completed, 40% of state health departments had received accreditation (ASTHO, 2017).

Relationship to 10 Essential Health Services

Surveys of state public health agencies indicate that, in general, most states perform public health activities falling within each of the 10 essential services, although it is difficult to evaluate this assessment because public health services and activities are not organized by the essential services.

Most services are specific to a health problem, population, and/or behavior. HIV/AIDS, STDs, foodborne diseases, waterborne diseases, maternal and child health, emergency preparedness, injuries, childhood immunizations, smoking, obesity, and nutrition are common organizational groupings of public health services and activities. In each case, the 10 essential services may (or may not) be relevant or provided.

For example, it is not clear whether HIV/AIDS programs are assessed (or should be assessed) on whether they offer all 10 essential services for the population they serve: monitor, diagnose, and investigate health problems related to HIV/AIDS in the community; inform, educate, and empower people with HIV/AIDS; mobilize community partnerships to solve their problems; develop policies and plans to support HIV/AIDS patients' health efforts; enforce laws and regulations to protect people with HIV/AIDS; link people with HIV/AIDS to needed personal health services if otherwise unavailable; ensure a competent workforce to meet HIV/AIDS patients' needs; evaluate services for people with HIV/AIDS; and research innovative solutions to their health problems. Further, it would be difficult to determine if all essential services were provided to people with HIV/AIDS because some essential services might be within the scope of the HIV/AIDS program and others might be within the responsibility of a crosscutting unit such as communications or epidemiology.

Also, it is difficult to compare across states on the essential services, because even though two states may conduct performance evaluations, the scope and depth of the evaluations undertaken may vary significantly, and the states may prioritize performance evaluation very differently. Further, there are few data showing whether the form of essential service provided was tailored to the particular needs of the population, or whether, for example, it was performed in response to a federal categorical grant without a particular need in the community.

In summary, state public health is a complex network of services and practices, reflecting the differences between states in their resources and values. The origin of this variation is federalism, the form of government in the United States that requires the federal and state governments to share power.

LOCAL PUBLIC HEALTH

The implementation and delivery of many, if not most, public health services occur at the local level—usually city, county, or region. LHDs are on the front line of control of communicable diseases and noncommunicable hazardous exposures, as well as informing and educating communities about public health issues. However, local public health organizations collaborate with state and federal public health agencies and depend a great deal on their resources—data, skilled personnel, funds, and so forth. In most states, the state and local public health agencies form a very connected system. The state may not provide direct services but offers a higher level of technical expertise at the research and policy level, which the LHD carries out.

NACCHO is the only organization dedicated to serving LHDs, which NACCHO defines as administrative or service units of local or state government "concerned with health, and carrying some responsibility for the health of a jurisdiction smaller than the state" (NACCHO, 2020a, p. 12).

There are enormous variations between LHDs, as we will discuss. It is almost true that if you have seen one LHD, you have seen one LHD. They differ among states and, within states, on organization, governance, services offered, and implementation strategies. Not surprisingly, a major factor driving variation is the size of the population served. There are approximately 2,800 total LHDs in the United States (NACCHO, 2020a). The majority (61%) of LHDs serve jurisdictions with 50,000 or fewer people, and 39% of LHDs serve jurisdictions with fewer than 25,000 people. However, most people are located in larger jurisdictions. LHDs serving large urban centers—departments in jurisdictions with 500,000 or more people—constitute only 6% of nationwide LHDs yet serve 52% of the U.S. population (NACCHO, 2020a). See **Figure 3.9**.

Organization and Governance

Nearly every state's population is served by LHDs (regional, county, municipal). The only exception is Rhode Island, which does not have any local or regional health agencies. Rather, the state health department operates on behalf of local public health, and there are no administrative or service units with responsibility for the health of a substate jurisdiction (NACCHO, 2020a).

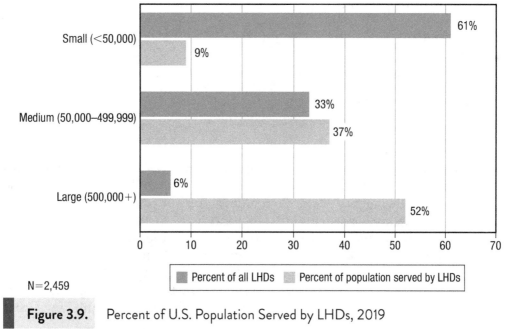

N=2,459

Figure 3.9.   Percent of U.S. Population Served by LHDs, 2019

LHD, local health department.

Source: National Association of County and City Health Officials. (2020). *2019 national profile of local health development.* https://www.naccho.org/uploads/downloadable-resources/Programs/Public-Health-Infrastructure/NACCHO_2019_Profile_final.pdf

The governance structure of LHDs is categorized according to their relationship with the state government:

- Centralized—all LHDs in the state are units of local government.
- Decentralized—all LHDs in the state are units of state government.
- Shared—all LHDs in the state are governed by both state and local authorities.
- Mixed—LHDs in the state have more than one governance type.

In 2019, 30 states were decentralized. All LHDs in Florida, Georgia, and Kentucky had shared governance. All LHDs in Arkansas, Delaware, Hawaii, Mississippi, New Mexico, and South Carolina were units of the state health agency that is, centralized. Rhode Island has no substate health units, and the remaining 10 states had a mixed governance structure (NACCHO, 2020a).

Another factor differentiating LHDs is whether there is an associated board of health. Boards of health can be advisory or governing. The majority (70%) of LHDs have boards of health, and most of these have *governing* boards (71%). LHDs serving large populations (over 500,000 persons) are most likely **not** to have an associated board of health (43%). LHDs with local governing authority—centralized—are most likely to have a *governing* board of health (63%; NACCHO, 2020a). See **Figure 3.10.**

The functions of boards of health are:

- Oversight,
- Policy development,
- Legal authority,
- Continuous improvement,
- Resource stewardship, and
- Partner engagement.

Most local boards of health have oversight authority (75%), which entails ulti-mate responsibility for performance through leadership and guidance including hiring and firing the agency head. Policy development functions, including en-suring that policies are consistent with laws and rules, are held by 66% of boards of health. Legal authority includes such functions as adopting public health reg-ulations and imposing or enforcing quarantine or isolation orders. About 61% of boards of health hold this authority. About 47% of boards of health have resource stewardship functions including approving the LHD budget, setting and impos-ing fees, imposing taxes for public health, or requesting a public health levy. Other

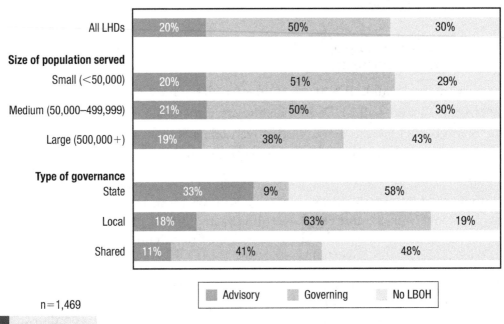

Figure 3.10.   LHDs With Local Board of Health by Size of Population Served and Type of Governance, 2019

LBOH, local board of health; LHD, local health department.

Source: National Association of County and City Health Officials. (2020). *2019 national profile of local health development.* https://www.naccho.org/uploads/downloadable-resources/Programs/Public-Health-Infrastructure/ NACCHO_2019_Profile_final.pdf

functions of boards of health are continuous improvement (49%) and responsi-bility to build and strengthen community partnerships (47%; NACCHO, 2020a).

Partnerships and Collaboration

Partnerships and collaboration with organizations including health care systems, colleges and universities, local businesses, nonprofit community organizations, and other government agencies are essential to the success of LHDs, as these ex-ternal relationships increase the visibility and extend the resources of the LHD, improving their effectiveness. **Figure 3.11** presents an interesting trajectory of this activity. There was a decline in external partnerships of all kinds between 2008 and 2016, which quickly rose after that.

Workforce

The workforce is the heart and soul of any organization, and public health orga-nizations are no exception. Thus, there are some concerning trends in the public health workforce. The estimated number of full-time equivalent LHD workers nationwide decreased steadily between 2008 and 2016, with a slight increase af-ter that. Overall, however, the LHD workforce, in full-time equivalents (FTEs), decreased by approximately 16%, from 166,000 in 2008 to 136,000 in 2019. At the same time, the population increased by 8% (NACCHO, 2020b). **Figure 3.12** doc-uments this decline by size of population.

The median number of FTEs in a U.S. LHD is 17, ranging from a median of six for departments serving a population of fewer than 25,000 people, to a median of 456 FTEs for departments serving more than a million people. The median number of local public health department FTEs per 10,000 persons served is 4.1 (NACCHO, 2020a).

A decrease in registered nurses is particularly significant since these health professionals play a critical role in the public health workforce, particularly in small and medium LHDs. Unfortunately, the number of registered nurses in public health has been declining. A NACCHO survey in 2019 found a decrease in registered nurses in LHDs of approximately 36%—from 33,200 in 2008 to 21,200 in 2019. Many LHDs had difficulty filling nursing positions as a result of barriers such as geographic location and noncompetitive pay. This shortage of nurses was expected to affect LHDs' capacity to maintain effective programs that meet community needs such as clinical services (i.e., immunization, ma-ternal and child health, and screening for high blood pressure, diabetes, blood lead, and communicable diseases; NACCHO, 2020b). See **Figure 3.13**.

The head of most LHDs is a full-time employee (94%), and this percentage has increased from 86% in 2008. The highest educational level for heads of local public health departments was doctoral degree (14%), master's degree (49%), followed by bachelor's degree (29%), and associate degree (8%). Heads with doctoral degrees are most often found in LHDs serving 500,000 people or more (56%). Twenty-six percent of LHD heads with less than 3 years' experience have a degree in public health, and 6% have a medical degree. In contrast, 31% of

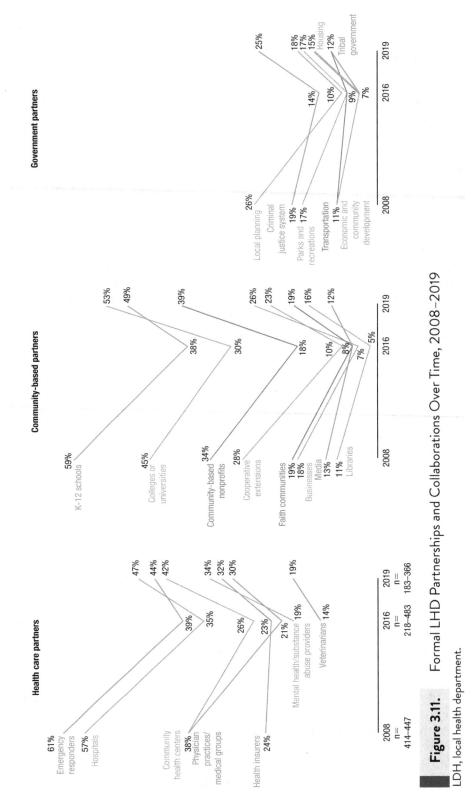

Figure 3.11. Formal LHD Partnerships and Collaborations Over Time, 2008–2019

LDH, local health department.

Source: National Association of County and City Health Officials. (2020). *2019 national profile of local health development.* https://www.naccho.org/uploads/downloadable
-resources/Programs/Public-Health-Infrastructure/NACCHO_2019_Profile_final.pdf

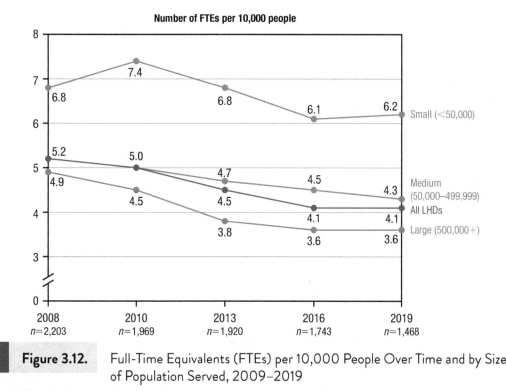

Number of FTEs per 10,000 people

Small (<50,000)

Medium (50,000–499,999)

All LHDs

Large (500,000+)

2008 *n*=2,203   2010 *n*=1,969   2013 *n*=1,920   2016 *n*=1,743   2019 *n*=1,468

Figure 3.12.   Full-Time Equivalents (FTEs) per 10,000 People Over Time and by Size of Population Served, 2009–2019

Source: National Association of County and City Health Officials. (2020). *2019 national profile of local health development.* https://www.naccho.org/uploads/downloadable-resources/Programs/Public-Health-Infrastructure/NACCHO_2019_Profile_final.pdf

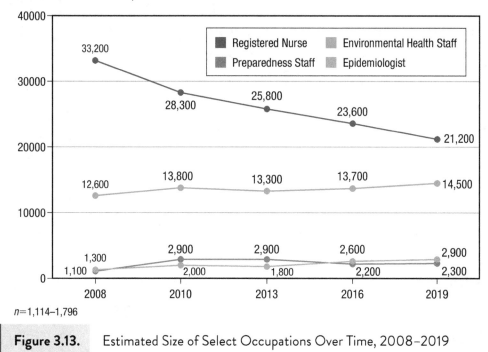

n=1,114–1,796

Figure 3.13.   Estimated Size of Select Occupations Over Time, 2008–2019

Source: National Association of County and City Health Officials. (2020). *2019 national profile of local health development.* https://www.naccho.org/uploads/downloadable-resources/2019-Profile-Workforce-and-Finance-Capacity.pdf

more experienced heads have an advanced public health degree, and 9% a medical degree.

- Two thirds of LHD heads are female, and since 2008, the percentage of female top executives has increased steadily, from 56% in 2008 to 66% in 2019.
- Fewer than 10% of top executives are Hispanic/Latino or a race other than White, and this percentage has remained about the same since 2008.
- Almost two thirds of top executives are 50 or older, and one quarter are 60 or older. Eleven percent are younger than 40. Since 2008, the proportion of top executives in their 50s has declined. Meanwhile, the proportions of both older (60+) and younger (less than 50) top executives have grown (NACCHO, 2020a).

The composition of the public health workforce overall is seen in **Table 3.4**. The largest portion of the workforce is administrative or clerical personnel (23,100 FTEs), the second-largest portion is environmental health worker (14,500 FTEs), followed by business and financial operations staff (8,900 FTEs). See **Table 3.4**.

Table 3.4. Estimated Number of Full-Time Equivalents (FTEs) in Select Occupations, 2019

Occupation	Number of FTEs	95% Confidence Intervals	
Agency leadership	5,800	5,500	6,100
Animal control worker	1,000	800	1,200
Behavioral health staff	6,700	4,500	8,900
Business and financial operations staff	8,900	5,900	11,900
Community health worker	5.600	4.300	6,300
Environmental health worker	14,500	12,500	16,500
Epidemiologist/statistician	2,900	2,000	3,800
Health educator	7,500	5,100	9,900
Information systems specialist	2,200	1,300	3,100
Laboratory worker	2,100	1,500	2,700
Licensed practical or vocational nurse	3,600	1,900	5,400
Nursing aide and home health aide	2,200	1,800	2,600
Nutritionist	5,100	4,700	5,500
Office and administrative support staff	23,100	20,800	25,500
Oral health care professional	2,200	1,900	2300
Preparedness staff	2,300	2,100	2,400

(continued)

Table 3.4. Estimated Number of Full-Time Equivalents (FTEs) in Select Occupations, 2019 (continued)

Occupation	Number of FTEs	95% Confidence Intervals	
Public health physician	1,300	900	1,600
Public information professional	600	550	700
Registered nurse	21,200	18,800	23,700

$n = 1,110–1,129$

Source: National Association of County and City Health Officials. (2020). *2019 national profile of local health development*. https://www.naccho.org/uploads/downloadable-resources/Programs/Public-Health-Infrastructure/NACCHO_2019_Profile_final.pdf

The composition of each LHD's workforce varies by size of the population served (see **Figure 3.14**). The smallest departments often consist only of a public health manager, secretary, environmental health worker, and nurse. Next to be added are typically emergency preparedness staff, a health educator, and a nutritionist. Nearly all of the largest departments have physicians, behavioral and environmental health scientists, epidemiologists, and information specialists, whereas these positions are rare in departments serving fewer than 100,000 people (NACCHO, 2020a).

Services and Activities

As with the other characteristics examined, there is wide variation in the activities and services offered by LHDs. The clinical programs and services offered directly are:

- Immunization,
- Screening for diseases/conditions,
- Treatment for communicable diseases,
- Maternal and child health services, and
- Other clinical services.

Childhood and adult immunizations, tuberculosis, HIV/AIDS, STD screening and treatment, and WIC administration were the clinical services most often offered by LHDs. See **Figure 3.15** (NACCHO, 2020a).

Population-based programs and services provided directly by LHDs are:

- Epidemiology and surveillance;
- Population-based primary prevention;
- Regulation, inspection, and/or licensing;
- Other environmental health services; and
- Other population-based services.

Among the surveillance and epidemiology activities, communicable/infectious disease, environmental health, maternal and child health, and syndromic

<10,000	10,000–24,999	25,000–49,999	50,000–99,999
4 Total FTEs	**8 Total FTEs**	**14 Total FTEs**	**28 Total FTEs**
1 Registered nurse	2 Registered nurses	3.8 Registered nurses	6 Registered nurses
1 Office and administrative support staff	2 Office and administrative support staff	3 Office and administrative support staff	5 Office and administrative support staff
0.9 Agency leadership	1 Agency leadership	1 Agency leadership	1 Agency leadership
	1 Environmental health worker	1.4 Environmental health workers	3 Environmental health workers
		0.6 Health educator	1 Health educator
		0.5 Preparedness staff	1 Preparedness staff
		0.2 Nutritionist	1 Nutritionist
			1 Business and financial operations staff

100,000–249,999	250,000–499,999	500,000–999,999	1,000,000+
60 Total FTEs	**119 Total FTEs**	**238 Total FTEs**	**480 Total FTEs**
10 Registered nurses	17 Registered nurses	29.5 Registered nurses	48 Registered nurses
10 Office and administrative support staff	18.5 Office and administrative support staff	30.8 Office and administrative support staff	75 Office and administrative support staff
3 Agency leadership	6 Agency leadership	7.5 Agency leadership	10 Agency leadership
7 Environmental health workers	14 Environmental health workers	25 Environmental health workers	36 Environmental health workers
2 Health educators	3 Health educators	6 Health educators	12 Health educators
1 Preparedness staff	2 Preparedness staff	3 Preparedness staff	5 Preparedness staff
2 Nutritionists	4.1 Nutritionists	8 Nutritionists	19 Nutritionists
2 Business and financial operations staff	4 Business and financial operations staff	8 Business and financial operations staff	21 Business and financial operations staff
0.5 Epidemiologist	1 Epidemiologist/statistician	3 Epidemiologists/staticians	8 Epidemiologists/statisticians
0.1 Public health physician	1 Public health physician	1 Public health physician	3 Public health physicians
	2.4 Community health workers	6.5 Community health workers	14 Community health workers
	1 Information systems specialist	2 Information systems specialists	5 Information systems specialists
	1 Public information professional	1 Public information professional	1 Public information professional
	0.2 Licensed practical or vocational nurse	2 Licensed practical or vocational nurses	4 Licensed practical or vocational nurses
		1.8 Laboratory workers	10 Laboratory workers
		1 Behavioral health staff	2.7 Oral health care staff

n=1,114–1,468

Figure 3.14.   Staffing Patterns in Median Full-Time Equivalents (FTEs) at Local Health Departments (LHDs) by Size of Population Served, 2019

Source: National Association of County and City Health Officials. (2020). *2019 national profile of local health development.* https://www.naccho.org/uploads/downloadable-resources/Programs/Public-Health-Infrastructure/NACCHO_2019_Profile_final.pdf

surveillance were most frequently provided. Primary prevention activities that were most often offered were tobacco, nutrition, and chronic disease programs. Among regulatory, inspection and licensing activities, food service, schools/daycare, septic systems, and recreational water were most likely to be programs offered by LHDs. Other frequently offered population-based programs were food safety education and public health nuisance abatement. See **Figure 3.16.**

Program/service	% of LHDs
Immunization	
Childhood immunizations	88%
Adult immunizations	88%
Screening for diseases/conditions	
Tuberculosis	86%
Other STDs	70%
HIV/AIDS	62%
High blood pressure	56%
Body mass index (BMI)	52%
Diabetes	39%
Cancer	31%
Cardiovascular disease	25%
Treatment for communicable diseases	
Tuberculosis	83%
Other STDs	52%
HIV/AIDS	46%

Program/service	% of LHDs
Maternal and child health services	
Women, Infants, and Children (WIC)	68%
Early and periodic screening, diagnosis, and treatment	38%
Well child clinic	30%
Prenatal care	30%
Other clinical services	
Oral health	30%
Home health care	15%
Substance abuse	15%
Behavioral/mental health	12%
Comprehensive primary care	11%

n=1,226–1,461

Figure 3.15.   Clinical Programs and Services Provided Directly by Local Health Departments (LHDs) in the Prior Year, 2019

Source: National Association of County and City Health Officials. (2020). *2019 national profile of local health development.* https://www.naccho.org/uploads/downloadable-resources/Programs/Public-Health-Infrastructure/NACCHO_2019_Profile_final.pdf

Program/service	% of LHDs
Epidemiology and surveillance	
Communicable/infectious disease	90%
Environmental health	84%
Maternal and child health	70%
Syndromic surveillance	65%
Chronic disease	51%
Behavioral risk factors	47%
Injury	37%
Population-based primary prevention	
Tobacco	78%
Nutrition	75%
Chronic disease programs	60%
Physical activity	59%
Opioids	45%
Injury	40%
Substance abuse (other than opioids)	37%
Mental illness	18%

Program/service	% of LHDs
Regulation, inspection, and/or licensing	
Food service establishments	78%
Schools/daycare	72%
Septic systems	68%
Recreational water (e.g., pools, lakes, beaches)	66%
Body art (e.g., tattoos, piercings)	58%
Private drinking water	56%
Children's camps	55%
Hotels/motels	55%
Lead inspection	52%
Campgrounds and recreational vehicles	49%
Health-related facilities	42%
Tobacco retailers	41%
Food processing	41%
Public drinking water	37%
Housing (inspections)	33%
Milk processing	11%

Program/service	% of LHDs
Other environmental health services	
Food safety education	78%
Public health nuisance abatement	72%
Vector control	55%
Indoor air quality	32%
Hazmat response	23%
Land use planning	19%
Air pollution	19%
Radiation control	16%
Noise pollution	16%
Other population-based services	
School health	37%
Laboratory services	33%
School-based clinics	29%
Animal control	17%
Emergency medical services	4%

n=1,136–1,466

Figure 3.16.   Population-Based Programs and Services Provided Directly by Local Health Departments (LHDs) in the Prior Year, 2019

Source: National Association of County and City Health Officials. (2020). *2019 national profile of local health development.* https://www.naccho.org/uploads/downloadable-resources/Programs/Public-Health-Infrastructure/NACCHO_2019_Profile_final.pdf

The availability of the clinical and population-based services varies with the size of the population served. Not surprisingly, larger LHDs offer much more than small units. However, to state that the LHD does not provide a service either directly or through contract does not necessarily indicate that those services are not publicly available within a jurisdiction. In some cases, another local government agency, a state agency, or an NGO may provide the service.

FUNDING PUBLIC HEALTH

Funding for the public health system comes mainly from public sources: taxes and other monies, such as fees, collected by the government at the federal, state, and local levels. However, there are many challenges to measuring public health funding in the United States (Sensenig, 2007). Chief among them is the difficulty of defining what government activities constitute public health services. "There is no clear-cut, universally accepted definition of government public health care services" (Sensenig, 2007, p. 103). Also, the distinction between health and public health services is not clear in the classification of budget categories. Finally, the government must collect expenditure data according to the Classification of the Functions of Government (COFOG), which is an international system developed by the United Nations.

Though not perfect, the **National Health Expenditure Accounts (NHEA)** provide an authoritative and well-accepted estimate of the size of public health funding. The NHEA are the official estimates of total health care spending in the United States including estimates of *public health spending*. CMS has provided the NHEA annually since 1960. The NHEA categories include expenditures for health care goods and services, public health activities, government administration, the net cost of health insurance, and investment related to health care.

The NHEA definition of public health is not comprehensive:

> In addition to funding the care of individual citizens, government is involved in organizing and delivering publicly provided health services such as epidemiological surveillance, inoculations, immunization/vaccination services, disease prevention programs, the operation of public health laboratories, and other such functions. In the NHEA, spending for these activities is reported in government public health activity. Funding for health research and government purchases of medical structures and equipment are reported in their respective categories. Government spending for public works, environmental functions (air and water pollution abatement, sanitation and sewage treatment, water supplies, and so on), emergency planning and other such functions are not included. (CMS, 2021, p. 27)

Despite the definition's weaknesses for public health, using the NHEA has the benefit of placing public health funding in the context of total health expenditures and the advantage of historical comparison.

As discussed earlier in the chapter, most federal government *public health activity* derive from the DHHS, especially the FDA and the CDC. Since the 9/11 attacks, there have been two additional sources of substantial public health funding: the Public Health and Social Services Emergency Fund—part of the DHHS Departmental Management Budget—and the Department of Homeland Security. Additionally, in response to the COVID-19 pandemic, funding was increased to the Public Health and Social Services Emergency Fund and the CDC. In the 2020 NHEA, data from the President's Budget was the primary source for estimating this increased federal public health spending, along with congressional budget justifications and treasury reports (CMS, 2021).

> There are two basic data sources used in estimation of government public health activity. Federal spending is taken from annual budget documents prepared by the various agencies and summarized in the budget of the U.S. (Executive Office of the President, 1960-2020). State and local government spending is estimated using data from the quinquennial (5-year) Census of Governments (U.S. Census Bureau, 1957, 1962, 1967, 1972, 1977, 1982, 1987, 1992, 1997, 2002, 2007, 2012, and 2017) and from its annual survey of state and local government finances (U.S. Census Bureau, 1960–2019). (CMS, 2021, p. 28)

Within the NHEA budget, public health spending in 2020 was about 5% of the $4.1 trillion budget. See **Figure 3.17**.

The NHEA also provide information about the growth of public health spending since 1960. The two major budget categories in the NHEA's National Health Expenditures are Health Consumption Expenditures and Investment. Within Health Consumption Expenditures are Personal Health Care, Government Administration and Net Cost of Health Insurance, and Government Public Health Activities. Since 1960, the public health expenditures have increased from $4 billion to $105 billion in 2019 and $223.7 billion in 2020. Per capita expenditures have also increased since 1960 from $2 to $320 in 2019 and $680 in 2020. Despite increases in spending—actual and per capita—public health expenditures remained a small portion of total health care spending from 1960 through 2019. For example, in 1960, Public Health Activities accounted for 1.4% of National Health Expenditures. That percent rose to almost 3% in 1990 and hovered around 3% until 2019. In 2020, that percent was 5.4%. See **Table 3.5**.

The change in public health expenditures between 2019 and 2020 is related to the COVID-19 pandemic, which affected all aspects of the National Health Expenditures. The NHEA tell us that, overall, U.S. health care spending increased 9.7% to $4.1 trillion in 2020, a much faster rate than the 4.3% increase in 2019.

THE NATION'S HEALTH DOLLAR ($4.1 TRILLION), CALENDAR YEAR 2020: WHERE IT WENT

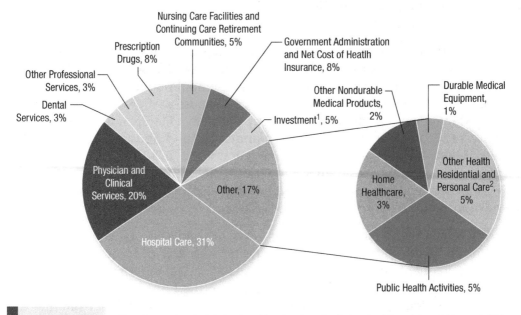

Figure 3.17.   The Nation's Health Dollar ($4.3 trillion), Calendar Year 2021: Where It Went

[1] Includes noncommercial research and structure and equipment.
[2] Includes expenditures for residential care facilities, ambulance providers, medical care delivered in nontraditional settings (such as community centers, senior citizen centers, schools, and military field stations), and expenditures for Home and Community Wavier programs under Medicaid.

Note: May not equal 100% due to rounding.

Source: Centers for Medicare & Medicaid Services, Office of the Actuary, National Health Statistics Group. (2021). *The nation's health dollar ($4.3 trillion), calendar year 2021: Where it went.* https://www.cms.gov/files/document/nations-health-dollar-where-it-came-where-it-went.pdf

Gross domestic product (GDP) declined 2.2% in 2020, leading to a sharp increase in the share of the overall economy related to health care spending—from 17.6% in 2019 to 19.7% in 2020. A 36% increase in federal expenditures for health in 2020, in response to the COVID-19 pandemic, was the major reason for the acceleration in health spending. Furthermore, growth was not linked to patient care, but to increased federal public health activity, to aid for health care providers through the Provider Relief Fund and Paycheck Protection Program loans, as well as increased federal Medicaid funding. These additional funds had a tremendous impact on growth of the entire health care sector, including public health:

> When spending associated with federal public health and other federal programs (which includes the Provider Relief Fund and Paycheck Protection Program loans) is excluded, total national health expenditures increased just 1.9 % in 2020. This was a function of less use of medical goods and services in 2020. (CMS, 2021b, p. 1)

Federal Public Health Funding

The federal public health budget is used for two purposes: (a) to fund federal activities and (b) to fund state and local activities by returning federal money to states. Categorical grants are the method most used by the CDC to fund state public health efforts. Categorical grants are program-focused, restricted to specific program use, and cannot be used to support broader or core public health responsibilities. Some categorical funding is based on population, some based on demonstrated need, and others are awarded competitively (Levi et al., 2007).

Federal categorical and block grants may be criticized because they require states to engage in activities mandated by particular grant program requirements rather than in accordance with the needs of the particular population being served. That is, because federal funding is available for one kind of program, a state may dedicate resources to that program area to obtain funds, even if the program does not align with the priorities dictated by the health needs of the state. Although this is not true of every federal grant program—the Preventive Health and Health Services Block Grant mentioned earlier, for example, allows for considerable flexibility in how the funds are used—the large proportion of state health department resources that come from the federal government should be kept in mind when considering state health department budgets. In effect, not all dollars available to the state health department are created equal—they are not all part of a general pool that can be simply allocated in accordance with the state's health needs and priorities. The availability of state sources of funding may therefore be critical in financing essential services in a manner that is consistent with the state's needs and priorities.

There is wide variation in the amount of state resources expended by state public health departments.

State Public Health Funding

As discussed previously, public health financing in the United States derives from a complex web of intergovernmental relationships at the federal, state, and local levels. Other than sharing common legal frameworks and federal funding opportunities, each state government is organized very differently, with its own priorities and organizational structure, when it comes to public health. As such, a comprehensive, up-to-date, and accurate summary of public health financing is difficult (Sensenig, 2007; Turnock & Atchison, 2002).

For example, while California had approximately 50% more people than Texas in 2003, its government was nearly three times as large in terms of expenditures. However, Texas spent four times more on public health than California, mostly because of the greater amount of federal funding received by Texas. Subtracting the entry of federal funds, Texas's appropriated funds were still 45% more than California, and as a proportion of total state expenditures, much larger. Overall, California spent $14.70 per person on population health in 2003, and Texas spent $99.30 per person. Most of Texas's public health spending went for chronic disease control and support for health behavior change, using federal funds (Milbank Memorial Fund, 2005).

Table 3.5. National Health Expenditures; Aggregate and Per Capita Amounts, Annual Percent Change and Percent Distribution: Selected Calendar Years 1960–2021

Item	1960	1970	1980
National Health Expenditures	$27.1	$74.1	$253.2
Health Consumption Expenditures	24.6	66.3	232.7
Personal Health Care	23.1	62.4	214.3
Government Administration and Net Cost of Health Insurance	1.1	2.6	11.9
Government Public Health Activities	0.4	1.4	6.4
Investment	2.6	7.7	20.6
U.S. Population[1]	186	210	230
Gross Domestic Product[2]	$542.4	$1,073.3	$2,857.3
National Health Expenditures		10.6%	13.1%
Health Consumption Expenditures		10.4	13.4
Personal Health Care		10.4	13.1
Government Administration and Net Cost of Health Insurance		9.4	16.4
Government Public Health Activities		13.8	16.9
Investment		11.7	10.3
U.S. Population[1]		1.2	0.9
Gross Domestic Product[2]		7.1	10.3
National Health Expenditures	100.0%	100.0%	100.0%
Health Consumption Expenditures	90.5	89.5	91.9
Personal Health Care	85.3	84.2	84.6
Government Administration and Net Cost of Health Insurance	3.9	3.5	4.7
Government Public Health Activities	1.4	1.8	2.5
Investment	9.5	10.5	8.1
National Health Expenditures	$146	$353	$1,099
Health Consumption Expenditures	132	316	1,010
Personal Health Care	124	297	930
Government Administration and Net Cost of Health Insurance	6	12	52
Government Public Health Activities	2	6	28
Investment	14	37	89
National Health Expenditures as a Percent of Gross Domestic Product	5.0%	6.9%	8.9%

[1]U.S. Bureau of the Census. Census resident-based population less armed forces overseas and population of outlying areas.
[2]U.S. Department of Commerce, Bureau of Economic Analysis.

Note: Numbers and percents may not add to totals because of rounding. Dollar amounts shown are in current dollars. Percent changes are calculated from unrounded data.

Source: Centers for Medicare & Medicaid Services, Office of the Actuary, National Health Statistics Group; U.S. Department of Commerce, Bureau of Economic Analysis; and U.S. Bureau of the Census.

1990	2000	2010	2019	2020
Amount in Billions				
$718.7	$1,366.0	$2,589.6	$3,757.4	$4,144.1
670.2	1,280.3	2,437.5	3,563.3	3,950.1
611.9	1,156.5	2,180.5	3,173.1	3,367.0
38.3	80.7	181.4	283.2	344.9
20.0	43.0	75.7	107.1	238.3
48.6	85.7	152.1	194.1	193.9
Millions				
254	282	309	328	329
Amount in Billions				
$5,963.1	$10,251.0	$15,049.0	$21,381.0	$21,060.5
Average Annual Percent Change from Previous Year Shown				
11.0%	6.6%	3.9%	4.2%	10.3%
11.2	6.7	3.9	4.4	10.9
11.1	6.6	3.6	5.1	6.1
12.4	7.8	9.3	−4.1	21.8
12.0	8.0	2.0	7.7	122.5
9.0	5.8	3.3	2.2	−0.1
1.0	1.1	0.8	0.5	0.3
7.6	5.6	3.9	4.1	−1.5
Percent Distribution				
100.0%	100.0%	100.0%	100.0%	100.0%
93.2	93.7	94.1	94.8	95.3
85.1	84.7	84.2	84.4	81.2
5.3	5.9	7.0	7.5	8.3
2.8	3.2	2.9	2.8	5.7
6.8	6.3	5.9	5.2	4.7
Per Capita Amount				
$2,835	$4,845	$8,381	$11,456	$12,591
2,643	4,541	7,889	10,865	12,002
2,413	4,102	7,057	9,675	10,230
151	286	587	863	1,048
79	153	245	326	724
192	304	492	592	589
Percent				
12.1%	13.3%	17.2%	17.6%	19.7%

When trying to understand the financing of public health departments and public health activities in particular, one should not assume that the numbers across states are comparable. Whereas Rhode Island has no LHDs, other states are organized with all LHDs independent from the state health departments. These differences mean per capita spending is not comparable, because funding may be at the local rather than the state level or vice versa. In addition, states may differ in the amount they appropriate for public health through taxation and fees, but they may also vary in the amount of "pass-through" funding that they obtain from the federal government (Milbank Memorial Fund, 2005).

Nationwide, state health departments obtain funding from federal, state, and other sources. Of these, the federal government provides the most funding—about 53% of total state expenditures on public health between 2015 and 2018. The largest federal contributors to state public health departments were the Department of Agriculture, followed by the CDC, HRSA, and other DHHS programs. Together, these agencies accounted for about 45% of state public health funding. State sources were the second largest source of funding for state public health departments—providing about 28% of their budgets. About 70% of state funding was from the General funds. See **Figure 3.18** (ASTHO, 2020). Note that funding declined, overall, and from both federal and state sources.

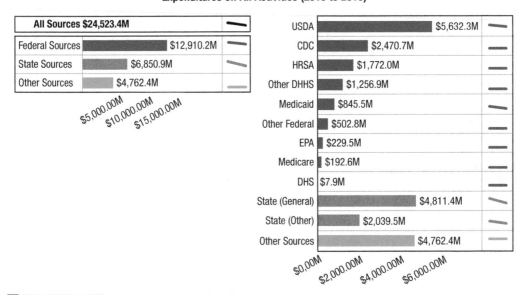

Expenditures: All States
Expenditures on All Activities (2015 to 2018)

Figure 3.18.   Expenditures on All Activities, 2015 to 2018

CDC, Centers for Disease Control and Prevention; DHHS, Department of Health and Human Services; DHS, Department of Homeland Security; EPA, Environmental Protection Agency; HRSA, Health Resources and Services Administration.

Source: Association of State and Territorial Health Officials. (n.d.). *Profile of state and territorial public health.* https://www.astho.org/topic/public-health-infrastructure/profile/#finance

There was tremendous variability between the states in amount and source of their public health funding. For example, Illinois received over half of its funding from the state and had virtually no other sources of funds except the state and federal governments. Their federal funding was predominantly from the CDC—69% of the federal allocation. See **Figure 3.19**.

In contrast, Tennessee received no state or other funds for public health. All funding was from the Department of Agriculture (39.5%), HRSA (39%), the CDC (13.5%), and other DHHS agencies. Tennessee's overall budget was $273.9 million during 2015 to 2018. However, New Jersey received most of its public health funding of $1,327.6 million from other sources (45.8%)—neither state nor federal. Their second source of funding was the federal government, and most of that was from the Medicaid program (55%). See **Figure 3.20**.

Local Public Health Funding

LHDs obtain funding from a combination of sources that includes local funds, state-direct funds, clinical sources such as from categorical grants, federal-direct funds, Medicaid and Medicare funds, and fees. One fourth of LHD revenues come from local sources, and 21% come from state sources. Thirteen percent of LHD revenues are payments for clinical services (Medicare, Medicaid, private insurers, or patient personal fees). See **Table 3.6**.

Annual per capita revenue sources illustrate the diversity of LHDs. The source of funding and the amount given depends on the governance structure of the local

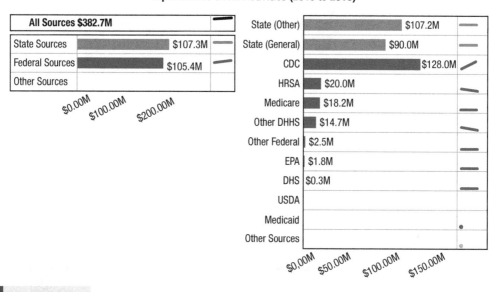

Figure 3.19.   Expenditures: Illinois

Source: Association of State and Territorial Health Officials. (n.d.). *Profile of state and territorial public health.* https://www.astho.org/topic/public-health-infrastructure/profile/#finance

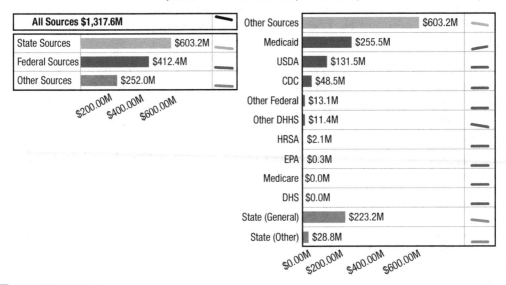

Figure 3.20. Expenditures: New Jersey

Source: Association of State and Territorial Health Officials. (n.d.). *Profile of state and territorial public health.* https://www.astho.org/topic/public-health-infrastructure/profile/#finance

Table 3.6. LHD Revenue Sources, 2019	
Source	**Percent**
Local sources	25
State sources	21
Federal pass-through	16
Federal direct	11
Medicaid/Medicare	10
Non clinical fees/fines	8
Other	5
Private health insurance	2
Private foundations	1
Patient fees	1

Sources: National Association of County & City Health Officials. (2020). *2019 national profile of local health departments.* https://www.naccho.org/uploads/downloadable-resources/Programs/Public-Health-Infrastructure/NACCHO_2019_Profile_final.pdf

health department. For example, on average, state-governed health departments receive only $3 per person from local sources, whereas locally governed departments receive $21 per person, and those with a shared governance structure receive $15 per person. Health departments that are locally controlled obtain far less money from the state and from Medicaid and Medicare funds than departments that are units of the state. As a result, they depend more heavily on local funds and fees.

Size of the population served also influences per capita funding. In general, LHDs serving fewer than 50,000 people have the highest per capita funding, compared to the LHDs serving larger populations. Degree of urbanization impacts funding. Urban LHDs receive substantially less funding per capita than rural departments. For example, federal direct and pass-through funding is $10 per capita for urban LHDs and $19 for their rural counterparts. Finally, census region differentiates funding levels per capita. Local funding is lowest in the South ($14/capita) and highest in the Midwest ($21/capita). State funding is lowest in the Northeast ($7/capita) and highest in the West ($33/capita). See Table 3.7.

Table 3.7. Median and Mean Annual per Capita Revenue Sources, by LHD Characteristics

	Local		State		Federal Direct and Pass-Through		Clinical[a]	
	Median	Mean	Median	Mean	Median	Mean	Median	Mean
All LHDs	$11	$18	$6	$14	$3	$13	$4	$13
Size of population served								
Small (<50,000)	$3	$20	$7	$16	$9	$17	$3	$18
Medium (50,000–499,995)	$9	$14	$6	$10	$8	$10	$3	$8
Large (500,000+)	$9	$19	$6	$11	$10	$19	$2	$7
Type of governance								
State	$1	$3	$5	$9	$8	$12	$4	$6
Local	$13	$21	$5	$12	$8	$13	$3	$12
Shared	$12	$15	$13	$26	$14	$24	$8	$25
Degree of urbanization								
Urban	$10	$17	$5	$9	$7	$10	$2	$6
Rural	$12	$19	$9	$19	$11	$19	$9	$21

(continued)

Table 3.7. Median and Mean Annual per Capita Revenue Sources, by LHD Characteristics (*continued*)

	Local		State		Federal Direct and Pass-Through		Clinical[a]	
	Median	Mean	Median	Mean	Median	Mean	Median	Mean
Census region								
Northeast	$18	$18	$2	$7	$1	$3	$0	$2
Midwest	$21	$21	$4	$3	$8	$13	$5	$16
South	$14	$14	$9	$16	$10	$17	$6	$19
West	$19	$19	$7	$33	$15	$25	$2	$7

n=365–510
[a]Includes Medicaid/Medicare, private health insurance, and patient personal fees.

Source: National Association of County and City Health Officials. (2020). *2019 national profile of local health departments*. https://www.naccho.org/uploads/downloadable-resources/Programs/Public-Health-Infrastructure/NACCHO_2019_Profile_final.pdf

Federal, state, and local government expenditures do not tell the entire story of public health spending in local areas. Depending upon the community, support for public health endeavors comes from community partners including the health department, other social and human service agencies, primary care providers, hospitals, businesses, community groups, schools, churches, volunteer organizations, and citizens themselves. There are no rules governing contributions from these partners. Much depends upon the local economy, market forces, political views, geography, and existing public health infrastructure (Barry et al., 1998, p. 31).

CHAPTER SUMMARY

The "public" public health system in the United States is complex and vast—encompassing multiple federal agencies, departments of health in every state and territory, and about 3,000 LHDs. As Ashish Jha, White House COVID-19 Response Coordinator for the Biden administration, said, "We have a very complicated form of government in America which is because we have a complicated country . . . (as a result), the ability to move policy resides at lots of different levels. If you want to try to move it all in one direction, you have to coordinate and bring people along" (Hutto, 2023, para. 8). The federal DHHS and USDA provide much of the funding for the system, as a whole, through major programs such as Medicare, Medicaid, and the Nutrition Program for Women, Infants, and Children (WIC).

Public health was tested as never before during the COVID-19 pandemic. The pandemic highlighted the impact of continued underfunding of public health around the country. Moreover, it led to threats not experienced before in this era:

"As health departments tackle the largest pandemic in modern history, the workforce is strained, resources are redirected to the response, essential services are disrupted, and leaders are faced with political pressures ranging from firings to death threats" (NACCHO, 2020a, p. 2). These are problems that continue to have an effect on the public health system and those who work in it.

We also note three trends within the public health system that are reorganizing public health activities and reallocating funding:

- Emphasis on health information systems including the collecting, processing, sharing, and using data for evidence-based policy-making.
  - The Public Health Data Modernization Initiative is an example. Another is the Nationwide Health Information Network (NHIN) exchange. The NHIN exchange is broadly defined as the set of standards, specifications, and policies that enable the secure exchange of health information over the internet. This program provides a foundation for the exchange of health information across diverse entities, within communities and across the country (Office of the National Coordinator for Health Information Technology, 2022).
- Appreciation of the interdependence and intertwining of health problems and their causes and the need for collaboration across organizations and disciplines in order to be effective.
  - One Health is an example of this approach, and it provides a template for the prevention and control of other health problems, beyond those of infectious diseases.
  - "Successful public health interventions require the cooperation of human, animal, and environmental health partners. Professionals in **human health** (doctors, nurses, public health practitioners, epidemiologists), **animal health** (veterinarians, paraprofessionals, agricultural workers), **environment** (ecologists, wildlife experts), and **other areas of expertise** need to communicate, collaborate on, and coordinate activities. Other relevant players in a One Health approach could include law enforcement, policymakers, agriculture, communities, and even pet owners. No one person, organization, or sector can address issues at the animal-human-environment interface alone" (NCEZID, 2022a, para. 6).
- Necessity of national preparedness for all kinds of emergencies, from pandemics to environmental disasters, that require teams ready to provide medical care, housing, food, and other necessities that are needed to preserve life. The recent development and funding of the Administration for Strategic Preparedness and Response (ASPR) as one of the operating divisions within the DHHS confirms the priority that preparedness has become. Furthermore, state and LHDs have joined in setting preparedness as a priority for their work (ASTHO, 2017, 2020; NACCHO, 2020a, 2020b).

DISCUSSION QUESTIONS

Q: What is the lead public health agency at the federal level, and what are its major activities and responsibilities?

Q: How does this federal public health agency interact with the state departments of health?

Q: What agency is responsible for the Medicare program? Medicaid program? SCHIP?

Q: What are the sources of funding for state departments of health?

Q: Discuss the degree of and why there is variation in public health services from state to state.

DATA SOURCES

For Chapter 3, the following sources of data can provide a deeper understanding of the agencies that administer the public health system in the United States:

- The DHHS Budget

  The DHHS contains so many programs that provide public health services to the nation, among them the CDC, the Administration for Children and Families, the FDA, and the CMS. Within these agencies are multiple divisions and programs, for example, the NCHS in CMS and the Temporary Assistance for Needy Families (TANF) program in the Administration for Children and Families. The DHHS budget is a window into these agencies and their divisions—how they are organized, what services or programs they provide, and how much they expend on each. Importantly, the budget provides a basis for comparing priorities within and between each agency. A good starting point for such an exploration is the DHHS Budget in Brief for Fiscal Year 2022, which contains the overall budget for DHHS and budgets for its agencies and their divisions. The Budget in Brief is also available for prior years, permitting a look at changes in priorities. You can begin your investigation here: https://www.hhs.gov/sites/default/files/fy-2022-budget-in-brief.pdf

- ASTHO Profiles

  ASTHO is the major professional organization for state public health officials, supporting their work and development of public health policy. Membership is comprised of 59 chief health officials from each of the 50 states, Washington, DC, five U.S. territories, and three Freely Associated States.

  The ASTHO Profiles of State and Territorial Public Health are a wealth of information about public health at the state level, and they can be used to assess and compare public health priorities and resources across states. The profiles include a description of the public health structure, governance, and priorities; workforce; services and programs; leadership; and finance in each state and in the nation overall. ASTHO prepared a profile in 2007, 2010, 2012, and 2016. An exploration of state public health can begin with the 2016 ASTHO Profile of State and Territorial Public Health, Volume 4: https://www.astho.org/globalassets/pdf/profile/profile-stph-vol-4.pdf

- NACCHO Profiles

NACCHO is the only organization dedicated to serving every LHD in the nation. The Profile study is the only longitudinal study of its kind focused on the infrastructure and practice of LHDs. The NACCHO profiles are a wealth of information about public health at the local "boots on the ground" level. The profiles include a description of the funding, staffing, governance, and activities of LHDs across the United States and provide a comprehensive view of LHD infrastructure and practice. NACCHO has prepared a profile every 3 years since 1990, and therefore, the profiles can be used to compare priorities, practices, and funding over time. An exploration of local public health can begin here with the 2019 National Profile of Local Health Departments: https://www.naccho.org/uploads/downloadable-resources/Programs/Public-Health-Infrastructure/NACCHO_2019_Profile_final.pdf

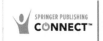 A robust set of instructor resources designed to supplement this text is located at **http://connect.springerpub.com/content/book/978-0-8261-8615-7**. Qualifying instructors may request access by emailing **textbook@springerpub.com**.

REFERENCES

Administration for Children and Families. (2023). *Budget*. https://www.acf.hhs.gov/about/budget

Administration for Strategic Preparedness and Response. (2022). *About ASPR*. https://aspr.hhs.gov/Pages/Home.aspx

Agency for Healthcare Research and Quality. (2022). *Agency for healthcare research and quality: A profile*. https://www.ahrq.gov/cpi/about/profile/index.html

Association of State and Territorial Health Officials. (2009). *ASTHO profile of state and territorial public health* (Vol. 1). https://stacks.cdc.gov/view/cdc/51137

Association of State and Territorial Health Officials. (2017). *ASTHO profile of state and territorial public health* (Vol. 4). https://www.astho.org/globalassets/pdf/profile/profile-stph-vol-4.pdf

Association of State and Territorial Health Officials. (2020). *ASTHO profile of state and territorial public health* (Vol. 5). https://www.astho.org/topic/public-health-infrastructure/profile/

Baker, E. L., & Koplan, J. P. (2002). Strengthening the nation's public health infrastructure: Historic challenge, unprecedented opportunity. *Health Affairs, 21*, 15–27. https://doi.org/10.1377/hlthaff.21.6.15

Baker, E. L., Potter, M. A., Jones, D. L., Mercer, S. L., Cioffi, J. P., Green, L. W., Halverson, P. K., Lichtveld, M. Y., & Fleming, D. W. (2005). The public health infrastructure and our nation's health. *Annual Review of Public Health, 26*, 303–318. https://doi.org/10.1146/annurev.publhealth.26.021304.144647

Barry, M. A., Centra, L., Pratt, E. T. B. Jr., Carol, K., & Giordano, L. (1998). *Where do the dollars go? Measuring local public health expenditures.* The National Association of County and City Health Officials, the National Association of Local Boards of Health, and the Public Health Foundation to the Office of Disease Prevention and Health Promotion, Office of Public Health and Science, & U.S. Department of Health & Human Services.

Beitsch, L. M., Brooks, R. G., Grigg, M., & Menachemi, N. (2006). Structure and functions of state public health agencies. *American Journal of Public Health, 96*, 167–172. https://doi.org/10.2105/AJPH.2004.053439

California Health & Human Services Agency. (2022). *About us.* https://www.chhs.ca.gov/about/departments-and-offices/

Centers for Disease Control and Prevention. (2021a). *Public health professionals gateway. 10 essential public health services.* https://www.cdc.gov/publichealthgateway/publichealthservices/essentialhealthservices.html

Centers for Disease Control and Prevention. (2021b). *Data modernization initiative: Strategic implementation plan.* https://www.cdc.gov/surveillance/pdfs/FINAL-DMI-Implementation-Strategic-Plan-12-22-21.pdf

Centers for Disease Control and Prevention. (2022a). *National public health performance standards.* https://www.cdc.gov/publichealthgateway/nphps/index.html

Centers for Disease Control and Prevention. (2022b). *Public health data modernization.* https://www.cdc.gov/budget/documents/fy2021/fy2021-PHDM-factsheet.pdf

Centers for Disease Control and Prevention. (2023). *Original essential public health services framework.* https://www.cdc.gov/publichealthgateway/publichealthservices/originalessentialhealthservices.html

Centers for Medicare & Medicaid Services. (2011). *National health expenditures accounts: Definitions, sources, and methods, 2012.* http://www.cms.gov/Research-Statistics-Data-and-Systems/Statistics-Trends-and-Reports/NationalHealthExpendData/Downloads/dsm-12.pdf

Centers for Medicare & Medicaid Services. (2021). *National health expenditure accounts: Methodology paper, 2020.* https://www.cms.gov/files/document/definitions-sources-and-methods.pdf

Centers for Medicare & Medicaid Services. (2021b). *National health expenditures 2020 highlights.* https://www.cms.gov/files/document/highlights.pdf

Centers for Medicare & Medicaid Services. (2022). *About CMS.* https://www.cms.gov/About-CMS/About-CMS

Centers for Medicare & Medicaid Services, Office of the Actuary, National Health Statistics Group. (2013). *Budget of the United States government: Detailed functional tables, estimates for fiscal year 2013.* http://www.gpo.gov/fdsys/pkg/BUDGET-2009-PER/pdf/BUDGET-2009-PER-12-5-1.pdf

Centers for Medicare & Medicaid Services, Office of the Actuary, National Health Statistics Group. (2021). *National health expenditures: Aggregate and per capita amounts, annual percent change and percent distribution: Calendar years 1960–2020.* https://www.cms.gov/Research-Statistics-Data-and-Systems/Statistics-Trends-and-Reports/NationalHealthExpendData/NationalHealthAccountsHistorical

Fee, E., & Brown, T. M. (2002). The unfulfilled promise of public health: Déjà vu all over again. *Health Affairs, 21*, 31–43. https://doi.org/10.1377/hlthaff.21.6.31

Hartsaw, K. (2009). Centers for disease control and prevention. In R. M. Mullner (Ed.), *Encyclopedia of health services research* (pp. 141–144). Sage.

Health Resources and Services Administration. (2021a). *Bureau of primary health care.* https://www.hrsa.gov/about/organization/bureaus/bphc

Health Resources and Services Administration. (2021b). *Bureaus & offices.* https://www.hrsa.gov/about/organization/bureaus

Health Resources and Services Administration. (2022, August). *Health center program: Impact and growth.* https://bphc.hrsa.gov/about-health-centers/health-center-program-impact-growth

Health Resources and Services Administration. (2023). *Bureau of primary health care.* https://bphc.hrsa.gov/

Health Resources and Services Administration, Bureau of Health Workforce. (2022). *Our work.* https://bhw.hrsa.gov/about-us

Hutto, E. (2023, February 24). *Ashish Jha on the end of the COVID-19 public health emergency.* MedPageToday. https://www.medpagetoday.com/opinion/faustfiles/103278

Indian Health Service. (2022). *Agency overview.* https://www.ihs.gov/aboutihs/overview/

Institute of Medicine. (1988). *The future of public health.* National Academy Press.

Institute of Medicine. (2003). *The future of the public's health in the 21st century.* National Academies Press.

Levi, J., Juliano, C., & Richardson, M. (2007). Financing public health: Diminished funding for core needs and state-by-state variation in support. *Journal of Public Health Management and Practice, 13*, 97–102. https://doi.org/10.1097/00124784-200703000-00004

Mays, G. P., Beitsch, L. M., Corso, L., Chang, C., & Brewer, R. (2007). States gathering momentum: Promising strategies for accreditation and assessment activities in multistate learning collaborative applicant states. *Journal of Public Health Management and Practice, 13*, 364–373. https://doi.org/10.1097/01.PHH.0000278029.33949.21

Mays, G. P., McHugh, M. C., Shim, K., Perry, N., Lenaway, D., Halverson, P. K., & Moonesinghe, R. (2006). Institutional and economic determinants of public health system performance. *American Journal of Public Health, 96*, 523–531. https://doi.org/10.2105/AJPH.2005.064253

McCarty, K. L., Nelson, G. D., Hodge, J. G., & Gebbie, K. M. (2009). Major components and themes of local public health laws in select U.S. jurisdictions. *Public Health Reports, 124*, 458–462. https://doi.org/10.1177/003335490912400317

Milbank Memorial Fund. (2005). *2002–2003 state health expenditure report*. Author.

National Association of County and City Health Officials. (2013). *Local health department job losses and program cuts: Findings from the 2013 profile survey*. Author.

National Association of County and City Health Officials. (2020a). *2019 National profile of local health departments*. https://www.naccho.org/uploads/downloadable-resources/Programs/Public-Health-Infrastructure/NACCHO_2019_Profile_final.pdf

National Association of County and City Health Officials. (2020b). *NACCHO's 2019 profile study: Changes in local health department workforce and finance capacity since 2008*. https://www.naccho.org/uploads/downloadable-resources/2019-Profile-Workforce-and-Finance-Capacity.pdf

National Center on Birth Defects and Developmental Disabilities. (2021). *What we do*. https://www.cdc.gov/ncbddd/aboutus/what-we-do.html

National Center for Chronic Disease and Health Promotion. (2022). *About the center*. https://www.cdc.gov/chronicdisease/center/index.htm

National Center for Emerging and Zoonotic Infectious Diseases. (2022a). *One health basics*. https://www.cdc.gov/onehealth/basics/index.html

National Center for Emerging and Zoonotic Infectious Diseases. (2022b). *SEDRIC: System for enteric disease response, investigation, and coordination*. https://www.cdc.gov/foodsafety/outbreaks/tools/sedric.html

National Center for Health Statistics. (2023). *National Center for Health Statistics*. https://www.cdc.gov/nchs/

National Center for Immunization and Respiratory Diseases. (2023). *About the Center*. Retrieved from https://www.cdc.gov/ncird/index.html

National Center for HIV, Viral Hepatitis, STD, and TB Prevention. (2023). *About the center*. https://www.cdc.gov/nchhstp/default.htm

National Institutes of Health. (2022). *About us*. https://www.nih.gov/about-nih

Occupational Safety and Health Administration. (2022). *About OSHA*. https://www.osha.gov/aboutosha

Office of the National Coordinator for Health Information Technology & Department of Health & Human Services. (2022). *Nationwide health information network exchange*. https://www.healthit.gov/sites/default/files/factsheets/nationwide-health-information-network-exchange.pdf

Passenger Cases 48 U.S. 283. (1849). https://supreme.justia.com/cases/federal/us/48/283/

Perlino, C. M. (2006). *Medicaid, prevention, and public health: Invest today for a healthier tomorrow*. American Public Health Association.

Public Health Accreditation Board. (2022). *About us*. https://phaboard.org/

Sensenig, A. L. (2007). Refining estimates of public health spending as measured in national health expenditures accounts: The United States experience. *Journal of Public Health Management and Practice, 13*, 103–114. https://doi.org/10.1097/00124784-200703000-00005

Tilson, H., & Berkowitz, B. (2006). The public health enterprise: Examining our twenty-first-century policy challenges. *Health Affairs, 25*, 900–910. https://doi.org/10.1377/hlthaff.25.4.900

Trust for America's Future. (2010). *Shortchanging America's health.* Author.

Trust for America's Health. (2020). *The impact of chronic underfunding on America's public health system: Trends, risks, and recommendations, 2020.* https://www.tfah.org/wp-content/uploads/2020/04/TFAH2020PublicHealthFunding.pdf

Turnock, B. J., & Atchison, C. (2002). Governmental public health in the United States: The implications of federalism. *Health Affairs, 21*, 68–78. https://doi.org/10.1377/hlthaff.21.6.68

U.S. Bureau of Labor Statistics. (2022). *About BLS.* https://www.bls.gov/

U.S. Department of Agriculture. (2022). *USDA FY 2022 budget summary.* https://www.usda.gov/sites/default/files/documents/2022-budget-summary.pdf

U.S. Department of Health & Human Services. (2022a). *About HHS.* https://www.hhs.gov/about/index.html

U.S. Department of Health & Human Services. (2022b). *Programs & services.* https://www.hhs.gov/programs/index.html

U.S. Department of Health & Human Services. (2022c). *Budget in brief: Fiscal year 2022.* https://www.hhs.gov/sites/default/files/fy-2022-budget-in-brief.pdf

U.S. Department of Health & Human Services, & Office of Disease Prevention and Health Promotion. (2022). *Healthy people.* https://health.gov/our-work/national-health-initiatives/healthy-people

U.S. Department of Health & Human Services, Public Health Functions Steering Committee, Office of Disease Prevention and Health Promotion, & Office of Public Health and Science. (1994). *Public health in America.* U.S. Department of Health & Human Services.

U.S. Department of Veterans Affairs. (2022). *Veterans health administration.* http://www.va.gov/health/

U.S. Environmental Protection Agency. (2021). *FY 2022: EPA budget in brief.* https://www.epa.gov/sites/default/files/2021-05/documents/fy-2022-epa-bib.pdf

U.S. Environmental Protection Agency. (2022). *Laws and executive orders.* https://www.epa.gov/laws-regulations/laws-and-executive-orders

U.S. Food and Drug Administration. (2018). *What we do.* https://www.fda.gov/about-fda/what-we-do#mission

Van Wave, T. W., Scutchfield, F. D., & Honoré, P. A. (2010). Recent advances in public health systems research in the United States. *Annual Review of Public Health, 31*, 283–295. https://doi.org/10.1146/annurev.publhealth.012809.103550

4

Infectious Disease Control

LEARNING OBJECTIVES

Students will learn . . .

1. The significance of infectious diseases to morbidity and mortality, historically and in the present.

2. The basic approach of the federal public health system toward infectious disease control.

3. How the public health system monitors infectious disease outbreaks and trends.

4. How the public health infrastructure responds to infectious disease outbreaks and new infectious diseases.

5. The public health role in developing vaccines and the success of immunizations in controlling infectious diseases.

Until the 20th century, infectious diseases were the greatest threat to human health, worldwide, and they have affected every aspect of life throughout human history. Authors such as Zinsser (*Rats, Lice and History*, 1935) and McNeill (*Plagues and Peoples*, 1976) have traced the political, economic, social, and military consequences of infectious diseases in various historical times and places. Barreto and her colleagues (2006) summarize McNeill's exploration of the underappreciated part played by infectious diseases in the evolution of human civilizations:

> Plagues and cholera used to devastate significant proportions of the populations of the great European cities. In his classic *Plagues and Peoples*, McNeill analyses the importance of infectious diseases in the history of humanity and concludes that the role of infectious diseases in the set of factors that defined the course of the historical evolution of human civilisation has been underestimated, and considers that this role was as important as that of economic and military determinants. The importance that the occurrence of these diseases, principally in the form of epidemics, had in forming the dominant political, social, and theological opinion of the different human societies in medieval and

141

modern times was fundamental in the definition and adoption of many of the pathways that led to civilisation. (Barreto et al., 2006, p. 192)

The invention of the microscope early in the 1600s and its application by Robert Hooke—who described the fruiting structures of molds in 1665—and Antoni van Leeuwenhoek—who is credited with the discovery of bacteria in 1676—permitted the study of the microorganisms that cause infectious diseases and the subsequent development of measures to prevent and treat them. The success of methods to prevent and treat infectious diseases changed the reasons for death in developed countries—those with access to these methods. Therefore, beginning in the 20th century, chronic degenerative diseases and injuries became the dominant causes of mortality in developed countries. For example, the first three causes of death in 1900 in the United States were infectious diseases—pneumonia and influenza, tuberculosis, and diarrhea, enteritis, and ulceration of the intestines—accounting for 31.4% of all deaths. By 2019, the first three causes of death were diseases of the heart, malignant neoplasms (cancer), and unintentional injuries (accidents), and they were responsible for 50.2% of all deaths. Pneumonia and influenza were the only infectious diseases among the top ten causes of mortality in 2019, accounting for only 1.7% of deaths.

The change in predominance of cause of mortality from infectious diseases to chronic diseases occurred rapidly between 1900 and the 1930s. In 1901, heart disease moved from the fourth to the third leading cause of death, displacing diarrhea, enteritis, and ulceration of the intestines. Tuberculosis and pneumonia and influenza remained the top two causes, but by 1910, heart disease had become the first leading cause of death. Tuberculosis and pneumonia and influenza had moved to spots two and three. This ranking remained until 1918 to 1920, when pneumonia went to the top of the list during the 1918 influenza pandemic. However, by 1921, heart disease was again the first leading cause of death, and it has remained so through the present. Tuberculosis began dropping lower and lower on the top 10 list of leading causes of mortality until 1954, when it dropped below the leading 10. Pneumonia and influenza remained in second place until the end of the 1930s. Although they have remained among the top 10 causes ever since, they are now near the bottom of the list. The top three causes of death from the end of the 1930s to 2007 were heart disease, cancer, and cerebrovascular disease (stroke), displacing the infectious diseases (National Center for Health Statistics [NCHS], 2015). From 2007 to 2019, chronic lower respiratory disease and then unintentional injuries vied for the third spot. An infectious disease was not one of the three leading causes of death again until 2020, with the emergence of COVID-19. See Table 4.1.

Prevention and treatment of infectious diseases also resulted in a tremendous increase in life expectancy in developed countries. In the United States, for example, life expectancy rose between 1900 and 2017 for both men and women and Whites and Blacks. Life expectancy for Whites of both sexes rose in this period from 47.6 to 78.8 years. For Blacks of both sexes, the increase was from 33 to 75.3 years (see Table 4.2). These substantial gains in life expectancy were seen for both men and women in both racial groups. However, the greatest gain for each group

Table 4.1. Change in Three Leading Causes of Death From Infectious to Noninfectious Diseases, United States, 1900–2020

	1900	1901	1910	1918–1920	1921	1923	1933	1938	2008	2016	2020
1	PI	PI	**HD**	PI	**HD**	**HD**	**HD**	**HD**	**HD**	**HD**	**HD**
2	TB	TB	PI	**HD**	PI	PI	**CA**	**CA**	**CA**	**CA**	**CA**
3	DEU	**HD**	TB	TB	TB	**CA**	PI	**CVD**	**CLRD**	**UI**	COV

Infectious Diseases: COV, COVID-19; DEU, diarrhea, enteritis, and ulceration of the intestines; PI, pneumonia and influenza; TB, tuberculosis.

Noninfectious Diseases or Injuries: CA, cancer; CLRD, chronic lower respiratory disease; CVD, cerebrovascular disease (stroke); HD, heart disease; UI, unintentional injuries.

Sources: National Center for Health Statistics. (2015). Leading causes of death, 1900–1998. In *Historical data, 1900–1998*. https://www.cdc.gov/nchs/data/dvs/lead1900_98.pdf; Heron, M. (2012). Deaths: Leading causes for 2008. *National Vital Statistics Reports, 60*(6). https://www.cdc.gov/nchs/data/nvsr/nvsr60/nvsr60_06.pdf; Kochanek, K. D., Murphy, S. L., Xu, J., & Arias, E. (2017). Mortality in the United States, 2016. *NCHS Data Brief, 293*. https://www.cdc.gov/nchs/data/databriefs/db293.pdf; and Murphy, S. L., Kochanek, K. D., Xu, J. Q., & Arias, E. (2021). Mortality in the United States, 2020. *NCHS Data Brief, 427*. https://www.cdc.gov/nchs/products/databriefs/db427.htm

Table 4.2. Life Expectancy at Birth (in Years) by Sex and Race, 1900 to 2017

Year	White
	Both Sexes
1900	47.6
1950	69.1
2000	77.3
2017	78.8
Gain in Life Expectancy (in Years) by Sex and Race, 1900–2017	
1900	–
1950	21.5
2000	8.2
2017	1.5

Source: National Center for Health Statistics. (2021). Table 4, life expectancy at birth, age 65, and age 75, by sex, race, and Hispanic origin: United States, selected years 1900–2018. *Health, United States, 2019.* https://www.ncbi.nlm.nih.gov/books/NBK569311/table/ch3.tab4/

was between 1900 and 1950. About two thirds of the total number of years gained in life expectancy came by 1950. This was due largely to control of infectious diseases.

ARE INFECTIOUS DISEASES STILL A SERIOUS THREAT TO HUMAN HEALTH?

By the mid-20th century, many people would have answered "no" to this question, believing that infectious diseases were a health problem of the past. However, starting in the early 20th century, some scientists recognized the continuing threat of infectious diseases. René Dubos was a leader in this thinking. He was a microbiologist born in 1901, just as scientific methods were providing hope that infectious diseases could be prevented and treated. By mid-century, when vaccines and antibiotics were proving their worth at controlling deadly diseases such as tuberculosis, pneumonia, smallpox, diphtheria, and others, Dubos was one of the first to predict that antibiotics would develop bacterial resistance. Thus, he was one of the earliest proponents of continual vigilance and study of microorganisms (Dubos, 1959). In an article entitled "Rene Dubos, A Harbinger of Microbial Resistance to Antibiotics," Moberg writes:

> In the half century before antibiotics, the number of clinically useful drugs was limited (vitamins, a few hormones including insulin, arsenicals, and sulfonamides), and sporadic reports of resistance were considered negligible. However, the rapidity and magnitude with which antibiotics were introduced after 1942 set the stage for a large-scale problem with fatal consequences. In this regard, Dubos was timely and prescient in expecting great resistance.
>
> . . . This prediction was the first of many issued by Dubos over the following 40 years. Once he grasped that bacterial resistance should be expected, he set about to probe deeper and to anticipate consequences of this phenomenon. One result was that he continued to predict that antibiotics, along with the increasing array of chemical therapies, could treat and control acute cases, but they could never eliminate infectious diseases. (Moberg, 1999, pp. 560–561)

We know now that Dubos and others like him were right. Since the mid-20th century, AIDS (acquired immunodeficiency syndrome), COVID-19 (the coronavirus disease caused by SARS-CoV-2, which emerged in December 2019), antibiotic resistant strains of common infections (e.g., methicillin-resistant *Staphylococcus aureus* [MRSA], vancomycin-resistant *Enterococcus* [VRE], and multidrug-resistant *Mycobacterium tuberculosis* [MDR-TB]) have released us from the misconception that infectious diseases are not a continuing threat to human health.

KEY IDEA

Infectious disease organisms are continually mutating to survive in changing surroundings, and as a result, new diseases arise that have neither effective treatment nor vaccine.

COVID-19 is the most recent example of the potential impact of new infectious diseases. For lack of knowledge about how to prevent or treat COVID effectively, it changed the leading causes of death in the United States in 2020. For the first time since 1900, an infectious disease—COVID-19—became the third leading cause of death. In 1900, diarrhea, enteritis, and ulceration of the intestines accounted for 28,491 deaths (8.3% of all deaths that year). In 2020, the Centers for Disease Control and Prevention (CDC) attributed 345,323 deaths (10.3% of all deaths) to COVID-19. COVID-19 as a cause of death was preceded only by heart disease and cancer in 2020.

In addition to mortality, infectious diseases are the cause of significant morbidity and use of health care services. The number of new cases of various infectious diseases is substantial. See **Table 4.3** for the number of new cases for selected infectious diseases in 2017 and 2018 (NCHS, 2019). Chlamydia and gonorrhea are the most frequently reported:

- Chlamydia—1,708,569 and 1,758,668 case reports in 2017 and 2018, respectively
- Gonorrhea—555,608 and 583,405 case reports in 2017 and 2018, respectively

Table 4.3. New Cases of Selected Nationally Notifiable Diseases: United States, 2017–2018

	2017	2018
Acute hepatitis A viral infection	3,365	12,474
Acute hepatitis B viral infection	3,409	3,322
Acute hepatitis C viral infection	4,225	4,768
Diphtheria	–	1
Haemophilus influenzae, invasive	5,548	5,573
Lyme disease	42,743	33,666
Measles (rubeola)	120	375
Meningococcal disease	353	327
Mumps	6,109	2,515
Pertussis (whooping cough)	18,975	15,609
Shigellosis	14,912	16,333
Spotted fever rickettsiosis	6,248	5,544
Tuberculosis	9,105	9,025
Poliomyelitis, paralytic	–	–

(continued)

Table 4.3. New Cases of Selected Nationally Notifiable Diseases: United States, 2017–2018 *(continued)*

	2017	2018
Rubella (German measles)	7	4
Salmonellosis, excluding typhoid fever	54,285	60,999
Sexually transmitted diseases		
Syphilis	101,584	115,045
• Primary and secondary	30,644	35,063
• Early, nonprimary and nonsecondary	34,013	38,539
• Unknown or late	35,992	40,137
• Congenital	935	1,306
Chlamydia	1,708,569	1,758,668
Gonorrhea	555,608	583,405
Chancroid	7	3

Source: National Center for Health Statistics. (2019). Selected nationally notifiable disease rates and number of new cases: United States, selected years 1950–2018. *Health, United States, 2019.* https://www.cdc.gov/nchs/data/hus/2019/010-508.pdf

Increased health care utilization due to infectious diseases is reflected in visits to physician offices and emergency departments. The number of visits to physician offices for infectious and parasitic diseases in 2018 was 7.2 million (Santo & Okeyode, 2018). There was also significant emergency department use:

- Number of emergency department visits with infectious and parasitic diseases as the primary diagnosis: 3.4 million; and
- Number of emergency department visits resulting in hospital admission with a principal hospital discharge diagnosis of infectious and parasitic diseases: 523,000 (Cairns et al., 2018).

Risky behaviors, overuse of antibiotics, and global migration are three causes of the increase in infectious disease threats, but we should not be surprised that these tiny beings are still with us and causing "trouble." As Moore (2007) expressively put it:

> The word "plague" would have sent a ripple of fear down the spines of the people in (Shakespeare's) audiences, and the fact that they had no knowledge of the agent that swept invisibly across continents, devastating populations and leaving families shattered and entire economies in tatters, only served to heighten the anxiety.
>
> We have come a long way since Shakespeare's sixteenth century. We know about bacteria, viruses, and microscopic protozoa. We can watch

the way that these tiny agents move into our bodies and damage our organs. We have a growing understanding of how our body mounts defensive strategies that fight off these invaders and have built some clever chemical that can help mount an assault on these bio-villains. In the middle of the twentieth century, as science was creating a new optimism, some serious commentators believed that the total eradication of nasty bacteria and viruses could be just a decade or so away. But it wasn't. Far from it. (p. 6)

ABOUT INFECTIOUS DISEASES

What Is an Infectious Disease?

An infectious disease is one caused by a microorganism or microbe that enters the body, multiplies, and damages cells. All microbes do not cause disease, but those that do are called pathogens. Microbes are categorized as bacteria, viruses, protozoa, fungi, prions, and parasites (National Academies of Sciences, Engineering, and Medicine [NASEM], 2022, paras. 4–9). And although we use the term microbe for all of them, the term is imperfect to describe the diversity, complexity, and number of organisms that cause infectious diseases.

> Microbes were so named because they were thought to only be visible with the help of a microscope. Yet, from a purely definitional standpoint, many fungi are exceptions to this rule, as are *Epulopiscium* bacteria. Another paradox is that both a virus that is 1/4000th the width of a strand of hair and a clearly visible bread mold are considered microbes. Fungi also include species like the honey fungus, which is the largest living thing on Earth by virtue of its vast underground filamentous networks that can stretch for miles. Clearly, there is wide variation in size and lifestyle, even within the same microbial group . . .
>
> Science's understanding of the microbial world has come a long way in the centuries since animalcules were first seen. They aren't considered little animals anymore, they are known to be the oldest occupants of Earth, and they significantly outnumber human beings and other eukaryotes. As knowledge of the microbial world has expanded, words like "microbe" or "microorganism" are still used as blanket terms that could refer to individuals from various groups, such as bacteria, fungi, viruses, or protozoa. (Hariharan, 2021, paras. 1 and 3)

How Do Infectious Disease Microbes Enter the Human Body?

Some infectious diseases are *contagious (or communicable)*, that is, they are spread from person to person (CDC, 2017). This can occur through direct person-to-person contact, through contact with infected body fluids, or by inhaling respiratory droplets or aerosols breathed out by someone who is infected.

Other infectious diseases are not contagious. These pathogens enter the body through contact with contaminated soil, water, or food or through contact with animals, for example, from bites by infected mosquitoes or ticks. Following is a very brief description of each category of infectious microbes and some of the diseases they cause in humans (NASEM, 2022):

- Viruses are very small packets of genetic material surrounded by a protein shell. They can only reproduce when they enter living cells. In humans, viruses cause influenza, COVID-19, HIV, measles, the common cold, rabies, and many other diseases.
- Bacteria are single-celled organisms that may live inside other organisms or on their own. Unlike viruses, they do not need a host to reproduce, but can reproduce inside the body. Although many bacteria are helpful to human health, some cause disease. Human diseases caused by bacteria include tuberculosis, tetanus, Lyme disease, and some types of food poisoning.
- Protozoa are single-celled organisms that do not have cell walls. They reproduce by splitting into two. Protozoa enter the body through contaminated food or water or via insect bites. Human diseases caused by protozoa include malaria, giardia, and toxoplasmosis.
- Fungi can be microscopic or very large. They reproduce mainly by making spores, and human contact with the spores causes illness. Diseases caused by fungi in humans include yeast infections, athlete's foot, and histoplasmosis.
- Prions are not living organisms, but microscopic particles of protein. Human diseases caused by prions include bovine spongiform encephalopathy (BSE) in cattle (also known as mad cow disease), chronic wasting disease in deer and related animals, and Creutzfeldt–Jakob disease (CJD) in humans.
- Parasitic worms, called helminths, include tapeworms, flukes, and roundworms. These organisms complete part of their lifecycle by living inside other organisms. Their eggs or larvae enter the body through contaminated food or water, penetration of the skin, insect bites, or contact with contaminated surfaces. Parasitic worms often grow and develop in the intestines, resulting in malnutrition. Schistosomiasis, also called bilharzia, is an example of an infectious disease caused by a blood fluke. Onchocerciasis, also known as river blindness, is caused by the roundworm.

Control and Prevention of Infectious Diseases

Today, both primary and secondary prevention methods are important tools used to control and prevent infectious diseases. The methods used for primary prevention include traditional surveillance, sanitation, vaccination, and quarantine. Secondary prevention relies on treatment including use of antimicrobial drug therapy and development of new therapies in response to novel infectious diseases as well as antimicrobial resistance among existing strains. Although the methods for preventing and treating infectious diseases are, in general, the same as in the past, great improvements in these methods have resulted because of advances in microbiology, information and communication systems, and laboratory techniques. Following is a description of public health practices related to infectious disease control and prevention, which continues to be an essential piece of public health in the United States and throughout the world.

Surveillance (or Monitoring) of Infectious Diseases

Case surveillance is the foundation of public health practice aimed at controlling infectious diseases in human populations. Surveillance is required to understand disease spread and to select appropriate measures to control outbreaks. Case surveillance occurs when a public health agency at the local, state, or national level collects information about a case or person diagnosed with a disease or condition that is considered threatening to the population (CDC, National Notifiable Diseases Surveillance System [NNDSS], 2021b). Surveillance information is based on these case reports, which are provided to the CDC's **NNDSS**:

> A surveillance case definition is a set of uniform criteria used to define a disease for public health surveillance. Surveillance case definitions enable public health officials to classify and count cases consistently across reporting jurisdictions. Surveillance case definitions are not intended to be used by healthcare providers for making a clinical diagnosis or determining how to meet an individual patient's health needs.
>
> While the list of reportable conditions varies by state, the Council of State and Territorial Epidemiologists (CSTE) has recommended that state health departments report cases of selected diseases to CDC's National Notifiable Diseases Surveillance System (NNDSS). Every year, case definitions are updated using CSTE's Position Statements. They provide uniform criteria of national notifiable infectious and noninfectious conditions for reporting purposes. (CDC, NNDSS, 2021a, paras. 1 and 2).

Thus, a major component of the public health effort to control and prevent infectious disease outbreaks is the NNDSS. The history of this program began in the 19th century when Congress authorized the U.S. Marine Hospital Service (forerunner of today's Public Health Service [PHS]) in 1878. The purpose of the Marine Hospital Service was to collect reports from U.S. consuls overseas about the common infectious diseases of the time—cholera, smallpox, plague, and yellow fever. These reports were used to determine if quarantine measures should be instituted to prevent the emergence and spread of disease in the United Sates. In 1879, Congress appropriated funds to collect and publish these notifiable diseases weekly. In 1893, the reporting was expanded by Congress to include information from states and municipalities, and by 1928, all states, the District of Columbia, Hawaii, and Puerto Rico were reporting 29 infectious diseases to the Surgeon General (CDC, 1996).

DID YOU KNOW?

Fifty years ago, morbidity statistics published each week were accompanied by the statement "No health department, state or local, can effectively prevent or control

(continued)

disease without knowledge of when, where, and under what conditions cases are oc-curring." These statistics appeared under the heading "Prevalence of Disease—United States" in each issue of *Public Health Reports* printed by the PHS, Office of the Surgeon General (Division of Public Health Methods; see pp. 533–536).

In 1949, the collection, compilation, and publication of these morbidity statistics was transferred to the National Office of Vital Statistics, which produced the *Weekly Morbidity Report*. In 1952 the publication was renamed *Morbidity and Mortality Weekly Report*, and responsibility for the publication was transferred to CDC in 1961. (CDC, 1996, p. 1)

Table 4.4. Reportable or Notifiable: What's the Difference?

Reportable Diseases and Conditions	Notifiable Diseases and Conditions
Each state or territory sets local laws and rules for which diseases and conditions must be reported.	• The Council of State and Territorial Epidemiologists and the CDC identify the list of notifiable diseases and conditions.
Health care professionals, laboratories, hospitals, and other providers must tell public health departments when a person is diagnosed.	• States voluntarily inform the CDC when a person meets certain criteria to become a case.
Public health departments collect information about the person and how they became ill.	• Case records do not contain personally identifiable information.
This information is used to locate the source of an outbreak and prevent spread.	• The CDC uses data to monitor, measure, and alert individual communities or the nation to outbreaks and other public health threats.
The list of diseases and conditions can change every year.	• The list of about 120 diseases and conditions is updated every year.

Source: Centers for Disease Control and Prevention, & National Notifiable Diseases Surveillance System. (2022). *What is case surveillance?* https://www.cdc.gov/nndss/about/index.html

In addition to the Notifiable Diseases and Conditions, there are Reportable Diseases and Conditions. The differences are outlined in **Table 4.4**.

In summary, the NNDSS collects data from state and local authorities about selected notifiable infectious diseases. The states report cases to the CDC voluntarily. Currently, reporting is mandated only at the state level through state legislation or regulation. In general, all states report the internationally quarantinable diseases, which include cholera, plague, and yellow fever, to comply with the World Health Organization's (WHO) International Health Regulations. The CDC, in collaboration with the CSTE, updates the list of notifiable diseases annually. The results of the NNDSS are published weekly in the *Morbidity and Mortality Weekly Report* (*MMWR*) and annually in a year-end summary. See the partial list of notifiable infectious diseases for 2022 in **Table 4.5** (CDC, NNDSS, 2021c).

Table 4.5. Current and Past Notifiable Conditions, United States, Selected Years Between 2005 and 2022

Code	Event Name	2005	2010	2015	2020	2021	2022
10560	AIDS	YES					
10350	Anthrax	YES	YES	YES	YES	YES	YES
10530	Botulism, foodborne	YES	YES	YES	YES	YES	YES
11020	Campylobacteriosis			YES	YES	YES	YES
	Cancer		YES	YES	YES	YES	YES
10470	Cholera	YES	YES	YES	YES	YES	YES
11065	Coronavirus disease 2019 (COVID-19)				YES	YES	YES
10680	Dengue fever/dengue		YES	YES	YES	YES	YES
11704	Dengue-like illness				YES	YES	YES
10040	Diphtheria	YES	YES	YES	YES	YES	YES
11630	Ebola hemorrhagic fever (replaced event code 11647, Viral Hemorrhagic Fevers)			YES	YES	YES	YES
10070	Encephalitis, post-chickenpox						
10080	Encephalitis, post-mumps						
10050	Encephalitis, primary						
11560	Enterohemorrhagic *Escherichia coli* (EHEC) O157:H7. (As of January 1, 2006, EHEC codes 11560, 11562, and 11564 were retired and a new code for Shiga toxin–producing *Escherichia coli* [see code 11563] should be used for reporting.)	YES					
	Foodborne disease outbreaks			YES	YES	YES	YES

(continued)

Table 4.5. Current and Past Notifiable Conditions, United States, Selected Years Between 2005 and 2022 (continued)

Code	Event Name	2005	2010	2015	2020	2021	2022
11570	Giardiasis	YES	YES	YES	YES	YES	YES
10280	Gonorrhea	YES	YES	YES	YES	YES	YES
11610	Hantavirus infection, non–Hantavirus pulmonary syndrome			YES	YES	YES	YES
10110	Hepatitis A, acute	YES	YES	YES	YES	YES	YES
10100	Hepatitis B, acute	YES	YES	YES	YES	YES	YES
10105	Hepatitis B, chronic	YES	YES	YES	YES	YES	YES
10101	Hepatitis C, acute	YES	YES	YES	YES	YES	YES
50248	Hepatitis C, perinatal infection				YES	YES	YES
10562	HIV infection, adult	YES	YES	YES	YES	YES	YES
10561	HIV infection, pediatric	YES	YES	YES	YES	YES	YES
11723	Invasive pneumococcal disease (condition name revised January 2010 from "Streptococcus pneumoniae, invasive disease" to "invasive pneumococcal disease")		YES	YES	YES	YES	YES
11712	Keystone virus disease				YES	YES	YES
11632	Lassa fever (replaced event code 11647, viral hemorrhagic fevers)			YES	YES	YES	YES
32010	Lead poisoning		YES	YES	YES	YES	YES
10490	Legionellosis	YES	YES	YES	YES	YES	YES
11080	Lyme disease	YES	YES	YES	YES	YES	YES
10130	Malaria	YES	YES	YES	YES	YES	YES

Code	Condition							
10140	Measles, total	YES	YES	YES	YES	YES	YES	YES
10150	Meningococcal disease	YES	YES	YES	YES	YES	YES	YES
10180	Mumps	YES	YES	YES	YES	YES	YES	YES
	Pesticide poisoning/pesticide-related illness and injury		YES	YES	YES	YES	YES	
10440	Plague	YES	YES	YES	YES	YES	YES	YES
10410	Poliomyelitis, paralytic	YES	YES	YES	YES	YES	YES	YES
10340	Rabies, animal	YES	YES	YES	YES	YES	YES	YES
10460	Rabies, human	YES	YES	YES	YES	YES	YES	YES
10250	Rocky Mountain spotted fever (nomenclature change; see spotted fever rickettsiosis)	YES						
10200	Rubella	YES	YES	YES	YES	YES	YES	YES
50267	*Salmonella enterica* typhi (*S. typhi*) infection		YES	YES	YES	YES	YES	YES
11000	Salmonellosis (retired as of January 1, 2018)	YES	YES	YES				
50265	Salmonellosis (excluding *S. typhi* infection and *S. paratyphi* infection)			YES	YES	YES	YES	YES
10575	Severe acute respiratory syndrome-associated coronavirus (SARS-CoV) disease	YES	YES	YES	YES	YES	YES	YES
11800	Smallpox	YES	YES	YES	YES	YES	YES	YES
10250	Spotted fever rickettsiosis	YES	YES	YES	YES	YES	YES	YES
11717	*Streptococcus pneumoniae*, invasive disease <5 years	YES						
10316	Syphilis, congenital syndrome	YES	YES	YES	YES	YES	YES	YES
10311	Syphilis, primary	YES	YES	YES	YES	YES	YES	YES

(continued)

Table 4.5. Current and Past Notifiable Conditions, United States, Selected Years Between 2005 and 2022 *(continued)*

Code	Event Name	2005	2010	2015	2020	2021	2022
10320	Syphilis, unknown duration or late				YES	YES	YES
10210	Tetanus	YES	YES	YES	YES	YES	YES
10220	Tuberculosis	YES	YES	YES	YES	YES	YES
10240	Typhoid fever (retired as of January 1, 2019)	YES	YES	YES			
11663	Vancomycin-intermediate *Staphylococcus aureus* (VISA)	YES	YES	YES	YES	YES	YES
11665	Vancomycin-resistant *Staphylococcus aureus* (VRSA)	YES	YES	YES	YES	YES	YES
	Waterborne disease outbreaks		YES	YES	YES	YES	YES
10660	Yellow fever	YES	YES	YES	YES	YES	YES
50224	Zika virus disease, congenital				YES	YES	YES
50223	Zika virus disease, noncongenital				YES	YES	YES
50222	Zika virus infection, congenital				YES	YES	YES
50221	Zika virus infection, noncongenital				YES	YES	YES

Source: National Notifiable Diseases Surveillance System. (2021). *Current and past notifiable conditions.* https://ndc.services.cdc.gov/event-codes-other-surveillance-resources/

The table also shows the change in notifiable diseases since 2005. For instance, botulism, cholera, diphtheria, and hepatitis A, acute, have been on the list continuously since 2005. In contrast, the Zika virus disease and infection were added in 2020, as were keystone virus disease and dengue-like illness. The full list is available at: Current and past notifiable conditions; https://ndc.services.cdc.gov/event-codes-other-surveillance-resources/

Methods for Controlling and Preventing Infectious Diseases

The information gained from surveillance and reporting allows counties, cities, and states to make informed decisions and implement policies to control infectious diseases, including:

- Insect and other animal control,
- Food handling measures,
- Immunization programs,
- Sexually transmitted disease tracking and treatment, and
- Water purification.

There are three basic strategies to combat infectious diseases once they are detected, and these involve both primary (before infection occurs) and secondary prevention:

1. Prevent disease from occurring in uninfected individuals through vaccine development and administration.
2. Develop treatments to assist recovery of individuals who become infected by the disease. This is secondary prevention using the tools and knowledge of health care.
3. Prevent exposure of uninfected persons to the infectious disease organism.

Methods to prevent exposure of the uninfected depend upon the organism's route of entry into the human body—physical contact with an infected person, air, water, food, or animals such as insects. When spread is through human contact and a disease is contagious, quarantine of cases or barriers between the infected and noninfected persons such as masks and gloves may be employed. When spread is through water, water purification, monitoring, and remediation are required. When spread is foodborne, food safety practices and their enforcement are needed. Spread through animal contact requires varied strategies depending upon the specifics of the contact and the animal. Or there may be a combination of these means for pathogens to enter the human body.

In the United States, the center of infectious disease control efforts—prevention of disease, disability, and death—is the Centers for Disease Control and Prevention (CDC). Three centers within the CDC are particularly important (CDC, 2021):

- National Center for HIV, Viral Hepatitis, STD, and TB Prevention (NCHHSTP):
  The NCHHSTP is focused on HIV infection/AIDS, non-HIV retroviruses, viral hepatitis, other sexually transmitted diseases, and tuberculosis.

- National Center for Immunization and Respiratory Diseases (NCIRD):
  The NCIRD directs its efforts on immunization and respiratory and related diseases.
- National Center for Emerging and Zoonotic Infectious Diseases (NCEZID):
  The NCEZID focuses on diseases that have been around for many years, emerging diseases, and zoonotic diseases.

Emerging infections are those that have increased recently or are threatening to increase in the near future (CDC, 2017). These infections could be:

- Completely new (e.g., Bourbon virus, which was recently discovered in Kansas);
- Completely new to an area (e.g., chikungunya in Florida);
- Reappearing in an area (e.g., dengue in south Florida and Texas); and
- Caused by bacteria that have become resistant to antibiotics (e.g., methicillin-resistant *Staphylococcus aureus* or MRSA) or drug-resistant tuberculosis (TB).

Zoonotic diseases (also known as zoonoses) are caused by microbes that spread between animals and people. They are a growing concern to public health and health care professionals: "Zoonotic diseases are very common, both in the United States and around the world. Scientists estimate that more than six out of every 10 known infectious diseases in people can be spread from animals, and three out of every four new or emerging infectious diseases in people come from animals" (NCEZID, 2021, para. 3).

Concepts Essential for Infectious Disease Control and Prevention

The following concepts aid public health professionals and policymakers in developing effective strategies for control and prevention of infectious diseases (van Seventer & Hochberg, 2017). When an individual—or host—is exposed to an infectious organism, the result of that exposure depends upon the relationship between characteristics of the organism—infectivity, pathogenicity, and virulence—and the susceptibility to infection of the individual. Both physical and social behavioral factors determine the host's vulnerability to exposure.

Infectivity, Pathogenicity, and Virulence. Infectivity is the probability that an infectious organism will infect an individual, if exposed to the organism. *Pathogenicity* refers to the ability of an organism to cause disease in the individual, given infection. *Virulence* is the probability of causing severe disease among those infected by the organism. Virulence reflects structural and/or biochemical properties of an infectious organism. Infectivity and pathogenicity can be measured by the *attack rate*, that is the number of exposed individuals who develop disease (number infected/number exposed). Virulence is often measured by the *case fatality rate*, that is the proportion of infected individuals who die from the disease (number deaths/number infected).

Healthy Carriers. Healthy carriers are infected persons who remain asymptomatic, but can transmit the infectious organism to others. They pose a significant problem to infectious disease control.

Host Susceptibility. The ability of an individual who has been exposed to a disease organism to resist infection or limit disease as a result of their biological makeup is termed *host susceptibility*. Both innate, genetic factors and acquired factors such as the immunity that develops following disease exposure or vaccination influence susceptibility. Susceptibility is also altered by age, stress, pregnancy, nutritional status, and underlying diseases. "An *immune host* is someone protected against a specific pathogen (because of previous infection or vaccination) such that subsequent infection will not take place or, if infection does occur, the severity of disease is diminished. The duration and efficacy of immunity following immunization by natural infection or vaccination varies depending upon the infecting agent, quality of the vaccine, type of vaccine (i.e., live or inactivated virus, subunit), and ability of the host to generate an immune response" (van Seventer & Hochberg, 2017, p. 24).

Disease Frequency and Extent. Identifying the occurrence and extent of an infectious disease within a specific geographic area or population are essential to disease control. Relevant concepts include:

- *Sporadic disease,* which is a disease that occurs occasionally and unpredictably.
- *Endemic disease,* which is a disease that occurs with predictable regularity. Endemic diseases can be categorized by their frequency as holoendemic (extreme), hyperendemic (high), mesoendemic (moderate), or hypoendemic (low).
- An e*pidemic,* which is an often sharp, increase in disease cases above a baseline level. An epidemic may be an endemic disease that has increased substantially or a disease that was not previously found in the population or area.
- A *pandemic* is an epidemic that occurs in a large geographic region—encompassing many countries or continents, or extending worldwide.

Prevalence and Incidence. Two measures essential for disease control are *prevalence* and *incidence*. Prevalence is the proportion of individuals who have a particular disease, at a given point in time (*point prevalence*) or during a specified time period (*period prevalence*). In contrast, incidence is a measure of the proportion of *new* cases of a disease in a population during a specific time period.

Herd Immunity. "*Herd immunity* refers to population-level resistance to an infectious disease that occurs when there are enough immune individuals to block the chain of infection/transmission. As a result of herd immunity, susceptible individuals who are not immune themselves are indirectly protected from infection" (van Seventer & Hochberg, 2017, p. 27). See **Figure 4.1**.

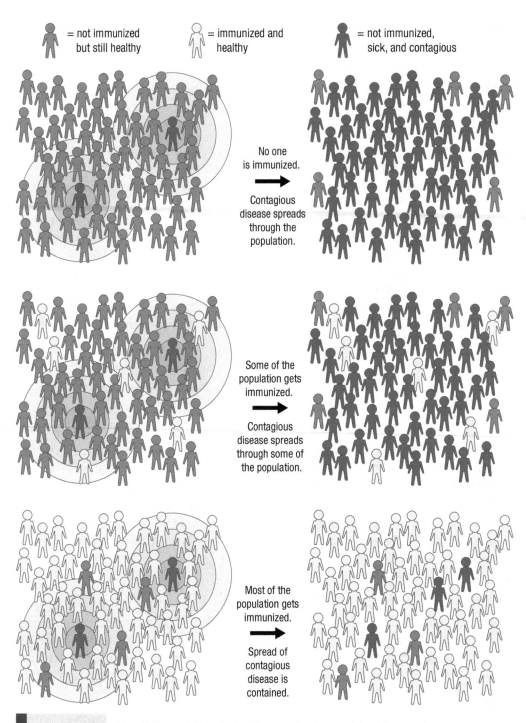

Figure 4.1.　The Effect of Population Immunization on Herd Immunity

Source: Van Seventer, J. M., & Hochberg, N. S. (2017). Principles of infectious diseases: Transmissions, diagnosis, prevention, and control. *International Encyclopedia of Public Health, 6,* 22–39. https://doi.org/10.1016/B978-0-12-803678-5.00516-6

INVESTIGATING AN INFECTIOUS DISEASE OUTBREAK*

There are several fundamental steps necessary to conduct an investigation of an infectious disease outbreak. They are:

- Verify the diagnosis of the disease that is suspected or under investigation;
- Establish the existence of an outbreak of disease or an epidemic;
- Characterize the distribution of disease cases by the variables of person, place, and time;
- Develop a hypothesis that can explain the observed distribution of cases; and
- Institute control measures as early as possible.

Verify Diagnosis

To verify the diagnosis of an outbreak of disease, the epidemiologist considers several factors.

- Laboratory tests may be used in a diagnosis of the disease. The investigator must make certain that the results are reliable by having the test confirmed by a trustworthy laboratory or repeated by another laboratory to confirm the original diagnosis. In each state, there is a diagnostic laboratory that is approved for this purpose.
- Use clinical criteria when the laboratory results are not entirely reliable or may not be available in a timely fashion. Some illnesses may be very mild or not apparent in laboratory tests. Similarly, there may be other unrelated illnesses that may be part of the initial count of cases in the outbreak investigation.
- Epidemiologic criteria may be added to the laboratory information and to the clinical criteria to further restrict the number of cases that are under investigation. For example, during the 1976 investigation of Legionnaires' disease in Philadelphia, there was no laboratory test available to confirm the clinical suspicion of the illness. Consequently, a clinical diagnosis of a respiratory illness with a fever was created. Because the clinical definition of a febrile respiratory illness was so broad as to include a very large number of unrelated cases, an additional component in the epidemiologic investigation was added to the case definition: An individual needed to have specific clinical findings and also to have attended the American Legion Convention in Philadelphia or entered one of the hotels where the convention itself was held during a specific period. This additional information helped restrict the suspect cases to determine and make a more accurate count of cases.

*We wish to acknowledge and thank the late Mahfouz H. Zaki, MD, MPH, DrPH, former distinguished university professor of Preventive Medicine and Public Health at Downstate Medical Center in Brooklyn and adjunct professor of Preventive Medicine at State University of New York at Stony Brook, for his contributions to this section, including Figures 4.2 through 4.4.

DID YOU KNOW?

In 1976, over 4,000 people from the Pennsylvania chapter of the American Legion convened to celebrate America's bicentennial in Philadelphia at the Bellevue-Stratford Hotel. The convention lasted about 4 days. After the attendees returned home, many began to sicken and eventually 34 died. The cause of their illness was *Legionella*, which was discovered after a vigorous search by scientists from the Centers for Disease Control and Prevention (CDC) following the outbreak in Philadelphia. The illness eventually became known as Legionnaires' disease. *Legionella* bacteria are found naturally in freshwater environments, like lakes and streams, but threaten health when they grow and spread in human-made building water systems like showerheads and sink faucets, structures that contain water and a fan as part of centralized air cooling systems, and hot water tanks and heaters. The disease is spread when people breathe small water droplets contaminated by *Legionella*. The number of cases of Legionnaires' disease reported to the CDC has been rising since 2000. Health departments reported nearly 10,000 cases of Legionnaires' disease in the United States in 2018 (CDC, 2021b).

Establish Existence of Outbreak

If an outbreak or an epidemic is considered an unusual occurrence of the disease in a defined population during a specific period, it must be documented. It could be a common disease in an unusual segment of the population (e.g., pneumonia in persons who attended the 1976 American Legion Convention in Philadelphia) or an unusual disease in a common segment of the population (e.g., the occurrence of a specific form of pneumonia caused by *Pneumocystis carinii* in young homosexual men), which was seen as a common factor in HIV-infected individuals in the early days of the AIDS epidemic in the 1980s. When trying to establish the existence of an outbreak of disease or an epidemic, epidemiologists do the following:

- Identify unreported or unrecognized cases that may be part of the specific outbreak of disease. These additional cases may be found by surveying hospitals, laboratories, physicians, and family and friends of the known cases.
- Determine the population at risk for developing the disease in question. This may be a specific classroom of children, or the entire school, or a much larger community of people.
- Compare the incidence of new cases of the disease in the population now with the previous period, using the case count as a numerator and the population at risk as the denominator. Take into consideration seasonal variations, while comparing the incidence of new cases with the same period in previous years.

Characterize Distribution of Cases by Person, Place, and Time

Understanding the cause of an outbreak results from the proper analysis of the distribution of cases by time, place, and person.

Person

The variable person can be used to compare the characteristics of the population contracting the disease to the characteristics of the population without the disease.

Place

The variable place can be used to detect a source of infection by identification of spatial clustering of cases. Cases can be plotted by the place where the individuals reside, work, or attend school, or by any other geographic location. Because clustering of cases may only reflect population density, maps should be drawn comparing the rates of outbreak in different geographic areas.

Time

The variable time is used to begin the construction of an epidemic curve, which is a graph showing the distribution of cases (on the *y*-axis) by the date of onset of the illness in hours, days, weeks, or months (on the *x*-axis). The shape of this curve may suggest either a common source outbreak or person-to-person transmission. A point source of exposure is suggested if all cases occur within one incubation period of the disease (i.e., the time in which the disease was incubating before signs and symptoms of disease occurred). Common source outbreaks of disease result from the exposure of individuals to the same causal factor or pathogen(s) including contaminated water, milk, food, or in other ingested, consumed, inhaled, or absorbed substances. Exposure to a contaminated source may be temporary or continuous. In the case of instantaneous or temporary contamination, transmission occurs in the following fashion (see **Figure 4.2**).

One characteristic feature of a temporary or instantaneous common source epidemic (sometimes called *point source*) is that all cases occur during a period that covers the range of one incubation period (see **Figure 4.3**). This pattern can be observed only if secondary cases do not result from the primary case.

Common source outbreaks differ from contact, or progressive, outbreaks whereby infection is transmitted from a patient or a carrier to one or more susceptibles, characterized by the epidemic diagram in **Figure 4.4**.

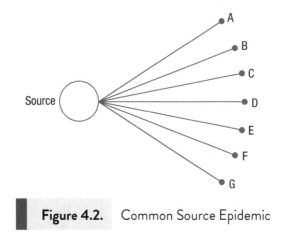

Figure 4.2.   Common Source Epidemic

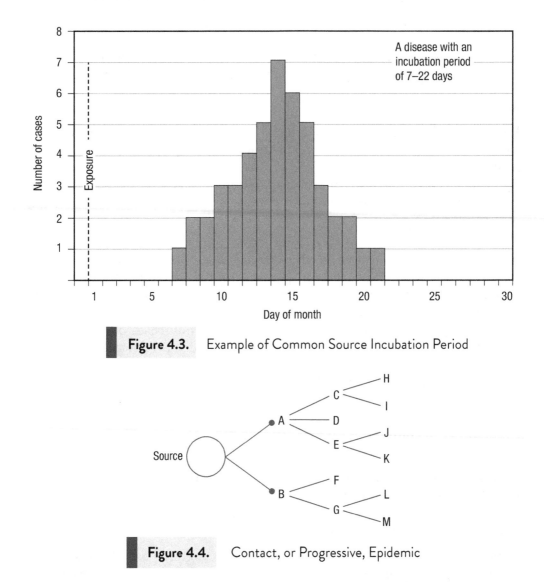

Figure 4.3. Example of Common Source Incubation Period

Figure 4.4. Contact, or Progressive, Epidemic

The shape of the epidemic curve in contact or progressive outbreak depends on the infectivity of the pathogen, its ability to survive outside of the human host, the proportion of susceptibles in the community, and the length of the carrier state. Cases that occur over several different incubation periods suggest either person-to-person transmission or a continuing common source of exposure and outbreak. If the incubation period of the disease is known, the curve indicates the probable time and possible source of the infection. If the time of exposure can be determined, the incubation period of the disease can be identified.

If the time of exposure is known, the incubation period can be used to establish a diagnosis in a foodborne disease outbreak. For example, if there is a chemical food poisoning due to the ingestion of copper, the incubation period can be measured in minutes. Staphylococcal food poisoning has an onset in 1 to 6 hours. Other foodborne bacteria that cause disease outbreaks are *Bacillus cereus*, with an incubation period of 10 to 16 hours; *Salmonella*, with an incubation period of 6 to 72 hours; and *Shigella*, with an incubation period of 24 to 48 hours.

Develop and Test the Hypothesis

In developing a hypothesis, the unusual or odd case may be extremely helpful. The exceptions frequently provide important information and may help explain the source of an infection, the mode of disease transmission, or the normal background of the disease. The following procedure is standard:

- Demonstrate the differences in the attack rates of people who were exposed and not exposed to the source of infection. The cases must be shown to be exposed more often to the risk factor than the group of individuals, known as the *controls*, who are not ill.

- Apply statistical tests to the data to indicate statistical differences between cases and controls.

- Collect clinical and environmental specimens if they are available for processing in an appropriate laboratory.

- If the laboratory data do not support the epidemiologic data, ignore the laboratory data.

- Formulate a conclusion based on all pertinent evidence and the results of the hypothesis testing.

- A final report describing all aspects of the investigation should be prepared.

Institute Control Measures

Institute control measures as early as possible in the outbreak investigation to prevent further occurrence of illness. Control or intervention measures are directed at one of the conditions or events in the infectious disease process. The control measures selected depend on the disease under consideration. For example, if a contaminated food is a suspected source of the infection, remove that food and submit to testing.

INFECTIOUS DISEASE CASE STUDIES

The following case studies illustrate public health practices related to selected infectious diseases. These include pandemic influenza, hepatitis B, *Salmonella*, and childhood infectious diseases that are vaccine-preventable. We end with a discussion of COVID-19 and the issues faced by public health professionals as they sought to prevent infectious disease morbidity, mortality, and disability in the face of a novel viral pandemic.

Case Study: Pandemic Influenza

Pandemic influenza, by definition, is a *global public health emergency*. It is a rare but recurring global outbreak of a new (novel) influenza A virus, which is able to infect people easily and spread from person to person in an efficient and sustained way. Global influenza pandemics occurred on three occasions in the century just passed. In 1918, the Spanish influenza (H1N1) pandemic killed an estimated 50 million people worldwide. A second influenza pandemic, known as the Asian influenza (H2N2), occurred in 1957. It resulted in an estimated 2 million deaths worldwide. A third pandemic in 1968, known as the Hong Kong influenza (H3N2), killed more than 1 million people. The 1918 Spanish influenza is believed by many to have caused more illness and death than any other disease in human history. As a comparison, COVID-19 has resulted in about 6.46 million deaths worldwide between January 2020 and August 2022 (WHO, 2022d).

Influenza pandemics are *rare* but *recurrent* events that meet three criteria:

- Result from a new influenza virus that emerges in a population that has little or *no* immunity,
- Cause *severe* illness and death in humans, and
- Require *sustained* human-to-human transmission by respiratory droplet (i.e., by coughing and sneezing).

An influenza pandemic is significantly different from seasonal influenza. Seasonal influenza occurs each year with some variation and causes approximately 36,000 deaths annually in the United States alone. There is a vaccine available every year, which may prevent infection or ameliorate illness in most people. Unlike the seasonal flu viruses, pandemic strains can infect multiple organs. An aberrant immune response known as a cytokine storm is responsible the pathophysiology of pandemic influenza (Flaherty, 2012; NCIRD, 2022).

Whether there are large numbers of deaths from pandemic influenza is determined primarily by four factors:

- Number of people infected (incidence and prevalence);
- Virulence of the virus (case fatality rate);
- Pathogenicity and infectivity (attack rate);
- Vulnerability of the affected populations (host susceptibility); and
- Effectiveness of preventive measures, such as isolation, quarantine, antiviral medications, and vaccines, if available.

The social and economic disruption in all countries affected can be tremendous. High rates of absenteeism in the workplace and in schools can be expected, as well as significant disruption in essential services and supplies of food, transportation, education, communications, and energy (**Figure 4.5**).

Control and Prevention of Pandemic Influenza

Formerly known as Global Influenza Surveillance Network (GISN), WHO's Global Influenza Surveillance and Response System (GISRS) is a critical component of preparedness throughout the world for pandemic influenza. The GISRS enables WHO to recommend twice annually the content of the influenza vaccine for the subsequent influenza season. More than 250 million doses of influenza vaccine are produced annually which contain WHO-recommended influenza

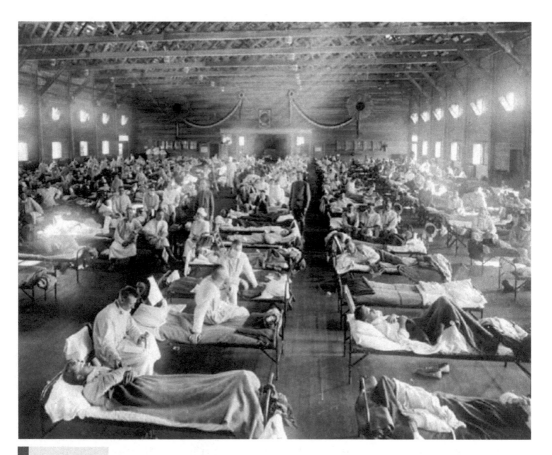

Figure 4.5.   In 1918, Influenza Victims Crowded into an Emergency Hospital at Fort Riley in Kansas

Source: Defense Health Agency, National Museum of Health and Medicine, Influenza Primary Resources. (2023). *Emergency hospital during 1918 influenza pandemic, Camp Funston, Kansas.* https://medicalmuseum.health .mil/assets/documents/education/nmhm_flu_content_presentation.pdf

strains. Frequent updating of the influenza vaccine content is necessary as influenza viruses are permanently evolving. Only a vaccine whose virus strains match the circulating influenza viruses will protect recipients efficiently from influenza disease and death.

The WHO Influenza Surveillance Network serves also as a global alert mechanism for the emergence of influenza viruses with pandemic potential. Its activities have contributed greatly to the understanding of influenza epidemiology. The network was established in 1952, after a WHO Expert Committee recommended that through an international network of laboratories, WHO would be able to advise WHO Member States as to "what influenza control measures are useful, useless or harmful." Since then, GISRS has grown:

- As of January 2022, GISRS has grown to include 148 National Influenza Centres (NICs), seven WHO Collaborating Centers (CCs), four Essential Regulatory Laboratories, and 13 H5 Reference Laboratories. These organizations form an interactive and complementary global operation.

- Between 2014 and 2019, GISRS tested an average of 3.4 million specimens every year. This rose to 6.7 million tests annually for influenza and 44.2 million tests for SARS-CoV-2 in 2020 and 2021.
- GISRS members share around 20,000 influenza virus samples every year to WHO CCs and regularly update the weekly influenza situation based on laboratory and disease surveillance reporting through the FluNet and FluID systems, thus allowing WHO to distribute timely risk assessments and alerts to countries.
- Based on GISRS surveillance, WHO has been recommending suitable viruses for inclusion in annual seasonal vaccines since 1973. Since 1998, GISRS has made biannual recommendations for seasonal influenza vaccine compositions for the northern and southern hemispheres. (WHO, 2022b, paras. 4–7)

As the countries of the world, including the United States, plan for pandemic influenza, preparedness efforts revolve around the following:

- Enhanced surveillance and early identification of cases in humans with isolation and contact tracing, and quarantine for exposed individuals to decrease transmission to others;
- Communication and education of health care professionals and the public about the seriousness of the situation;
- Implementation of infection-control measures and the provision of quality medical and supportive care;
- Maintenance of emergency and essential community services; and
- Outbreak control via the use of antiviral treatments, prophylaxis, and vaccination, if available.

Local health departments have been included in planning for a pandemic flu over the years. In recent years, there has also been greater collaboration between local health departments and other local governmental departments as part of overall disaster preparedness. This has allowed the departments of health to work more closely with the police, fire, rescue, and emergency services, local hospitals and physicians, and various other public safety units. It is believed that any major effort to respond to this threat will require a strong local response.

To respond to a pandemic influenza, vaccine manufacturers need the capability to develop and produce large quantities of new vaccines within months and not the 8 to 10 years that is needed today. This will entail making huge investments in new technologies to produce vaccines rapidly. Developing a cell-culture–derived vaccine instead of depending on chicken egg embryos; creating a library of clinical grade vaccine strains that are now appearing; new microdiagnostic laboratory assays; refining production methods to reduce the time and cost of making vaccines; and boosting an immune response after a single dose of a nasal spray vaccine would all be major contributions to an effective response to a pandemic influenza. Traditional public health methods to control an outbreak may include isolation and quarantine of infected persons, which may be ineffective after a short period.

Recent literature raised important questions regarding the implication of resistance to antiviral agents for the management of influenza and for planning a response to a possible pandemic (Hayden, 2006). Because of the high levels of resistance to amantadine and rimantadine detected among influenza A viruses, the CDC recommended in 2006 that neither drug be used for the treatment or chemoprophylaxis of influenza A infections (CDC, 2006b). Given that the two most important medical interventions—vaccines and antiviral medications—may likely be in short supply, federal, state, and local efforts need a strong community education program on methods of infection control. It is recommended that all communities be targeted for infection control education, including minority, low-income, and immigrant populations.

Public health officials believe that it is of paramount importance that federal and state-level governments invest in the local infrastructure. Appropriate activities include enhanced funding for local medical research institutions, local hospitals, physicians, nurses, educators and other professionals, and devoting substantial resources to local emergency and public health systems. Pandemic influenza is rare, but the probability of its recurrence is still substantial.

Case Study: Hepatitis B

One of the notifiable infectious diseases monitored by the NNDSS is hepatitis B—acute, chronic, and perinatal. Hepatitis B is an example of a viral infection that is transmitted to an uninfected person through exposure to bodily fluids of infected individuals. Needlestick injuries, tattooing, piercing, and exposure to infected blood and other body fluids including saliva and menstrual, vaginal, and seminal fluids can spread the disease. Sexual transmission is prevalent in unvaccinated persons with multiple sexual partners. "In highly endemic areas, hepatitis B is most commonly spread from mother to child at birth (perinatal transmission) or through horizontal transmission (exposure to infected blood), especially from an infected child to an uninfected child during the first 5 years of life" (WHO, 2022, para. 5). It is common for infants who are infected by their mothers or infected before 5 years old to develop chronic hepatitis B.

The hepatitis B viral (HBV) infection attacks the liver and can cause acute and chronic hepatitis. Chronic hepatitis B can lead to cirrhosis, liver cancer, liver failure, and premature death. It is the cause of up to 80% of hepatocellular carcinoma (primary liver cancer). Worldwide, almost 300 million people were estimated to be living with chronic hepatitis B infections in 2019, with 1.5 million new infections occurring each year. There were estimated to be 820,000 deaths in 2019 from hepatitis B infection. Risk for chronic infection is related to age at infection: approximately 90% of infected infants become chronically infected, compared with 2% to 6% of adults.

Persons with chronic HBV infection are often asymptomatic and may not be aware that they are infected, yet are capable of infecting others. About 25% of adults who become carriers as children die from liver cancer or cirrhosis caused by the infection. Chronic infection is responsible for most HBV-related morbidity and mortality, including chronic hepatitis, cirrhosis, liver failure, and hepatocellular carcinoma (CDC, 2009; WHO, 2022).

Control and Prevention of Hepatitis B

The hepatitis B vaccine is safe and effective according to WHO, and has been available in the United States since 1982 (WHO, 2013b). Since then, the control of perinatal infection has been a crucial part of the evolving vaccination strategy of the Advisory Committee on Immunization Practices (ACIP). The CDC, American Academy of Pediatrics (AAP), and the ACIP recommend maternal identification through screening and newborn prophylaxis, which can significantly reduce neonatal infection and potential sequelae. Preventing perinatal HBV transmission is an integral part of the national strategy to eliminate hepatitis B in the United States. National guidelines call for the following:

- Universal screening of pregnant women for HBsAg during each pregnancy;
- Case management of HBsAg-positive mothers and their infants;
- Provision of immunoprophylaxis for infants born to infected mothers, including hepatitis B vaccine and hepatitis B immune globulin [sic];
- Routine vaccination of all infants with the hepatitis B vaccine series, with the first dose administered at birth. (CDC, 2012a)

To accomplish the goal of eliminating perinatal hepatitis B transmission, many local health departments administer the Perinatal Hepatitis B Prevention Program in coordination with the CDC (2013c). As an example, New York State Public Health Law requires the completion of the following steps if a pregnant woman is hepatitis B surface antigen (HBsAg)-positive:

Reporting of the Case

- Physicians report to the County Department of Health's Perinatal Hepatitis B Prevention Program.
- Diagnostic laboratories report to the County Department of Health's Perinatal Hepatitis B Prevention Program.
- Labor and delivery hospitals report to the County Department of Health's Perinatal Hepatitis B Prevention Program.
- County Department of Health reports to New York State Department of Health (NYSDOH).

Management of the Case

- *Isolation.* Blood, body fluid, and tissue precautions are indicated for a pregnant woman who is HBsAg-positive and for her infant.
- *Investigation.* Case investigations are performed to determine the source of infection and exposure to the infant—sexual, needle sharing, and household contacts.

- *Laboratory Work and Follow-Up.* Follow-up is needed regarding HBsAg status of the mother and her infant, including follow-up laboratory work to determine the success of treatment for infants who complete the hepatitis B vaccine series.
- *Counseling.* HBsAg-positive individuals shall be counseled in measures to prevent the spread of hepatitis B transmission to household, sexual, and needle-sharing contacts.
- *Referral.* Individuals diagnosed as hepatitis B carriers should be referred to their private physicians for disease management.

Management of the Contacts

- *Investigation.* Case investigation is performed to determine the exposure to household, sexual, and needle-sharing contacts.
- *Laboratory Testing and Follow-Up.* Identified household, sexual, and needle-sharing contacts should be tested for the presence of HBV, and vaccine offered if indicated by their physicians.
- *Infants.* The purpose of maternal screening and intervention is to prevent the development of hepatitis B infection among infants born to mothers who are HBsAg-positive.

Case Study: Childhood Vaccinations

Childhood vaccinations are an essential public health strategy for maintaining a healthy population of children, adolescents, and adults free of infectious diseases. The CDC's Advisory Committee on Immunization Practices (ACIP) provides a list of childhood vaccinations recommended for all children. By age 6 years, a child immunized according to schedule will have received the vaccines listed in Table 4.6. This schedule is recommended by the ACIP, and approved by the CDC, AAP and American Academy of Family Physicians (AAFP; NCIRD, 2022).

The **National Immunization Survey (NIS)**, sponsored by the NCIRD, monitors immunization coverage among children in the United States (NCIRD, 2020).

Table 4.6. Vaccine-Preventable Diseases Recommended for Children Birth Through 6 Years, United States

Disease	Vaccine	Disease Spread by	Disease Complications
Chickenpox	Varicella	Air, direct contact	Infected blisters, bleeding disorders, encephalitis (brain swelling), pneumonia (infection in the lungs), death
Diphtheria	DTaP[a]	Air, direct contact	Swelling of the heart muscle, heart failure, coma, paralysis, death

(continued)

Table 4.6. Vaccine-Preventable Diseases Recommended for Children Birth Through 6 Years, United States (*continued*)

Disease	Vaccine	Disease Spread by	Disease Complications
Haemophilus influenzae type b	Hib	Air, direct contact	Meningitis (infection of the covering around the brain and spinal cord), intellectual disability, epiglottitis (life-threatening infection that can block the windpipe and lead to serious breathing problems), pneumonia (infection in the lungs), death
Hepatitis A	HepA	Direct contact, contaminated food or water	Liver failure, arthralgia (joint pain), kidney, pancreatic, and blood disorders, death
Hepatitis B	HepB	Contact with blood or body fluids	Chronic liver infection, liver failure, liver cancer, death
Influenza (flu)	Flu	Air, direct contact	Pneumonia (infection in the lungs), bronchitis, sinus infections, ear infections, death
Measles	MMR[b]	Air, direct contact	Encephalitis (brain swelling), pneumonia (infection in the lungs), death
Mumps	MMR[b]	Air, direct contact	Meningitis (infection of the covering around the brain and spinal cord), encephalitis (brain swelling), inflammation of testicles or ovaries, deafness, death
Pertussis (whooping cough)	DTaP[a]	Air, direct contact	Pneumonia (infection in the lungs), death
Polio	IPV	Air, direct contact, through the mouth	Paralysis, death
Pneumo-coccal	PCV13	Air, direct contact	Bacteremia (blood infection), meningitis (infection of the covering around the brain and spinal cord), death
Rotavirus	RV	Through the mouth	Severe diarrhea, dehydration, death
Rubella	MMR[b]	Air, direct contact	Very serious in pregnant women—can lead to miscarriage, stillbirth, premature delivery, birth defects
Tetanus	DTaP[a]	Exposure through cuts in skin	Broken bones, breathing difficulty, death

[a]DTaP combines protection against diphtheria, tetanus, and pertussis.
[b]MMR combines protection against measles, mumps, and rubella.

Source: National Center for Immunization and Respiratory Diseases. (2022b). *Recommended vaccinations for infants and children.* https://www.cdc.gov/vaccines/schedules/easy-to-read/child-easyread.html

The basic goal for children from birth through 35 months is completion of the *combined 7-vaccine series*, which provides immunization against diphtheria, pertussis, tetanus, poliovirus, measles, mumps, rubella, hepatitis B, hemophilus influenza B, chicken pox, and pneumococcal infections.

The NIS survey results for the *combined 7-vaccine series* among children aged 35 months by birth year 2011 through 2017 indicate that, overall, about 75% of the children were vaccinated for the *combined 7-vaccine series*. Vaccination rates were higher for fewer than 7 vaccines administered. For example, 93.2% of 35-month-old children born in 2011 had at least one dose of the MMR vaccine and that percent was 94.6% for children born in 2018. The likelihood of being fully or partially vaccinated varied by income, insurance coverage, and race/ethnicity, with children living below 400% of the federal poverty level, non-Hispanic Black children, and children without health insurance the least likely to been fully vaccinated by 35 months old (Hill et al., 2021). Detailed child vaccination coverage by race/ethnicity and poverty is available in *Health, United States 2020–2021*, Table VaxCh (NCHS, 2022).

Immunization Successes

The long-term benefits of wide-scale immunizations of children are clear, as can be observed in the following table, which displays the peak number of prevaccine annual cases for many infectious diseases compared to their number in 2017 (see Table 4.7).

Table 4.7. The Impact of Vaccines on the 2017 Incidence of Selected Infectious Diseases in the United States

Disease	Peak Cases in Prevaccine Era (year)	Cases in 2017 (*n*)	Disease Reduction (%)
Smallpox	110,672 (1920)	0	100
Diphtheria	30,508 (1936)	0	100
Measles (nonimported)	763,094 (1958)	99	99.99
Mumps	212,932 (1964)	6,109	97.13
Rubella	488,796 (1964)	7	100.00
Congenital rubella syndrome	20,000 (1964–65)	5	99.98
Pertussis	265,269 (1934)	18,975	92.85
Polio (paralytic)	21,269 (1952)	0	100
Tetanus	601 (1948)	33	94.51

Source: Rodrigues, C. M. C., & Plotkin, S. A. (2020). Impact of vaccines; health, economic and social perspectives. *Frontiers in Microbiology, 11*, 1526. https://doi.org/10.3389/fmicb.2020.01526

Not only are more children being protected from diseases through vaccinations, but vaccinations also result in cost savings. **Table 4.8** shows the cost savings and death rates associated with childhood vaccination programs compared to non-vaccination programs (Zhou et al., 2005).

Unvaccinated Children

The percentage of children fully vaccinated, however, is threatened by a number of factors including access to vaccination sites and COVID-19, during which utilization of medical care declined for children and adults. Another concern is vaccine hesitancy and exemptions. In 1991, less than 1% of children were exempted from childhood vaccinations by states and localities. By 2004, nearly 2.5% of children were exempted. Currently, there are medical and religious exemptions in nearly all states. Personal exemptions, on the other hand, exist in 18 states, including Texas, Utah, Ohio, Michigan, and Minnesota (Immunize.org, 2021). This situation has led to more clusters of childhood diseases that were previously rare and is becoming an increasingly serious public health risk to many unvaccinated children and immunocompromised individuals of all ages.

Unvaccinated children are susceptible to serious illnesses, such as measles, polio, diphtheria, hepatitis, meningitis, and rubella. In addition, they present a danger to others who may not be fully protected. Herd immunity is the concept that if enough people are vaccinated against a disease, there is little opportunity for the disease organism to multiply and spread. In this way, even people who are not able to be vaccinated are still protected. Herd immunity fails when too many people in a population opt out of being vaccinated. Personal or philosophical exemptions are considered potentially dangerous and bad public health policy (Omer et al., 2006).

Measles is a recent example of resurgence of a vaccine-preventable infectious disease in the United States. A recent study identifies the causes for resurgence, which include vaccine hesitancy:

> Despite the overall reduction in the percentage of imported cases of ·measles in the US over the past two decades, pockets of internal transmission of the disease following importation via increasing number of outbreaks in unvaccinated subpopulations, reinforced by vaccine hesitancy, account for the increasing incidence rates of the disease in the US. Taking a step further on the current control measures to control indigenous transmission through efficient vaccination coverage in at-risk subpopulations and among international US travellers, improved disease surveillance and rapid outbreaks containment are essential in curbing the resurgence of measles in the US. (Dimala et al., 2021, p. 9)

Vaccine hesitancy, the choice of individuals or their caregivers to delay or decline vaccination, can lead to overall lower levels of herd immunity. Outbreaks of measles in the United States, including a large 2014 measles outbreak at an amusement park in California, highlight the phenomena of vaccine refusal and associated

Table 4.8. Health and Economic Outcomes for Selected Vaccine-Preventable Diseases With and Without a Vaccination Program

	Without Vaccination Program				Prevented or Saved by Vaccination Program			
	Cases (No.)	Deaths (No.)	Direct Costs[a]	Total Cost[a]	Cases (No.)	Deaths (No.)	Direct Costs[a]	Total Cost[a]
Diphtheria	247,214	24,721	2,358	24,930	247,212	24,721	2,358	24,930
Tetanus	153	23	8	29	146	22	8	28
Pertussis	2,662,307	1,049	2,265	3,668	2,614,874	1,008	2,193	3,545
Hib	17,530	663	1,434	2,696	17,469	661	1,430	2,689
Polio	60,974	723	2,084	4,890	60,974	723	2,084	4,890
Measles	3,493,722	2,795	2,646	5,875	3,433,036	2,794	2,645	5,874
Mumps	2,100,718	11	936	1,459	2,095,917	11	934	1,456
Rubella	1,786,334	14	88	381	1,784,030	14	88	380
Congenital rubella syndrome	616	68	115	173	602	66	112	169
Hepatitis B	232,001	3,427	168	1,272	207,353	3,024	149	1,121
Varicella	3,788,807	70	205	1,184	3,160,391	57	173	993
Total	14,330,376	33,564	12,307	46,557	13,622,004	33,101	12,174	45,075

[a]Costs are rounded and given in millions of US dollars.

Hib, *Haemophilus influenzae* type b.

Source: Zhou, F., Santoli, J., Messonnier, M., Yusuf, H., Shefer, A., Chu, S., & Harpaz, R. (2005). Economic evaluation of the 7-vaccine routine childhood immunization schedule in the United States, 2001. *Archives of Pediatric and Adolescent Medicine, 159*(12). http://www.317coalition.org/documents/more resources16.pdf.

increased risk for vaccine-preventable diseases among both nonvaccinated and fully vaccinated (but not fully protected) individuals (Phadke et al., 2016).

Following is a commentary written by Paul Offit and published in *The Wall Street Journal* in 2007, discussing the problem of unvaccinated children. It is just as timely today as it was in 2007.

Fatal Exemption: Relationship Between Vaccine Exemptions and Rates of Disease

Commentary by Paul Offit, MD, Chief of Division of Infectious Diseases, Children's Hospital of Philadelphia. Published in The Wall Street Journal, *January 20, 2007.*

Last month [October 2006] the *Journal of the American Medical Association (JAMA)* published a study that received little attention from the press and, as a consequence, the public. The study examined the incidence of whooping cough (pertussis) in children whose parents had chosen not to vaccinate them; the results were concerning.

Vaccines are recommended by the Centers for Disease Control and Prevention (CDC) and professional societies, such as the American Academy of Pediatrics. But these organizations can't enforce their recommendations; only states can do that—usually when children enter day care centers and elementary schools—in the form of mandates. State vaccine mandates have been on the books since the early 1900s; but aggressive enforcement of them didn't occur until much later, born from tragedy.

In 1963 the first measles vaccine was introduced in the United States. Measles is a highly contagious disease that can infect the lungs causing fatal pneumonia, or the brain causing encephalitis. Before the measles vaccine, measles caused 100,000 American children to be hospitalized and 3,000 to die every year. In the early 1970s, public health officials found that states with vaccine mandates had rates of measles that were 50 percent lower than states without mandates. As a consequence, all states worked toward requiring children to get vaccines. Now every state has some form of vaccine mandates.

But not all children are subject to these mandates. All fifty states have medical exemptions to vaccines, such as a serious allergy to a vaccine component. Forty-eight states also have religious exemptions; Amish groups, for example, traditionally reject vaccines, believing that clean living and a healthy diet are all that are needed to avoid vaccine preventable diseases. And twenty states have philosophical exemptions; in some states these exemptions are easy to obtain, by simply signing your name at the bottom of a form; and in others they're much harder, requiring notarization, annual renewal, a signature from a local health official, or a personally written letter from a parent.

The *JAMA* study examined the relationship between vaccine exemptions and rates of disease. The authors found that between 1991 and 2004 the percentage of children whose parents had chosen to exempt them from vaccines increased by 6% per year, resulting in a 2.5-fold increase. This increase occurred almost solely in states where philosophical exemptions were easy to obtain. Worse, states with easy-to-obtain

---

(continued)

philosophical exemptions had twice as many children suffering from pertussis—a disease that causes inflammation of the windpipe and breathing tubes, pneumonia, and, in about twenty infants every year, death—than states with hard-to-obtain philosophical exemptions.

The finding that lower immunization rates caused higher rates of disease shouldn't be surprising. In 1991 a massive epidemic of measles in Philadelphia centered on a group that chose not to immunize its children; as a consequence nine children died from measles. In the late 1990s, severe outbreaks of pertussis occurred in Colorado and Washington among children whose parents feared pertussis vaccine. And in 2005 a 17-year-old unvaccinated girl, unknowingly having brought measles back with her from Romania, attended a church gathering of 500 people in Indiana and caused the largest outbreak of measles in the United States in 10 years; an outbreak that was limited to children whose parents had chosen not to vaccinate them. These events showed that for contagious diseases like measles and pertussis it's hard for unvaccinated children to successfully hide among herds of vaccinated children.

Some would argue that philosophical exemptions are a necessary pop-off valve for a society that requires children to be injected with biological agents for the common good. But as anti-vaccine activists continue to push more states to allow for easy philosophical exemptions one thing is clear, more and more children will suffer and occasionally die from vaccine preventable diseases.

When it comes to issues of public health and safety we invariably have laws. Many of these laws are strictly enforced and immutable. For example, we don't allow philosophical exemptions to restraining young children in car seats or smoking in restaurants or stopping at stop signs. And the notion of requiring vaccines for school entry, while it seems to tear at the very heart of a country founded on the basis of individual rights and freedoms, saves lives. Given the increasing number of states allowing philosophical exemptions to vaccines, at some point we are going to be forced to decide whether it is our inalienable right to catch and transmit potentially fatal infections.

CHAPTER SUMMARY

The story of infectious diseases—their causes, detection, control, treatment, and prevention—are fundamental to public health's story. Basic public health concepts, such as incidence, prevalence, case fatality rate, herd immunity, and so forth, were developed through study of infectious diseases. The terms epidemic, pandemic, and endemic are fundamental to public health methods. Instances in which infectious diseases have been identified and controlled are among the most important of public health's successes and include cholera, smallpox, tuberculosis, polio, and so many others. The public health role in developing vaccines and the success of immunizations in controlling many infectious diseases cannot be overestimated. These public health successes have had a major impact on morbidity and mortality, historically and in the present. The public health infrastructure around control and prevention of infectious diseases, as well as the methods developed, are essential to the health of Americans.

DISCUSSION QUESTIONS

Q: What is herd immunity and how is it achieved?

Q: What is the difference between incidence and prevalence of a disease?

Q: How would an infectious disease outbreak be investigated?

Q: How successful have immunizations been in controlling infectious diseases?

Q: What are some of the factors that increase susceptibility to infectious diseases and how do they relate to the health impact pyramid?

Q: What is the disease burden of foodborne diseases in the United States?

DATA SOURCES

For Chapter 4, these sources of data can provide a deeper understanding of infectious disease control. The Centers for Disease Control and Prevention (CDC) has three centers that are central to surveillance and control of infectious diseases. Two of these centers collect data that are publicly available. Following are data sources from these centers:

- National Center for HIV, Viral Hepatitis, STD, and TB Prevention (NCHHSTP)

  The NCHHSTP is focused on HIV infection/AIDS, non-HIV retroviruses, viral hepatitis, other sexually transmitted diseases, and tuberculosis. NCHHSTP AtlasPlus is an interactive tool that gives users the ability to create customized tables, maps, and charts using nearly 20 years of CDC's surveillance data on HIV, viral hepatitis, STD, and TB. AtlasPlus also provides access to indicators on social determinants of health (SDOH) allowing users to view social and economic data in conjunction with surveillance data for each disease. Get started here: https://www.cdc.gov/nchhstp/atlas/about-atlas.html

- National Center for Immunization and Respiratory Diseases (NCIRD)

  NCIRD directs its efforts to immunization and respiratory and related diseases. The Influenza Division at CDC collects, compiles, and analyzes information on influenza activity year-round in the United States. FluView, a weekly influenza surveillance report, and FluView Interactive, an online application which allows for more in-depth exploration of influenza surveillance data, are updated each week. One topic from FluView Interactive is influenza-associated pediatric mortality, which can be explored here: https://gis.cdc.gov/GRASP/Fluview/PedFluDeath.html

A robust set of instructor resources designed to supplement this text is located at http://connect.springerpub.com/content/book/978-0-8261-8615-7. Qualifying instructors may request access by emailing **textbook@springerpub.com**.

REFERENCES

Barreto, M. L., Teixeira, M. G., & Carmo, E. H. (2006). Infectious diseases epidemiology. *Journal of Epidemiology and Community Health, 60*(3), 192–195. https://doi.org/10.1136/jech.2003.011593

Cairns, C., Kang, K., & Santo, L. (2018). *National hospital ambulatory medical care survey: 2018 emergency department summary tables*. National Center for Health Statistics. https://www.cdc.gov/nchs/data/nhamcs/web_tables/2018-ed-web-tables-508.pdf

Centers for Disease Control and Prevention. (1996). Historical perspectives notifiable disease surveillance and notifiable disease statistics—United States, June 1946 and June 1996. *Morbidity and Mortality Weekly Report, 45*(25), 530–536. https://www.cdc.gov/mmwr/preview/mmwrhtml/00042744.htm

Centers for Disease Control and Prevention. (2004). Diagnosis and management of foodborne illnesses: A primer for physicians and other health care professionals. *Morbidity and Mortality Weekly Report, 53*(RR-4), 1–33. https://pubmed.ncbi.nlm.nih.gov/15123984/

Centers for Disease Control and Prevention. (2005). Progress in reducing measles mortality–Worldwide, 1999–2003. *Morbidity and Mortality Weekly Report, 54*(8), 200–203. https://pubmed.ncbi.nlm.nih.gov/15744229/

Centers for Disease Control and Prevention. (2006a). New laboratory assay for diagnostic testing of avian influenza A/H5 (Asian Lineage). *Morbidity and Mortality Weekly Report, 55*(5), 127. https://pubmed.ncbi.nlm.nih.gov/16467779/

Centers for Disease Control and Prevention. (2006b). High levels of adamantane resistance among influenza A (H3N2) viruses and interim guidelines for use of antiviral agents—United States, 2005–2006 influenza season. *Morbidity and Mortality Weekly Report, 55*(2), 44–46. https://pubmed.ncbi.nlm.nih.gov/16424859/

Centers for Disease Control and Prevention. (2009). *Epidemiology and prevention of vaccine-preventable diseases* (11th ed.). Public Health Foundation.

Centers for Disease Control and Prevention. (2010). Recommended immunization schedules for persons aged 0 through 18 years–United States, 2010. *Morbidity and Mortality Weekly Report, 58*(51 & 52), 1–4. https://www.cdc.gov/mmwr/preview/mmwrhtml/mm5851a6.htm

Centers for Disease Control and Prevention. (2011). *Investigation of outbreak of infections caused by Salmonella Saintpaul*. http://www.cdc.gov/salmonella/saintpaul/jalapeno/

Centers for Disease Control and Prevention. (2012a). *Hepatitis B information for health professionals*. http://www.cdc.gov/hepatitis/HBV/

Centers for Disease Control and Prevention. (2012b). *Food safety: How many cases of food-borne disease are there in the United States?* http://www.cdc.gov/foodsafety/facts.html#howmanycases

Centers for Disease Control and Prevention. (2012c). *Investigation update: Outbreak of Salmonella typhimurium infections, 2008–2009 (final update).* http://www.cdc.gov/salmonella/typhimurium/update.html

Centers for Disease Control and Prevention. (2012d). *Multistate outbreak of Salmonella bredeney infections linked to peanut butter manufactured by Sunland, Inc.* https://www.cdc.gov/salmonella/bredeney-09-12/index.html

Centers for Disease Control and Prevention. (2012e). *Prevention and treatment of avian influenza A viruses in people.* http://www.cdc.gov/flu/avianflu/prevention.htm

Centers for Disease Control and Prevention. (2013a). *National notifiable diseases surveillance system.* http://wwwn.cdc.gov/nndss/script/history.aspx

Centers for Disease Control and Prevention. (2013b). *2013 national notifiable infectious conditions.* http://wwwn.cdc.gov/nndss/script/conditionlist.aspx?type=0&yr=2013

Centers for Disease Control and Prevention. (2013c). *Viral hepatitis—funded partners: Perinatal hepatitis B prevention coordinators.* http://www.cdc.gov/hepatitis/Partners/PeriHepBCoord.htm

Centers for Disease Control and Prevention. (2013d). *National immunization survey.* http://www.cdc.gov/nis/

Centers for Disease Control and Prevention. (2013e). *PulseNet.* http://www.cdc.gov/pulsenet/

Centers for Disease Control and Prevention. (2013f). *FoodNet.* http://www.cdc.gov/foodnet/

Centers for Disease Control and Prevention. (2013g). *The national outbreak reporting system.* http://www.cdc.gov/nors/about.html

Centers for Disease Control and Prevention. (2021a). *CDC's infectious disease national centers.* https://www.cdc.gov/ddid/centers.html

Centers for Disease Control and Prevention. (2021b). *Legionella (Legionnaires' disease and pontiac fever).* https://www.cdc.gov/legionella/about/causes-transmission.html

Centers for Disease Control and Prevention, National Center for Emerging and Zoonotic Infectious Diseases. (2017). *Who we are.* https://www.cdc.gov/ncezid/who-we-are/index.html

Centers for Disease Control and Prevention, National Center for Emerging and Zoonotic Infectious Diseases. (2021). *One health: Zoonotic diseases.* https://www.cdc.gov/onehealth/basics/zoonotic-diseases.html

Centers for Disease Control and Prevention, National Notifiable Diseases Surveillance System. (2021a). *Surveillance case definitions for current and historical conditions.* https://ndc.services.cdc.gov/

Centers for Disease Control and Prevention, National Notifiable Diseases Surveillance System. (2021b). *What is case surveillance?* https://www.cdc.gov/nndss/about/index.html

Centers for Disease Control and Prevention, & National Notifiable Diseases Surveillance System. (2021c). *Current and past notifiable conditions.* https://ndc.services.cdc.gov/search-results-year/

Centers for Disease Control and Prevention. (2023). *Leading causes of death, 1900–1998.* https://www.cdc.gov/nchs/data/dvs/lead1900_98.pdf

Dimala, C. A., Kadia, B. M., Nji, M. A. M., & Bechem, N. D. (2021). Factors associated with measles resurgence in the United States in the post-elimination era. *Scientific Reports, 11, 51.* https://doi.org/10.1038/s41598-020-80214-3

Dubos, R. (1959). *Mirage of health: Utopias, progress and biological change.* Harper and Brothers.

Flaherty, D. K. (Ed.). (2012). *Immunology for pharmacists.* Mosby.

Hariharan, J. (2021). *What counts as a microbe?* American Society for Microbiology. https://asm.org/Articles/2021/April/What-Counts-as-a-Microbe

Hayden, F. G. (2006). Antiviral resistance in influenza viruses—Implications for management and pandemic response. *New England Journal of Medicine, 354*(8), 785–788. https://doi.org/10.1056/NEJMp068030

Hill, H. A., Yankey, D., Elam-Evans, L. D., Singleton, J. A., & Sterrett, N. (2021). Vaccination coverage by age 24 months among children born in 2017 and 2018—National immunization survey-child, United States, 2018–2020. *Morbidity and Mortality Weekly Report, 70,* 1435–1440. https://doi.org/10.15585/mmwr.mm7041a1

Immunize.org. (2021). *State information.* https://www.immunize.org/laws/exemptions.asp

McNeill, W. H. (1976). *Plagues and peoples.* Anchor Books.

Moberg, C. L. (1999). René Dubos, A harbinger of microbial resistance to antibiotics. *Perspectives in Biology and Medicine, 42*(4), 559–580. https://doi.org/10.1353/pbm.1999.0011

Moore, P. (2007). *The essential handbook of epidemics, viruses and plagues.* Penguin Books.

National Academies of Sciences, Engineering, and Medicine. (2022). *Infectious disease.* https://www.nationalacademies.org/based-on-science/are-all-infectious-diseases-caused-by-viruses-and-bacteria

National Center for Health Statistics. (2019). Selected nationally notifiable disease rates and number of new cases: United States, selected years 1950–2018. In *Health, United States, 2019.* https://www.cdc.gov/nchs/data/hus/2019/010-508.pdf

National Center for Health Statistics. (2022). Vaccination coverage for selected diseases by age 24 months, by race and Hispanic origin, poverty level, and location of residence: United States, birth years 2010–2016. In *Health, United States 2020–2021.* https://www.cdc.gov/nchs/data/hus/2020-2021/VaxCh.pdf

National Center for Immunization and Respiratory Diseases. (2020a). *Pandemic influenza.* https://www.cdc.gov/flu/pandemic-resources/index.htm#:~:text=An%20influenza%20pandemic%20is%20a,an%20efficient%20and%20sustained%20way

National Center for Immunization and Respiratory Diseases. (2020b). Vaccination coverage among young children (0–35 months). *ChildVaxView.* https://www.cdc.gov/vaccines/imz-managers/coverage/childvaxview/index.html

National Center for Immunization and Respiratory Diseases. (2022a). *Measles cases and outbreaks.* https://www.cdc.gov/measles/cases-outbreaks.html

National Center for Immunization and Respiratory Diseases. (2022b). *Recommended vaccinations for infants and children.* https://www.cdc.gov/vaccines/schedules/easy-to-read/child-easyread.html

National Center for Immunization and Respiratory Diseases. (2022c). *Vaccines in the child and adolescent immunization schedule.* https://www.cdc.gov/vaccines/schedules/downloads/child/0-18yrs-combined-schedule-bw.pdf

National Institute of Allergy and Infectious Diseases. (2010). *Community immunity.* http://www.niaid.nih.gov/topics/Pages/communityImmunity.aspx

Occupational Safety and Health Administration. (2010). *Foodborne disease: Control and prevention.* http://www.osha.gov/SLTC/foodbornedisease/control.html

Offit, P. (2007). Fatal exemption: Relationship between vaccine exemptions and rates of disease. *Wall Street Journal.* http://online.wsj.com/news/articles/SB116925887913182362

Omer, S. B., Pan, W. K. Y., Halsey, N. A., Stokley, S., Moulton, L. H., Navar, A. M., Pierce, M., & Salmon, D. A. (2006). Nonmedical exemptions to school immunization requirements: Secular trends and association of state policies with pertussis incidence. *Journal of American Medical Association, 296*(14), 1757–1763. https://doi.org/10.1001/jama.296.14.1757

Phadke, V. K., Bednarczyk, R. A., Salmon, D. A., & Omer, S. B. (2016). Association between vaccine refusal and vaccine-preventable diseases in the United States: A review of masles and pertussis. *JAMA, 315*(11), 1149–1158. https://doi.org/10.1001/jama.2016.1353

Santo, L., & Okeyode, T. (2018). *National ambulatory medical care survey: 2018 national summary tables.* https://www.cdc.gov/nchs/data/ahcd/namcs_summary/2018-namcs-web-tables-508.pdf

United States Department of Agriculture, Food Safety and Inspection Service. (2014). *HACCP-based inspection models project.* http://www.fsis.usda.gov/wps/portal/fsis/topics/regulatory-compliance/haccp/haccp-based-inspection-models-project/history-HIMP/History-of-HIMP

Van Seventer, J. M., & Hochberg, N. S. (2017). Principles of infectious diseases: Transmissions, diagnosis, prevention, and control. *International Encyclopedia of Public Health, 6,* 22–39. https://doi.org/10.1016/B978-0-12-803678-5.00516-6

World Health Organization. (2012). *Stopping measles and rubella with one combined vaccine.* http://www.who.int/immunization/newsroom/measles_rubella/en/index.html

World Health Organization. (2022a). *Hepatitis B.* http://www.who.int/mediacentre/factsheets/fs204/en/

World Health Organization. (2022b). *Celebrating 70 years of GISRS (the global influenza surveillance and response system).* https://www.who.int/news/item/03-02-2022-2022-celebrating-70-years-of-gisrs-(the-global-influenza-surveillance-and-response-system)

World Health Organization. (2022c). *Hepatitis B.* https://www.who.int/en/news-room/fact-sheets/detail/hepatitis-b

World Health Organization. (2022d). *WHO coronavirus (COVID-19) dashboard.* https://covid19.who.int/

Zhou, F., Santoli, J., Messonnier, M., Yusuf, H., Shefer, A., Chu, S., & Harpaz, R. (2005). Economic evaluation of the 7-vaccine routine childhood immunization schedule in the United States, 2001. *Archives of Pediatric and Adolescent Medicine, 159*(12). http://www.317coalition.org/documents/more resources16.pdf

Zinsser, H. (1935). *Rats, lice and history.* Little, Brown and Company.

5 | Injury and Noninfectious Disease Control

LEARNING OBJECTIVES

Students will learn . . .

1. The significance of noninfectious diseases and injuries for mortality and morbidity in the United States.

2. The basic approach of the federal public health system to prevention and control of noninfectious diseases and injury.

3. The risk factors for childhood obesity and child and teen motor vehicle injuries.

4. Some important federal initiatives to reduce and prevent childhood obesity in communities.

5. Some important federal initiatives to reduce and prevent child and teen motor vehicle injuries in communities.

Infectious disease control has historical significance for public health—having provided many, if not most, of public health's early successes—and it remains a major component of public health practice today, as discussed in the previous chapter. However, the scope and practice of public health in the United States has steadily increased since the 19th century in response to changes in the health problems that have the greatest impact on morbidity and mortality.

In 2019, the 10 leading causes of death in the United States were noninfectious conditions or injuries, with the exception of influenza and pneumonia. Together, they account for about 72% of all deaths in 2019—64.2% noninfectious diseases and 7.8% injuries. See Table 5.1. The predominance of noninfectious diseases and injuries as leading causes of death has been evident for at least 40 years. In 1980, the 10 leading causes of death were the same as in 2019 with

Table 5.1. Leading Causes of Death and Number of Deaths: United States, 2019

All Races and Origins, Both Sexes, All Ages

Rank	Cause of Death[a]	Number of Deaths	Percent of Total Deaths
	All causes	2,854,838	100
1	Diseases of heart	659,041	23.1
2	Malignant neoplasms	599,601	21.0
3	**Unintentional injuries**	**173,040**	**6.1**
4	Chronic lower respiratory diseases	156,979	5.5
5	Cerebrovascular diseases	150,005	5.3
6	Alzheimer disease	121,499	4.3
7	Diabetes mellitus	87,647	3.1
8	Nephritis, nephrotic syndrome, and nephrosis	51,565	1.8
9	Influenza and pneumonia	49,783	1.7
10	**Suicide**	**47,511**	**1.7**

[a]See Notes at the end of this chapter for discussion of definitional issues related to comparing 1980 and 2019 causes of death.

Source: National Center for Health Statistics, National Vital Statistics System, Xu, J. Q., Murphy, S. L., Kochanek, K. D., & Arias, E. (2021). Deaths: Final data for 2019. *National Vital Statistics Reports, 70*(8). National Center for Health Statistics. https://www.cdc.gov/nchs/data/nvsr/nvsr70/nvsr70-08-508.pdf

two exceptions. Atherosclerosis was in the top 10 in 1980, but not in 2019, and only the 2019 list contains Alzheimer disease. Similarities between 2019 and 1980 also include:

- Diseases of the heart and malignant neoplasms were the top two causes of death in both 1980 and 2019.
- Suicide was the 10th leading cause of death in both years.
- Injuries accounted for a much smaller percent of death than noninfectious conditions in both 1980 and 2019.

However, there are some differences of note in the impact of each cause. Injuries actually accounted for a lower percentage of total deaths in 1980—6.7% of total deaths compared to 7.8% in 2019. Also, the two leading causes of death—diseases of the heart and malignant neoplasms—accounted for a smaller percent of deaths in 2019. In 2019, they were responsible for 44.1% of all deaths, compared to 59.1% in 1980. In addition, the percent of deaths due to diabetes rose from 1.7% in 1980 to 3.1% in 2019 (Xu et al., 2021). See **Table 5.2**.

Table 5.2. Leading Causes of Death and Number of Deaths: United States, 1980

All Races and Origins, Both Sexes, All Ages

Rank	Cause of Death[a]	Number of Deaths	Percent of Total Deaths
	All causes	1,989,841	100
1	Diseases of heart	761,085	38.2
2	Malignant neoplasms	416,509	20.9
3	Cerebrovascular diseases	170,225	8.5
4	**Unintentional injuries**	**105,718**	**5.3**
5	Chronic obstructive pulmonary diseases	56,050	2.8
6	Pneumonia and influenza	54,619	2.7
7	Diabetes mellitus	34,851	1.7
8	Chronic liver disease and cirrhosis	30,583	1.5
9	Atherosclerosis	29,449	1.5
10	**Suicide**	**26,869**	**1.4**

[a]See Notes at the end of this chapter for discussion of definitional issues related to comparing 1980 and 2019 causes of death.

Source: National Center for Health Statistics, National Vital Statistics System, Xu, J. Q., Murphy, S. L., Kochanek, K. D., & Arias, E. (2021). Deaths: Final data for 2019. *National Vital Statistics Reports*, 70(8). National Center for Health Statistics. https://www.cdc.gov/nchs/data/nvsr/nvsr70/nvsr70-08-508.pdf

Variation in Mortality by Age, Sex, and Race/ethnicity

Limiting discussion to overall mortality—that is, to all races and origins, both sexes, and all ages concurrently—conceals significant differences between groups. Knowing variations in cause of death by age, sex, and race/ethnicity are indispensable for understanding how to control chronic diseases and injuries. A review of 2019 mortality statistics suggests why this is so. Following are several examples of differences between men and women:

- In 2019, males had a higher relative burden of mortality from unintentional injuries, which was the third leading cause of death for this group, accounting for 7.6% of deaths, but the sixth leading cause for females, accounting for 4.4% of deaths.

- Suicide ranked eighth for males (2.5% of deaths) but was not ranked among the 10 leading causes for females. Chronic liver disease and cirrhosis was the ninth leading cause for males (1.9% of deaths), but it was not in the top 10 for females. (Heron, 2021, p. 9)

There are also significant differences in mortality by age. Death from unintentional injuries provides an example:

> The leading cause of death for the population aged 1–44 was unintentional injuries. The relative burden of mortality from this cause was far greater at younger ages, accounting for 38.1% of deaths for age group 10–24, 34.2% of deaths for age group 25–44, and 31.0% of all deaths for age group 1–9. In contrast, unintentional injuries was the third leading cause of death for age group 45–64 (9.0% of deaths), the sixth leading cause for age group 85 and over (2.9%), and the seventh leading cause for age group 65 and over (2.9%). (Heron, 2021, p. 10)

Substantial differences in mortality by race and ethnicity also exist. For example, Table 5.3 contains the percentage of total deaths from injuries by race and Hispanic origin. Of all race/ethnic groups, non-Hispanic American Indian/Alaska Natives have the highest burden of injury death—15.9% of total deaths due to unintentional accidents, suicide, and homicide. Persons of Hispanic origin have the next highest burden of injury death—12.4%. The group with the lowest burden of injury mortality is non-Hispanic Asians at 6.7% of total deaths due to accidents, suicide, and homicide. See Table 5.3.

Table 5.3. Percentage of Total Deaths From Injuries by Race and Hispanic Origin: United States, 2019

| | Race and Hispanic Origin | | | | |
Cause of Death	White[a] Percent of Total Deaths	Black[a] Percent of Total Deaths	American Indian/Alaska Native[a] Percent of Total Deaths	Asian[a] Percent of Total Deaths	Hispanic Percent of Total Deaths
Unintentional injuries (accidents)	5.7	6.2	11.3	4.4	8.9
Intentional self-harm (suicide)	1.7	0.9	3.0	1.9	2.0
Assault (homicide)	0.2	2.9	1.6	0.4	1.5
Total Percentage of Total Deaths	**7.6**	**10.0**	**15.9**	**6.7**	**12.4**

[a]Non-Hispanic.

Source: Heron, M. (2021). Deaths: Leading causes for 2019. *National Vital Statistics Reports, 70*(9), 1–114.

The differences in cause of death by age, sex, and race/ethnicity are startling and essential to understand as we seek to improve population health and limit premature death. Young people generally die from injuries—especially unintended injuries, but also the intentional injuries of homicide and suicide. Men are most at risk of early death from injury, and Native American and Blacks die from injuries of all kinds at a higher rate than Whites, Asians, and Hispanics. Understanding these differences is central to prevention and control of premature death and health promotion.

It should also be noted that, in 2020, the COVID-19 pandemic changed the leading causes of death when this infectious disease became the third leading cause, replacing injuries. However, it seems likely that COVID-19 will not remain there because of the effectiveness of vaccines and treatments, and that injuries and noninfectious diseases will retain their place as the overriding causes of death in the United States.

CONTROL AND PREVENTION OF INJURY AND NONINFECTIOUS DISEASE

Public health practices can be classified in the following way:

- Surveillance and research of a health problem; and
- Interventions to prevent and control a health problem.

Surveillance and research of health problems include the following types of activities:

- Provide information on incidence, prevalence, and risk factors;
- Conduct research on causes and consequences of the health problem;
- Evaluate effectiveness of interventions aimed at preventing and controlling the health problem; and
- Develop data systems necessary for surveillance and research.

Interventions to prevent and control health problems include the following activities:

- Educate population at risk and related persons on how to reduce risk of the health problem;
- Provide services for victims of the health problem, including screening, treatment, and supportive services; and
- Change social and/or physical environments to prevent health problems from occurring, which include advocacy and policy solutions.

The number of problems tackled within the area of injury prevention and noninfectious disease control is tremendous. The list includes noninfectious diseases such as:

- Arthritis,
- Cancer,

- Chronic kidney diseases,
- Chronic pain,
- Dementias,
- Diabetes,
- Drug and alcohol and tobacco addiction,
- Heart disease and stroke,
- Osteoporosis, and
- Respiratory diseases.

The list includes injuries, as

- Intentional injuries including self-harm (suicide) and violence against others; and
- Unintentional injuries including motor vehicle crashes, falls, drownings, and others.

Prevention efforts address underlying issues and strategic interventions such as:

- Child and adolescent development,
- Health communication,
- Nutrition and healthy eating,
- Overweight and obesity,
- Physical activity,
- Preventive health care, and
- Sleep.

Table 5.4 presents a partial list of the Centers for Disease Control and Prevention's (CDC) *National Health Initiatives, Strategies and Action Plans* for injury and noninfectious disease control. These initiatives establish and reflect the public health agenda for the nation. The list gives an indication of the scope, variety, and number of issues related to injuries and noninfectious diseases that are targeted by public health. Each is a planning document that establishes strategic priorities for addressing the nation's most pressing health problems. They can be used "to develop state or local plans, prioritize public health activities, inform funding proposals, and create other materials to ensure that public health efforts align with national goals" (CDC, 2022, para. 1).

The relevant centers within the CDC that address injury and noninfectious disease prevention are:

- National Center on Birth Defects and Developmental Disabilities (NCBDDD),
- National Center for Chronic Disease Prevention and Health Promotion (NCCDPHP),
- National Center for Environmental Health/Agency for Toxic Substances and Disease Registry, and
- National Center for Injury Prevention and Control (NCIPC).

Table 5.4. Strategies and Action Plans for Injury and Noninfectious Disease Control, Centers for Disease Control and Prevention, March 2, 2022

Alzheimer disease

- National Plan to Address Alzheimer Disease
- Healthy Aging in Action: Advancing the National Prevention Strategy
- The Healthy Brain Initiative: A National Public Health Road Map to Maintaining Cognitive Health

Chronic disease

- National Action Plan for Cancer Survivorship: Advancing Public Health Strategies
- National Public Health Agenda for Osteoarthritis

Environmental health

- Federal Action Plan to Reduce Childhood Lead Exposures and Associated Health Impacts
- President's Task Force on Environmental Health Risks and Safety Risks to Children

Heart disease and stroke

- The Public Health Action Plan to Prevent Heart Disease and Stroke: Ten-Year Update
- Million Hearts Initiative

Injury and violence prevention (child safety, highway safety, occupational safety, suicide, violence)

- Facing Addiction in America: The Surgeon General's Report on Alcohol, Drugs, and Health
- National Action Plan for Adverse Drug Event Prevention
- National Action Plan for Child Injury Prevention
- National Strategies for Advancing Bicycle Safety
- National Strategies for Advancing Child Pedestrian Safety
- National Strategy for Suicide Prevention: Goals and Objectives for Action
- National Strategy for Youth Preparedness Education: Empowering, Educating and Building Resilience
- Prevention Through Design National Initiative
- Toward Zero Deaths: A National Strategy on Highway Safety

Smoking and tobacco use

- E-cigarette Use Among Youth and Young Adults: A Report of the Surgeon General, 2016
- Ending the Tobacco Epidemic: A Tobacco Control Strategic Action Plan for the U.S. Department of Health and Human Services
- Surgeon General's Report on Smoking and Health, *The Health Consequences of Smoking—50 Years of Progress.*

Each of these centers is under the Deputy Director for Noninfectious Diseases—one of the five major divisions of the CDC. Two divisions are particularly relevant for the following discussion:

- Division of Unintended Injury Prevention within NCIPC, and
- Division of Nutrition, Physical Activity, and Obesity within NCCDPHP.

As a result of the wide range of problems related to control and prevention of injuries and noninfectious diseases, public health's response to each will not be discussed. Instead, we examine two childhood health problems that illustrate public health practice for injury and noninfectious disease control. These are:

- Motor vehicle injuries among children and teens, and
- Childhood obesity.

Our discussion of motor vehicle injuries and childhood obesity will focus on the CDC's efforts. The CDC often leads the state and local public health ventures intellectually and through provision of technical and financial resources such as cooperative agreements and block and categorical grants. However, we also discuss state and local activities, as these are the levels where surveillance and research occur and strategies and policies are implemented.

MOTOR VEHICLE INJURIES AMONG CHILDREN AND TEENS

The NCIPC, the CDC's lead division for injury prevention, reports the following statistics about the prevalence and cost, monetary and nonmonetary, of motor vehicle accidents.

- Unintentional injuries are one of the 10 leading causes of death in the United States for men and women of every age and racial/ethnic group. Unintentional injuries are **the leading cause of death** for persons aged 1 to 44 years old (Xu et al., 2021).
- Motor vehicle accidents are one of the foremost causes of unintentional injuries. Almost 41,000 people died in motor vehicle crashes in the United States in 2020 (NCIPC & CDC, 2022f).
- Motor vehicle accidents are a leading cause of years of potential life lost before age 75 (NCIPC & CDC, 2022d).
- Motor vehicle injuries are also a leading cause of morbidity. There were over 2.1 million emergency department visits for motor vehicle injuries in 2020 (NCIPC & CDC, 2022f). They are responsible for a major portion of all disabilities, which affect about 25% of all persons 18 to 64 years old and about 61% of persons 65 and over (NCHS & CDC, 2010; Table 5.5).
- Motor vehicle crashes are expensive, with one study estimating that in 2020 they cost the country over $430 billion a year in total costs including medical costs and cost of lives lost (NCIPC & CDC, 2022f).

Table 5.5. Initial Injury-Related Visits to Hospital Emergency Departments by Age, Sex, and Type of Injury, United States, 2005–2018

Sex and Age of Injured	Type of Injury	Average Annual Number of Initial Injury-Related Visits per 10,000 People			
		2005–2006	2007–2008	2013–2014	2017–2018
Male, under 18 years		1,346.6	1,216.8	1,236.6	1,345.9
	Unintentional	1,165.8	1,056.3	1,104.4	1,181.9
	Falls	361.5	345.0	354.1	439.0
	Motor vehicle traffic accident	94.8	70.0	48.9	71.0
Male, 18–24 years		1,729.5	1,547.4	1,435.4	1,153.9
	Unintentional	1,345.4	1,200.6	1,114.7	923.6
	Falls	215.2	207.7	152.4	129.1
	Motor vehicle traffic accident	261.6	245.8	235.4	185.9
Female, under 18 years		1,008.7	848.2	1,053.8	1,062.2
	Unintentional	851.1	745.3	904.8	925.3
	Falls	289.1	280.9	313.1	316.9
	Motor vehicle traffic accident	102.1	78.2	72.9	67.5
Female, 18–24 years		1,329.3	1,186.5	1,148.1	1,113.8
	Unintentional	1,010.5	921.0	924.5	806.6
	Falls	205.0	210.5		227.0
	Motor vehicle traffic accident	280.6	264.5	231.1	203.1

Source: National Center for Health Statistics & National Hospital Ambulatory Medical Care Survey. (2021). Initial injury-related visits to hospital emergency departments, by sex, age, and intent and mechanism of injury: United States, average annual, selected years 2005–2006 through 2017–2018. *Health, United States, 2020–2021*. https://www.cdc.gov/nchs/data/hus/2020-2021/InjEDVis.pdf

Vulnerability of Children and Teens

Children and teens are very vulnerable to motor vehicle injuries and death.

- In 2020, more than 607 children ages 12 years and younger died as occupants in motor vehicle crashes, and more than 63,000 were injured. In 2019, almost 2,400 teens (13–19 years) were killed in motor vehicle crashes in the United States, and about 258,000 were treated in emergency departments for motor vehicle crash injuries (NCIPC & CDC, 2022f).
- Motor vehicle crashes were the second leading cause of unintentional injury death for children 1 to 4 years old in 2020. They were the first leading cause of unintentional injury death for children and young adults—5 to 9, 10 to 14, and 15 to 24 years old—in 2020 (NCIPC & CDC, 2022a).

Not surprisingly, then, prevention of motor vehicle injuries and fatalities is a major public health activity in the United States, particularly focused on young people, and the CDC's NCIPC plays a leading role.

Core State Injury Prevention Program

The 1985 and 1989 Institute of Medicine and National Academy of Sciences reports contained a national call for a consolidated federal focus on injury prevention. The key goals were:

- Build an infrastructure;
- Bring the public health perspective to injury prevention; and
- Apply the same proven prevention techniques used for infectious disease transmission and chronic illness to reducing injury and its consequences (NCIPC & CDC, 2022c).

This call was answered by the CDC with its decision to fund and guide injury prevention programs nationwide through the NCIPC. The **Core State Injury Prevention Program (SIPP)** is one of these CDC efforts. It facilitates surveillance and prevention of injury and death for an array of types of injuries including motor vehicle crashes, traumatic brain injury, adverse childhood experiences, and local injury priorities (NCIPC & CDC, 2022c). The three Core SIPP goals are:

- Engage in surveillance activities.
- Strengthen strategic collaborations and partnerships.
- Conduct assessment and evaluation.

The activities of the Core SIPP to reduce risk factors and increase protective influences are evidence based and intended to prevent injuries and death. These activities include:

- Utilizing robust data and surveillance,
- Strengthening strategic collaborations and partnerships, and
- Conducting assessment and evaluation.

The program builds on the infrastructure established through previous iterations of the Core Violence and Injury Prevention Program (VIPP), which began in the early 2000s, and the Core State Violence and Injury Prevention Program (SVIPP), which followed it (NCIPC & CDC, 2022b).

As of 2022, Core SIPP supports 23 funded state partners to maintain and strengthen their injury and violence prevention programs with a focus on key components: building a solid infrastructure; collecting and analyzing data; designing, implementing and evaluating programs; providing technical support and training; and affecting behavior and knowledge. The 23 states are: Arizona, Colorado, Georgia, Hawaii, Illinois, Kentucky, Louisiana, Maryland, Massachusetts, Michigan, Minnesota, Nebraska, New York, North Carolina, Oklahoma, Ohio, Oregon, Rhode Island, Tennessee, Utah, Virginia, Washington, and Wisconsin.

Five of the 23 funded state partners serve as Regional Network Leaders and provide a structure for cross-state collaboration and assistance to all states within their designated regions. Together they address injury and violence prevention across all 50 states. RNLs develop partnerships with appropriate organizations and research centers, and also work with the CDC and each other to identify common issues and shape effective program infrastructure at the state, regional, and national level. Six of the 23 funded state partners participate in Surveillance Quality Improvement (SQI). They conduct injury data investigations supportive of promoting and advancing uniform injury case definitions, improving data quality, and advancing methodology (NCIPC & CDC, 2022b).

DID YOU KNOW?

Sources of Motor Vehicle Injury and Fatality Data
In addition to data that are developed by individual projects through Core SIPP and other programs, there are data that are applicable to all states and regions. First, fatal injury data are drawn from death certificate data from the *National Vital Statistics System*—deaths, death rates, and years of potential life lost (a measure of premature death) by specific causes of injury mortality and common causes of death. Second, national estimates of injuries treated in U.S. hospital emergency departments are from the National Electronic Injury Surveillance System—All Injury Program (NEISS-AIP)—nonfatal injuries and nonfatal injury rates. Third, violent death data are from the National Violent Death Reporting System (NVDRS)—violent incidents and deaths, death rates, and causes of injury mortality. These data are provided for 16 states only and are not nationally representative. Data are made available in WISQARS™ (Web-based Injury Statistics Query and Reporting System), an interactive database system that provides customized reports of injury-related data.

Prevention Policies and Practices

Beginning in the late 2000s, many projects were established with funding from Core SIPP and descriptions of them provides excellent examples of public health prevention practices related to injury. As with most public health interventions, initiatives were implemented at the state and local levels to ensure culturally appropriate communications and in other ways be responsive to local needs, preferences, and conditions. In terms of primary and secondary prevention, interventions can be grouped as follows:

- *Primary Prevention*
  - Educating population at risk and related persons on how to reduce risk of the health problem
  - Changing the social and/or physical environment to prevent health problems from occurring, including advocacy and policy solutions
- *Secondary and Tertiary Prevention*
  - Providing services for victims of a health problem, including screening, treatment, and supportive services

KEY IDEA

Two prevention and control initiatives aimed at reducing motor vehicle injuries among children and teens are *Child Passenger Safety* and *Teen Drivers*. We will discuss both initiatives—surveillance, research, policy, and program implementation.

As we will see, both the *Child Passenger Safety* and *Teen Drivers* initiatives emphasize primary prevention, particularly education. This does not mean that providing health care services, that is, secondary and tertiary prevention, does not occur at other levels—state and local—for children who have sustained motor vehicle injuries. Much of this care—including screening, diagnosis, and treatment of injury victims—is provided through public and private health insurance plans. Moreover, the provision of medical care for all people is a major goal of public health, and the general public health effort to ensure access to health care for all through support of health care reform will be discussed later in the chapter. The public health effort to ensure health care for all must be viewed as a component of motor vehicle injury interventions that is supported by public health.

Child Passenger Safety Program

The *Child Passenger Safety* program has been a major public health initiative since its inception in the 1970s. Motor vehicle crashes are one of the most common causes of child injury and death in the United States. In 2020, they accounted for one of every four unintentional child injury deaths, with 72% of these to child passengers. In 2020, 607 child passengers younger than 13 were killed in motor vehicle crashes, and more than 63,000 were injured. Public health efforts, including the *Child Passenger Safety* program, have had a positive effect. Child passenger injuries and death have greatly declined: In 2020, child passenger deaths were 56% lower than in 1975 (IIHS-HLDI, 2023a) due to efforts by public health partners to reduce the risk factors associated with child passenger deaths.

DID YOU KNOW?

Safety research has been the basis for the improvements in child passenger safety that we see today. Two investigations into the risk factors for child motor vehicle accidents are described here (CDC, 2012). These two studies and many others have provided the information base for public health efforts to prevent and control childhood motor vehicle accidents.

Children's Hospital of Philadelphia Study
Study: Interview with parents of children younger than 16 years involved in a motor vehicle crash.

   Main outcome measures: Typical use of child restraints, type of restraint in use at the time of the crash, parents' understanding of child restraint laws in their state, and parents' understanding of how the motor vehicle crash had affected the child's daily life.

   Findings: Children with one or more physical limitations after the crash accounts for 3.3%. Parents were more likely to report physical limitations among older children (7.6%) than younger children (1%). Children whose whiplash injuries were reported to have physical limitations after their injury accounts for 47%. Children who were not restrained optimally were nearly twice as likely as optimally restrained children to have physical limitations.

Alcohol-Impaired Driving and Children in the Household
Study: Second Injury Control and Risk Survey, a nationally representative cross-sectional telephone survey of adults.

   Main outcome measure: Alcohol-impaired driving by an adult with a child in the household.

   Findings: An estimated 2.5 million adult drivers with children living in their households reported that they had been a recent alcohol-impaired driver.

Risk Factors for Child Motor Vehicle Injuries and Fatalities

The risk factors for motor vehicle injuries and fatalities among children have been identified through the surveillance and research functions of the NCIPC's *Child Passenger Safety* program. They include the following:

A Drinking Driver
- Twenty-four percent of motor vehicle–related deaths among children ages 0 to 14 years involved a drinking driver.

- A higher proportion of children killed in a motor vehicle crash and riding with an alcohol-impaired driver were not restrained (56%), compared to 38% of children where the driver was not alcohol impaired.

Improper or No Use of Seat Belt or Booster Seat
- The rate of serious and fatal injuries to children can be reduced by half by using age- and size-appropriate car and booster seats.
- Restraint use among young children often depends on the driver's seat belt use. Almost 40% of children riding with unbelted drivers were themselves unrestrained.
- Child restraint systems are often used incorrectly. One study found that 72% of nearly 3,500 observed car and booster seats were misused in a way that could be expected to increase a child's risk of injury during a crash.

Placing Child in the Front Seat of a Motor Vehicle
- Riding in the back seat reduces the risk of serious injury to children under 16 by 40% (NCIPC & CDC, 2022a).

Prevention Policies and Practices for Child Motor Vehicle Safety

The principal interventions that have been supported by the research of the *Child Passenger Safety* initiative have concerned educating people about the need to use booster seats or seat belts; providing car seats themselves to people with children; and advocating for safety seat laws and their enforcement. There is strong evidence that child safety seat laws, safety seat distribution and education programs, communitywide education and enforcement campaigns, and incentive-plus-education programs are effective in increasing child safety seat use (NCIPC & CDC, 2022a).

Thus, educating parents to use car seats and seat belts for their children is a pervasive theme in the interventions used to prevent child passenger injuries. The program, *Protect the Ones You Love*, is an example. The *Child Passenger Safety* website contains materials that can be used in educational campaigns including information about the risk of injury and tips for parents about how to keep their child safe in a motor vehicle (CDC, 2023):

> We all want to keep our children safe and secure and help them live to their full potential. Knowing how to prevent leading causes of child injury, like road traffic injuries, is a step toward this goal. Every hour, 150 children between ages 0 and 19 are treated in emergency departments for injuries sustained in motor vehicle crashes. More children ages 5–19 die from crash-related injuries than from any other type of injury. Thankfully, parents can play a key role in protecting the children they love from road traffic injuries. . . .
>
> Prevention tips: One of the best protective measures you can take is using seat belts, child safety seats, and booster seats that are appropriate for your child's age and weight. (CDC, 2023, paras. 1–4)

However, education alone has not been found effective. The Task Force on Community Preventive Services (TFCPS, 2005, 2018) did not find evidence that education programs that provide information to parents, children, or professional groups about the importance of child safety seats and how to use them properly were effective when used alone. A caveat is that the task force also said that evidence was insufficient because the educational interventions evaluated in their studies varied widely and the small number of available studies produced inconsistent results. The task force did find, however, that incentive and education programs that reward parents for obtaining and correctly using child safety seats or directly reward children for correctly using safety seats are effective, and these programs also include educational components.

The TFCPS (2005, 2018) identified and rated the evidence on effectiveness for several interventions of this type. Child safety seat laws require children traveling in motor vehicles to be buckled into federally approved infant or child safety seats that are appropriate for the child's age and size. All states currently have child safety seat laws in place. The laws, which vary from state to state, specify the children they cover in terms of age, height, weight, or a combination of these factors. In 2005, the task force found the following improvements in child safety due to these laws:

- Child safety seat laws are effective in reducing fatal injuries to children by approximately 35%.
- These laws are also effective in reducing all injuries to children by approximately 17%.
- These laws are also effective in increasing child safety seat use by approximately 13 percentage points (TFCPS, 2005, p. 334).

These laws continue to have a positive effect on child safety today (TFCPS, 2018).

Other interventions that public health advocates for change are the social or physical environments to prevent childhood motor vehicle injuries and fatalities:

- Distribution and education programs provide free or low-cost child safety seats to parents, along with education about proper use of the seats. The idea behind such programs is that parents who cannot afford a safety seat or who have a poor understanding of the importance of the seat might be more likely to use it if they receive financial help in acquiring a safety seat and learn about the importance of using it (TFCPS, 2005, p. 335).
- Communitywide information and enhanced enforcement campaigns provide information about child safety seats and child automobile safety to an entire community (usually defined geographically). These campaigns use several approaches: mass media, publicity, safety seat displays in public places, and special law enforcement strategies, such as checkpoints, dedicated law enforcement officials, or alternative penalties (e.g., warnings instead of tickets; TFCPS, 2005, p. 337).

Child passenger deaths have declined steadily since they were identified in the 1970s as a public health problem that could be prevented. Further, the CDC and its partners continue to emphasize research that examines what interventions are the most effective at increasing consistent and correct use of child safety seats and booster seats. The agency seeks to improve strategies that increase child passenger safety (NCIPC & CDC, 2023; TFCPS, 2018). These include changes to the social and physical environment through a combination of laws, incentives, and community-wide education campaigns.

Teen Drivers Program

Another major public health initiative begun in the 1970s—*Teen Drivers* program— is aimed at reducing motor vehicle death and injury among teens. In 2020, motor vehicle crashes took an enormous toll on 13- to 19-year olds in the United States. There were about 2,800 teens killed and about 227,000 injured in motor vehicle crashes. This number is equivalent to about eight deaths and hundreds of injuries per day. It is also estimated that teen motor vehicle crashes resulted in about $40.7 billion in medical costs (NCIPC & CDC, 2022e). Efforts to decrease the burden of teen injury and death from motor vehicle crashes have had success. Despite the magnitude of death and injury occurring today, teenage crash deaths have declined substantially since 1975—71% among males and 61% among females (II-HS-HLDI, 2023b). Following is a description of the Teen Driver initiative and its findings.

Risk Factors for Teen Motor Vehicle Fatalities and Injuries

The risk factors for motor vehicle fatalities and injuries by teen drivers have been identified through the surveillance and research functions of the NCIPC's *Teen Driver* program (NCIPC & CDC, 2022e). They include the following:

Being 16 to 19 Years Old
- The risk of motor vehicle crashes is higher among 16- to 19-year-olds than among any other age group. Per mile driven, teen drivers ages 16 to 19 are three times more likely than older drivers to crash.

Male Teen
- The motor vehicle crash death rate for male drivers ages 16 to 19 years was three times as high as the death rate for female drivers in the same age group in 2020

Teen Driving With Teen Passengers
- The presence of teen passengers increases the crash risk of unsupervised teen drivers. This risk increases with the number of teen passengers.

- The presence of male teenage passengers increases the likelihood of risky driving behavior.

Newly Licensed Teen

- Crash risk is particularly high during the first year that teenagers are eligible to drive.

Inexperience

- Teens are more likely than older drivers to underestimate or not be able to recognize dangerous situations, as well as more likely to make critical errors that can lead to serious crashes.

Nighttime and Weekend Driving

- Nighttime driving is riskier than daytime driving for drivers of all ages, but particularly for teen drivers. Per miles driven, the fatal crash rate at night for teen drivers (ages 16–19 years) is about three times as high as for adult drivers (ages 30–59 years). About 44% of crash deaths among teens ages 13 to 19 occurred between 9 p.m. and 6 a.m., and 50% occurred on Friday, Saturday, or Sunday in 2020.

Not Using Seat Belts

- Not wearing a seatbelt is a risk factor. Among teen drivers and passengers 16 to 19 years of age who were killed in car crashes in 2020, 56% were not wearing a seat belt at the time of the crash.

Distracted Driving

- Distraction negatively affects driving performance for all drivers but can be especially dangerous for young, inexperienced drivers. In 2019, among U.S. high school students who drove, 39% texted or e-mailed while driving at least once during the prior 30 days.

Speeding

- Teens are more likely than older drivers to speed and to allow shorter distances from the front of one vehicle to the front of the next. About 35% of male drivers and 18% of female drivers (ages 15–20 years), involved in fatal crashes, were speeding.

Drinking Alcohol or Using Drugs

- Any amount of alcohol consumption before driving increases the risk of crashes among teen drivers, and their risk is greater than older drivers with the same concentration of alcohol. Drug use is also a risk factor.

Prevention Policies and Practices for Teen Motor Vehicle Safety

Similar to the *Child Passenger Safety* initiative, *Teen Drivers* also emphasizes education, and in addition, advocates for changes in the environment that will reduce the risk of injury and death among teen drivers. The CDC named motor vehicle injuries as one of its "Winnable Battles," meaning they believed that with targeted efforts and interventions, there could be a sizable impact on the injuries and deaths related to motor vehicles in the near future.

Common types of educationally oriented interventions to promote safe teen driving include school-based instructional programs, peer organizations, and social norming campaigns (Elder et al., 2005). They generally focus on prevention of driving after drinking (DD) and riding with drinking drivers (RDD). A review of the effectiveness of various kinds of programs summarized each type of program in 2005, which is still relevant in 2023:

> School-based instructional programs are a commonly used approach to addressing the problems of DD and RDD. These programs vary widely in their focus, with some targeting a variety of consequences of substance use and others more directly focused on problems related to alcohol-impaired driving. . . . Many of the more recent school-based programs to prevent DD and RDD are either explicitly theory-based or incorporate theory-based concepts and methods, such as peer intervention social deviance, educational inoculation, and risk skills training. . . .
>
> Social norming programs generally consist of ongoing, multiyear public information programs conducted on college campuses to reduce alcohol use, although they can also be conducted in other settings and for other target behaviors. The key objective is to provide students with more objective normative information regarding student alcohol consumption, thus reducing their misperceptions and ultimately changing their behavior.
>
> School-based peer organizations are groups of students, often with faculty advisors, who encourage other students to refrain from drinking, DD, and RDD. An example is Students Against Destructive Decisions (SADD), formerly called Students Against Drunk Driving. They include both didactic and interactive delivery, usually involving peer-to-peer delivery, but frequently involving outside experts as well. (Elder et al., 2005, pp. 290–294)

Educational programs may also focus on the parents' role in teen driving. For instance, *Parents Are the Key* materials help parents understand how to help their teens avoid motor vehicle crashes by improving parental management of the process of learning to drive. This includes developing a Parent–Teen Driving Agreement. These kinds of interventions encourage parental restrictions and oversight on newly licensed teen drivers (NCIPC & CDC, 2022e).

Interventions that target the larger social and physical environments include advocacy for building safer motor vehicles, enforcement of laws related to drunk driving, and changing community attitudes about teen driving. Regarding laws and law enforcement, lowering blood alcohol concentrations laws for young or inexperienced drivers; instituting sobriety checkpoints; and raising the minimum legal drinking age (MLDA) laws to 21 years of age (or maintain the age at 21 years) have all been found effective in reducing fatalities and injuries among teen drivers and their passengers (NCIPC & CDC, 2022e). These legal interventions are strongly advocated by public health.

A public health advocacy issue related to teen driving is the graduated driver licensing (GDL), a system of laws and practices that gradually introduce young drivers into the driving population (NCIPC & CDC, 2022e). Full licensing is delayed while the teen gets initial driving experiences under low-risk conditions. GDL is associated with reductions of 19% for injury crashes and 21% for fatal crashes among 16-year-olds. GDL systems exist in all U.S. states and the District of Columbia, but the strength of GDL laws varies by state. The best practice is a three-stage GDL that includes:

Stage 1: Learner's Permit
- Minimum age of 16 to obtain a learner's permit
- A requirement to have a learner's permit for at least 12 months
- At least 70 supervised practice hours

Stage 2: Intermediate/Provisional License
- No teen or young adult passengers
- Restrictions on nighttime driving (from 9 or 10 p.m. until 5 a.m., or sometimes longer)

Stage 3: Full Licensure
- Minimum age of 18 to obtain a full license

Success of Motor Vehicle Injury Prevention Efforts for Children and Teens

Have the public health efforts through Core SIPP and other projects funded by the CDC to reduce motor vehicle injuries among children and teens been successful? There is some evidence that suggests they have. First, a study of trends in motor vehicle deaths between 1999 and 2019 found a marked decline in deaths for both males and females 24 years and younger, beginning around 2000 and accelerating about 2005 (Spencer et al., 2021)—the period in which the NCIPC was increasing its efforts in injury control and prevention (NCIPC & CDC, 2022c; see **Figure 5.1** for males):

- In 1999, rates among males were highest for those aged 15 to 24 (35.0 per 100,000). By 2019, the rate for males aged 15 to 24 (19.0) was lower than that for males aged 25 to 64 (19.7) and 65 and over (21.8).
- Throughout the period, rates among males were lowest for those aged 0 to 14; rates decreased 56% from 4.5 in 1999 to 2.0 in 2019 (Spencer et al., 2021, p. 2).

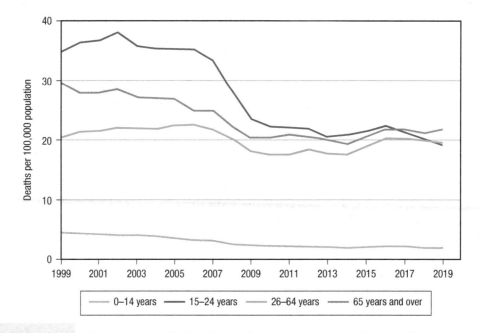

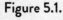

Figure 5.1.   Motor Vehicle Traffic Death Rates Among Males, by Age Group: United States, 1999–2019

[1] Stable trend from 1999 to 2006; significant decreasing trend from 2006 to 2010 ($p < .05$); stable trend from 2010 through 2019.

[2] Stable trend from 1999 to 2005; significant decreasing trend from 2005 to 2010 ($p < .05$); stable trend from 2010 through 2019.

[3] Significant increasing trend from 1999 to 2006; significant decreasing trend from 2006 to 2010; significant increasing trend from 2010 through 2019 ($p < .05$).

[4] Significant decreasing trend from 1999 to 2010, with varying rates of change ($p < .05$); stable trend from 2010 through 2019.

Source: Spencer, M. R., Hedegaard, H., & Garnett, M. (2021). Motor vehicle traffic death rates, by sex, age group, and road user type: United States, 1999–2019. *NCHS Data Brief*, (400). https://www.cdc.gov/nchs/data/databriefs/db400-H.pdf

For females, there are similar findings. Rates among females in 1999 were highest for those 15 to 24 years old and 65 years and over—15.7 and 15.8/100,000, respectively. However, the rates for women 15 to 24 had declined by 2019 to 8.2/100,000 population. Throughout the period, rates among females were lowest for those aged 0 to 14. These rates decreased 54% from 3.5 in 1999 to 1.7 in 2019. See **Figure 5.2.**

Second, another indication that public health efforts to reduce injury and death from motor vehicle crashes among young people met with success is found in trends in emergency department visits between 2005 and 2018 (NCHS & CDC, 2022b). There was a trend downward in visits for motor vehicle crashes among both men and women under 18 years old and 18 to 24 years old. See **Table 5.5.**

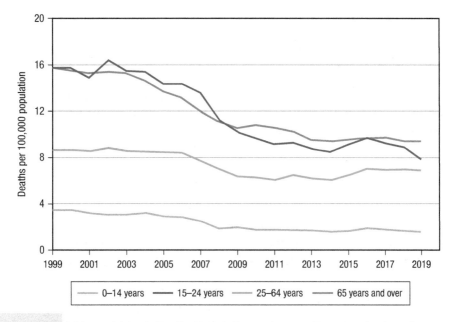

Figure 5.2.   Motor Vehicle Traffic Death Rates Among Females, by Age Group: United States, 1999–2019

[1] Stable trend from 1999 to 2004; significant decreasing trend from 2004 to 2014, with varying rates of change ($p < .05$); stable trend from 2014 through 2019.

[2] Stable trend from 1999 to 2004; significant decreasing trend from 2006 to 2010; significant increasing trend from 2010 through 2019 ($p < .05$).

[3] Stable trend from 1999 to 2006; significant decreasing trend from 2006 to 2010 ($p < .05$); stable trend from 2010 through 2019.

[4] Significant decreasing trend from 1999 to 2006 ($p < .05$); stable trend from 2006 through 2019.

Source: Spencer, M. R., Hedegaard, H., & Garnett, M. (2021). Motor vehicle traffic death rates, by sex, age group, and road user type: United States, 1999–2019. *NCHS Data Brief*, (400). https://www.cdc.gov/nchs/data/databriefs/db400-H.pdf

Many factors undoubtedly played a part in the reduction we see in fatalities and emergency department visits for motor vehicle injuries among children and teens. These could include improvements to motor vehicle safety such as air bags and laws that have discouraged alcohol-impaired driving. But did the Institute of Medicine's and the National Academy of Sciences' 1985 and 1989 reports calling for a consolidated federal focus on injury prevention, which was followed by the CDC's concerted focus on injury, spark the improvements we see? This is a question worth considering by people who hope to improve the health of populations through public action in the future.

CHILDHOOD OBESITY

Since the 1960s, childhood obesity has been seen as a worldwide health problem (Organization for Economic Cooperation and Development [OECD], 2011; International Association for the Study of Obesity [IASO], 2012, 2014). It is particularly concerning because of the many chronic conditions that are related to obesity, which include high blood pressure, high cholesterol, type 2 diabetes, breathing problems such as asthma and sleep apnea, and joint problems (DNPAO & CDC, 2022b).

By 2010, the IASO had determined the number of children who were overweight, including obese, globally (see **Figure 5.3**). The IASO estimated that over 200 million children 5 to 17 years of age were obese or overweight. The IASO reported that even while obesity rates vary by country, ranging from 5% in Africa to over 30% in the United States, childhood obesity had been on the rise since the 1960s and was a severe and growing threat to public health.

As noted in **Figure 5.3**, the United States had a serious childhood obesity problem in 2010, and this has continued through 2020. In 2017 to 2020, for children and adolescents aged 2 to 19 years, the prevalence of obesity was 19.7%, and obesity affected about 14.7 million children and adolescents (DNPAO & CDC, 2022b).

In the United States, the DNPAO is the CDC's lead division for obesity prevention and control. The DNPAO is at the forefront in the development of knowledge about obesity—its prevalence, incidence, risk factors, causes, and consequences. This information, then, is being used to develop prevention interventions—primary, secondary, and tertiary. The following description of public health practice related to the prevention and control of obesity is from the CDC's DNPAO (2022a), which again is the predominant actor in terms of agenda setting, surveillance and research, and source of funding to stimulate prevention strategies. The emphasis is on childhood obesity.

Health Consequences of Childhood Obesity

The increased number of obese children in the United States has resulted in an increased prevalence of serious medical conditions in this population. Diseases that were once considered adult problems are now being diagnosed in obese children including diseases of the kidneys, pancreas, heart, and circulatory system. Pediatricians have become accustomed to treating diseases in the child population that were previously prevalent only in adults, and the childhood obesity epidemic has changed the practice of pediatrics, such that pediatricians now commonly treat type 1 diabetes, hypertension, elevated cholesterol, and hyperlipidemia. Obese children have been found to have an increased risk of type 2 diabetes (Trevino et al., 2008).

The circulatory system of the obese child is also affected. Obese children are more likely than normal weight children to have elevated cholesterol, hypertension, and hyperlipidemia (Freedman et al., 2001). Hypertension, or high blood pressure, stresses the heart because the heart muscle has to work harder to pump blood throughout the body. Obesity in childhood increases the amount of time throughout the life span in which the heart is undergoing stress. Children who are obese also suffer from hyperlipidemia, an excess of fat in the blood, at a higher rate than nonobese children. The circulatory system expends more effort to move

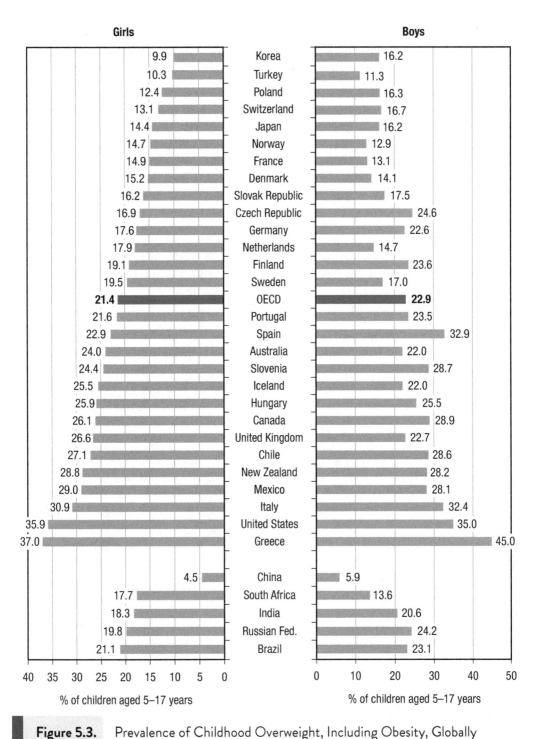

Figure 5.3. Prevalence of Childhood Overweight, Including Obesity, Globally

Source: Organization for Economic Development and Cooperation. (2011). *Obesity update 2012.* http://www.oecd
.org/health/49716427.pdf

blood through the body as a result of hyperlipidemia. These three disorders have a major effect on the heart later in the obese child's life. A child with these conditions will have an increased likelihood of adult heart and circulatory problems.

In addition to physical health problems, childhood obesity has a negative impact on social relationships and sense of well-being. Not surprisingly, research has found that obese children are at greater risk than their normal weight counterparts of having low social status in school (Friedlander et al., 2003; McNeely & Crosnoe, 2008). They are more likely to be the targets of bullying, teasing, and scorn, which have long-term emotional consequences including depression and low self-esteem (Moran, 1999).

Studies have also indicated that obese children maintain and increase their body mass index (BMI) scores in adulthood to become obese adults (Serdula et al., 1993). One study of students 13 to 20 years of age found that only 14.7% reduced their weight below the 95th percentile, which represents the obesity level (Gordon-Larsen et al., 2004). Another study found that approximately 80% of overweight children 10 to 15 years of age become obese by age 25 (Whitaker et al., 1997).

The adverse effects of obesity on child health, as well as the long-term, negative effects of childhood obesity on adult health, have motivated public health to seek solutions to the problem, as we will discuss next. The examples—provided from the recent past—exemplify the kinds of prevention and control programs and policies that have continued to be implemented in the United States.

Defining and Measuring Childhood Obesity

Overweight and obesity are defined by WHO as "abnormal or excessive fat accumulation that may impair health" (WHO, 2022). There are a number of methods of measuring obesity and overweight. These include skinfold thickness measurements (with calipers), underwater weighing, bioelectrical impedance, dual-energy x-ray absorptiometry (DXA), and isotope dilution. However, these methods are expensive and, in addition, need to be performed with expensive equipment by highly trained personnel. Further, many of them can be difficult to standardize across observers or machines, making comparisons across studies and time periods difficult and unreliable (DNPAO & CDC, 2022c).

As a result, the **BMI** is commonly used in studies of overweight and obesity in populations and individuals although it is not as accurate as more expensive measures of obesity and overweight. BMI is a simple index of weight-to-height that is calculated as the weight of an individual in kilograms divided by the square of the height in meters (kg/m^2). BMI provides the most useful population-level measure of overweight and obesity as it is the same for both sexes and for all ages of adults. However, it should be considered as a rough guide because it may not correspond to the same degree of fatness in different individuals (WHO, 2022, para. 3).

The current WHO Child Growth Standards, launched in April 2006, include BMI charts for infants and young children up to age 5. Additionally, WHO has developed Growth Reference Data for children 5 to 9 years. "It is a reconstruction of the 1977 National Center for Health Statistics (NCHS)/WHO reference and uses the original NCHS data set supplemented with data from WHO child growth standards sample for children up to age 5" (WHO, 2022).

The BMI is calculated for children and adults in the same way, but the criteria used to interpret the BMI for children and adolescents are different from those for adults. For children, overweight and obesity use age- and sex-specific growth charts. These growth charts are a series of percentile curves that illustrate the distribution of selected body measurements in children and have been used to track the growth of infants, children, and adolescents in the United States since 1977. See **Figure 5.4** for an example of a growth chart. The reasons for using

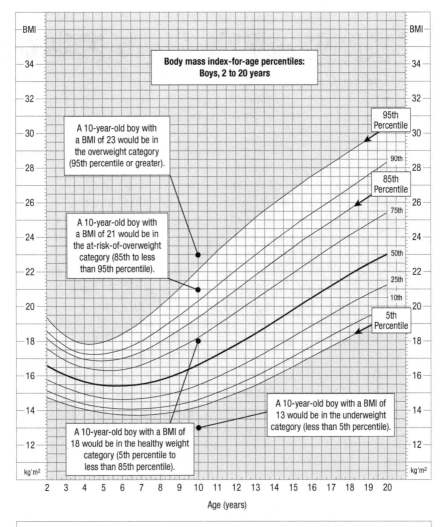

Figure 5.4.   Growth Chart With Body Mass Index for Boys, 2 to 20 Years

age- and sex-specific percentiles from growth charts to determine overweight and obesity in children are that the amount of body fat changes with age; and the amount of body fat differs between girls and boys.

In the United States, the CDC recommends the use of WHO growth standards to monitor growth for infants and children ages 0 to 2 years of age and the CDC growth charts for children age 2 years and older. Using these growth charts:

- Overweight is defined as a BMI at or above the 85th percentile and lower than the 95th percentile.
- Obesity is defined as a BMI at or above the 95th percentile for children of the same age and sex (DNPAO & CDC, 2022a).

DID YOU KNOW?

Sources of Childhood Obesity Data
As with other public health efforts, data systems are necessary to provide information about the incidence, prevalence, and risk factors for obesity; to conduct research on the causes and consequences of obesity; and to evaluate the effectiveness of interventions aimed at preventing and controlling obesity. Surveillance data for obesity are obtained from the National Health and Nutrition Examination Survey (NHANES), which is program of studies designed to assess the health and nutritional status of adults and children in the United States. It is unique in that it combines interviews and physical examinations. NHANES is a major program of the National Center for Health Statistics (NCHS).

About 5,000 persons are surveyed each year. The NHANES interview includes demographic, socioeconomic, dietary, and health-related questions. The examination component consists of medical, dental, and physiological measurements, as well as laboratory tests administered by highly trained medical personnel. NHANES findings are used to determine the prevalence of major diseases and risk factors for diseases and provide information to assess nutritional status and its association with health promotion and disease prevention. They are the basis for national standards for such measurements as height, weight, and blood pressure (NCHS & CDC, 2022a).

In addition to NHANES, some states continue to implement data-based programs developed by DNPAO, but discontinued at the federal level after 2011. These are two surveillance systems that are program based: Pediatric Nutrition Surveillance System (PedNSS) and Pregnancy Nutrition Surveillance System (PNSS). Both are used to monitor the nutritional status of low-income infants, children, and women in federally funded maternal and child health programs. PedNSS provides data on the prevalence and trends of nutrition-related problems. PNSS is used to identify risk factors associated with infant mortality and poor birth outcomes. The data sources for PedNSS and PNSS are existing data from the following public health programs for nutrition surveillance:

- Special Supplemental Nutrition Program for Women, Infants, and Children (WIC)
- Early and Periodic Screening, Diagnosis, and Treatment (EPSDT) Program (PedNSS only)

Risk Factors for Childhood Obesity

Based on the extensive surveillance and research conducted or sponsored by DNPAO, WHO, and other organizations, we know a great deal about the risk of childhood obesity in the United States, as we shall discuss now.

Age, sex, race/ethnicity, and socioeconomic status of children impact the risk of childhood obesity in America. Recent findings using NHANES data from 2017 to 2018 are revealing:

- The obesity rate among young people ages 12 to 19 is 21.2%, compared to 20.3% for youth ages 6 to 11 and 13.4% for the youngest group, ages 2 to 5.
- Obesity rates are higher among boys than girls.
- African Americans, Hispanics, and Native Americans have the highest rates of childhood obesity in the United States. Prevalence of obesity is 26.2% among Hispanic children, 24.8% among non-Hispanic Black children, 16.6% among non-Hispanic White children, and 9.0% among non-Hispanic Asian children (DNPAO & CDC, 2022b).
- By gender and race/ethnicity, obesity rates are higher for non-Hispanic Black girls (29.1%) and Hispanic boys (28.1%). Non-Hispanic Asian children had the lowest obesity rates across all races, with the rate among boys at 12.4% and for girls, 5.1% (Robert Wood Johnson Foundation, 2021, January 14).

In the United States, lower socioeconomic status is one of the most important risk factors for childhood obesity (see **Figure 5.5**). The association between socioeconomic status, race and ethnicity, and childhood obesity is highly related to nutrition: fewer healthy choices in supermarkets in low-income, minority neighborhoods; more eating at fast food restaurants because of convenience and availability; and the high cost of more nutritious, lower calorie foods. Hemmingsson (2018, p. 204) argues further that socioeconomic adversity is a "key upstream catalyst that sets the stage for critical midstream risk factors such as family strain and dysfunction, offspring insecurity, stress, emotional turmoil, low self-esteem, and poor mental health." These midstream risk factors, particularly stress and emotional turmoil, motivate calorie-dense junk food self-medication and subtle addiction, to relieve psychological and emotional discomfort.

In terms of specific food intake, longitudinal studies have found a strong association between obesity and sugar-sweetened beverage consumption. Some cross-sectional studies have found that other eating-related behaviors contribute to childhood overweight. These include buying lunch at school, eating supper while watching television or without family supervision, consuming less energy at breakfast or more at dinner, and missing breakfast (Moreno & Rodriguez, 2007).

Lack of physical activity is another important risk factor for childhood obesity. Coupled with poor eating habits, a sedentary life style is highly likely to lead to excessive weight gain. Time in front of the television and computer is particularly implicated (Hu et al., 2003; Robinson, 1998). The adverse effect of television

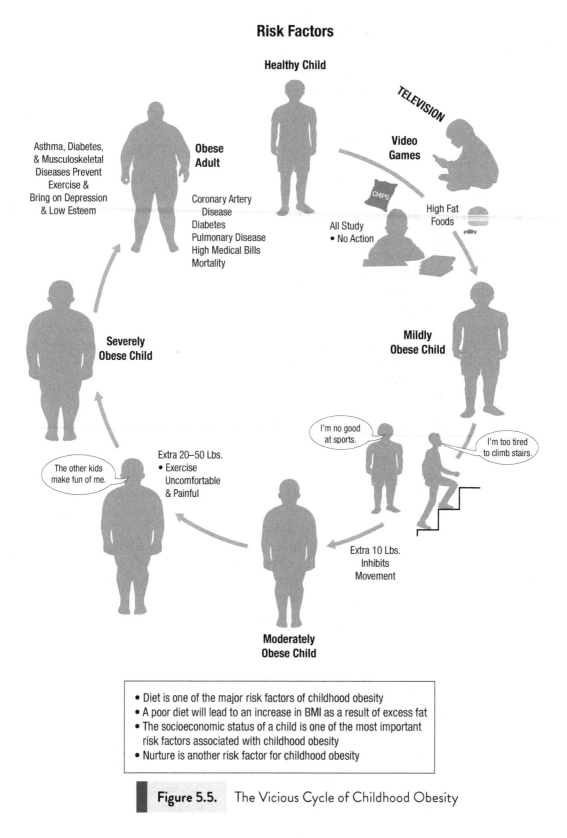

Figure 5.5.   The Vicious Cycle of Childhood Obesity

watching on physical activity is compounded by the accompanying exposure to advertising for poor food choices such as sweetened beverages and breakfast foods. Other technologies such as video games further reduce the time children in the United States spend in physical activity.

Parents and schools impact the risk of childhood obesity. Multiple studies have shown a strong correlation between childhood obesity and parental obesity. Children tend to learn their eating habits from their parents, and a child's risk of becoming obese doubles if one or both of the parents are obese (Fuemmeler et al., 2013). There may also be a familial link in that children of parents who were obese as kids tend to have high BMIs (Li et al., 2009). On the other hand, parents can influence children to eat healthily by setting an example and providing nutritious meals at home. In addition, schools can have a large impact on food choices, impacting childhood obesity for better or worse. A school cafeteria that provides a soda vending machine is enabling a child to make a poor choice.

Prevention Policies and Practices for Childhood Obesity

Under the **Nutrition, Physical Activity and Obesity Program (NPAO)**, a cooperative agreement between the DNPAO and 23 state health departments, interventions were developed to prevent and control childhood obesity. The NPAO's goal was to prevent and control obesity and other chronic diseases through healthful eating and physical activity. The state programs developed strategies to leverage resources and coordinate statewide efforts with multiple partners to address all of the following DNPAO principal target areas:

- Increase physical activity;
- Increase the consumption of fruits and vegetables;
- Decrease the consumption of sugar-sweetened beverages;
- Increase breastfeeding initiation, duration, and exclusivity;
- Reduce the consumption of high energy dense foods; and
- Decrease television viewing (CDC, 2014).

States were guided by the CDC's *Recommended Community Strategies and Measurements to Prevent Obesity in the United States: Implementation and Measurement Guide* (Keener et al., 2009). The strategies were aimed at changing the social and physical environments at the local level—a community-based approach to ensure that there were opportunities and incentives for all to obtain nutritious food and engage in physical activity, thereby addressing the underlying causes of obesity. The strategies did not rely on education alone. Rather, they were implemented through policy changes and partnerships with local organizations. As the authors write, "This product is the result of an innovative and collaborative process that seeks to reverse the U.S. obesity epidemic by transforming communities into places where healthy lifestyle choices are easily incorporated into everyday life. To reverse the obesity epidemic, we must change our physical and food environments to provide more opportunities for people to eat healthy foods and to be physically active on a daily basis" (Keener et al., 2009, p. ii). The 24 strategies, which the CDC recommended to encourage and support healthy lives, are contained in Appendix 5.1. Each strategy is illustrated by a community-based example of its implementation.

Success of Childhood Obesity Prevention Efforts

The problem of childhood obesity in the United States remains, although there have been successes. In 2014, the CDC found declines in obesity among low-income preschoolers in 19 of 43 states/territories examined. Twenty states and Puerto Rico held steady at their current rate, and obesity increased slightly in three states. Nevertheless, one in eight preschoolers is obese in the United States (DNPAO, 2019, December 6). See Figure 5.6.

A more recent study by Anderson et al. (2019) found some positive news and some negative news about childhood obesity in the United States. The findings—positive and negative—from their long-term study are as follows:

- The prevalence of childhood obesity in the United States more than tripled over the last four decades from 5% in 1978 to 18.5% in 2016.

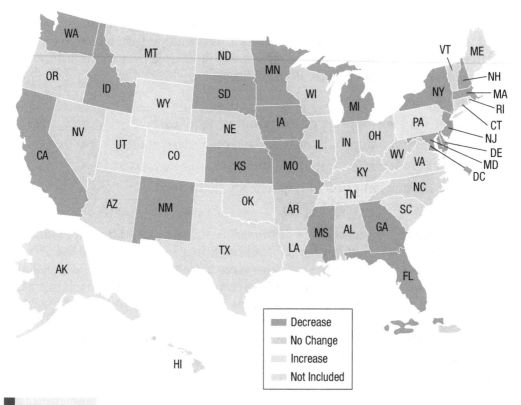

Figure 5.6.   Many States and U.S. Territories Are Showing Decreases in Childhood Obesity

- There is evidence of a slowing. After increasing from 0.4% to 0.7% per year between 1978 and 2004, the rate of increase slowed to 0.1% per year between 2004 and 2016.
- The prevalence of obesity increased steadily through approximately age 10, and levels were relatively unchanged after that.
- The prevalence of obesity varied by race, especially among children entering kindergarten, with Black and Hispanic children most likely to be obese.
- Overall and among all subgroups the rate of growth in obesity from kindergarten through third grade declined (Anderson et al., 2019).

Public health and its partners have been motivated to reduce childhood obesity because of its severely adverse effects on child health, as well as its long-term, negative impact on adult health. The examples here—provided from the recent past—exemplify the kinds of prevention and control programs and policies that have continued to be implemented in the United States. They involve counseling parents to increase child physical activity and nutritious food intake. They also consider access to physical activity and nutritious food in communities and how to improve these attributes in child environments. Individually, many programs have led to reductions in obesity among children. However, overall, the problem remains a serious one in the United States. Clearly, prevention efforts are still needed to sustain and expand gains made to reduce childhood obesity.

CHAPTER SUMMARY

Today, noninfectious diseases and injuries predominate as the leading causes of mortality and morbidity in the United States. Even though infectious diseases are historically significant to public health, the scope and practice of public health has steadily changed since the 19th century in response to the predominance of noninfectious diseases and injuries.

The basic public health approach to prevention and control of noninfectious diseases and injury begins with research to determine magnitude and risk factors, followed by development of policies and practices to address them. Implementation of policies is next, often at the local level, and finally evaluation of implementation to facilitate improvement in policies and practices.

Two of many health problems that concern public health are motor vehicle injuries among children and teens and childhood obesity. Both are significant causes of morbidity and mortality among young people. The response to them illustrates public health practice for injury and noninfectious disease control beginning with research about magnitude of the problems and their risk factors. In both cases, policies and practices include a great deal of education and public communication with young people themselves, as well as their parents and teachers. They also include changing social and legal environments. In the case of motor vehicle safety this entails providing seatbelts and car seats and enforcing their use; lowering blood alcohol concentrations laws for young or inexperienced drivers; instituting sobriety checkpoints; raising the MLDA laws to 21 years of age (or maintain the age at 21 years); speed limit enforcement; and the GDL system. For childhood obesity, policies are aimed at increasing physical activity among children and improving access to nutritious foods. These efforts have had some success as evidenced by declines in motor vehicle deaths and injuries among young people and a more recent downward trend in childhood obesity, though neither result is considered satisfactory as yet.

DISCUSSION QUESTIONS

Q: What is the disease burden of noninfectious diseases in the United States?

Q: What is the disease burden of injuries in the United States?

Q: Describe a community-based approach to reducing childhood obesity that emphasizes the bottom layer of the Health Impact Pyramid (socioeconomic factors).

Q: Describe a community-based approach to reducing childhood obesity that emphasizes changing the context to make individuals' default decisions healthy (Health Impact Pyramid, layer 2).

Q: Describe a community-based approach to reducing childhood obesity that emphasizes long-lasting protective interventions (Health Impact Pyramid, layer 3).

NOTES

1. The mortality statistics presented in this report were compiled in accordance with World Health Organization (WHO) regulations, which specify that member countries classify and code causes of death in accordance with the current revision of the *International Classification of Diseases (ICD)*. The *ICD* provides the basic guidance used in virtually all countries to code and classify causes of death. Effective with deaths occurring in 1999, the United States began using the 10th revision of this classification. In 2022, the *ICD-11* became the official version for reporting. For earlier years, causes of death were classified according to the revisions then in use:

   1979–1998, Ninth Revision; 1968–1978, Eighth Revision, adapted for use in the United States; 1958–1967, Seventh Revision; and 1949–1957, Sixth Revision. Changes in classification of causes of death due to these revisions may result in discontinuities in cause-of-death trends. Consequently, cause-of-death comparisons among revisions require consideration of comparability ratios and, where available, estimates of their standard errors.

DATA SOURCES

Surveillance, data collection, and data analysis are essential to understanding how to control and prevent injury and noninfectious disease. For Chapter 6, the following data sources are useful for increasing your knowledge about the prevalence, incidence, risk factors, and costs of many noninfectious diseases and types of injuries in the United States. Each database is a product of the Centers for Disease Control and Prevention (CDC).

- DNPAO Interactive Database. This interactive database provides national and state-level data about the health status and behaviors of Americans as well as environmental or policy supports. Categories include breastfeeding, fruits and vegetables, physical activity, sugar drinks, television watching, and obesity/weight. Data can be examined by demographic characteristics such as gender and race/ethnicity, as well as by state and year. The data come from multiple sources. You can begin your investigation here: https://www.cdc.gov/nccdphp/dnpao/data-trends-maps/

- Web-Based Injury Statistics Query and Reporting System (WISQARS). CDC's WISQARS™ is an interactive, online database that provides fatal and nonfatal injury, violent death, and cost of injury data. Researchers, the media, public health professionals, and the public can use WISQARS™ data to learn more about the public health and economic burden associated with unintentional and violence-related injuries in the United States. WISQARS was introduced in 2000. It enables exploration of injury data, maps, and visualizations. Begin your investigation here: https://www.cdc.gov/injury/wisqars/index.html

- National Health and Nutrition Examination Survey (NHANES). NHANES is a program of studies designed to assess the health and nutritional status of adults and children in the United States. The survey is unique in that it combines interviews and physical examinations. NHANES is the basis for many studies of obesity. The data can be accessed and analyzed directly, and an online tutorial is available. There is also an interactive dashboard with the capability of visualizing certain trends. Start here for your exploration: https://www.cdc.gov/nchs/nhanes/index.htm

- Behavioral Risk Factor Surveillance System (BRFSS). The BRFSS is the nation's premier source of information about health-related risk behaviors, chronic health conditions, and use of preventive health services. Begun in 1984, BRFSS now collects data in all 50 states as well as the District of Columbia and three U.S. territories. With about 400,000 completed telephone interviews with adults each year, it is the largest continuously conducted health survey in the world. Begin exploring here: https://www.cdc.gov/brfss/index.html

A robust set of instructor resources designed to supplement this text is located at **http://connect.springerpub.com/content/book/978-0-8261-8615-7.** Qualifying instructors may request access by emailing **textbook@springerpub.com.**

REFERENCES

Anderson, P. M., Butcher, K. F., & Whitmore-Schanzenbach, D. (2019). Understanding recent trends in childhood obesity in the United States. *Economics & Human Biology, 34,* 16–25. https://doi.org/10.1016/j.ehb.2019.02.002

Centers for Disease Control and Prevention. (2010). *Parents are key.* http://www.cdc.gov/ParentsAreTheKey/about/index.html

Centers for Disease Control and Prevention. (2012). *Injury prevention and control: Motor vehicle injuries.* http://www.cdc.gov/motorvehiclesafety/index.html

Centers for Disease Control and Prevention. (2013). *Progress on childhood obesity.* http://www.cdc.gov/vitalsigns/childhoodobesity/

Centers for Disease Control and Prevention. (2014). *Division of nutrition, physical activity and obesity.* State Nutrition, Physical Activity and Obesity Programs, Cooperative Agreement DP08-805. https://www.cdc.gov/nccdphp/dnpao/state-local-programs/pdf/dnpao-805-coorperative-agreement-web_tag508.pdf

Centers for Disease Control and Prevention. (2022). *National health initiatives, strategies & action plans.* https://www.cdc.gov/publichealthgateway/strategy/index.html

Centers for Disease Control and Prevention. (2023). *Buckle up.* https://www.cdc.gov/transportationsafety/seatbelts/states.html

Dehghan, M., Akhtar-Danesh, N., & Merchant, A. T. (2005). Childhood obesity, prevalence and prevention. *Nutrition Journal, 4*(24). https://doi.org/10.1186/1475-2891-4-24

Division of Nutrition, Physical Activity, and Obesity & Centers of Disease Control and Prevention. (2021). *WISQARS: Leading causes of death visualization tool.* https://wisqars.cdc.gov/data/lcd/home

Division of Nutrition, Physical Activity, and Obesity & Centers of Disease Control and Prevention. (2022a). *About child and teen BMI.* https://www.cdc.gov/healthyweight/assessing/bmi/childrens_bmi/about_childrens_bmi.html

Division of Nutrition, Physical Activity, and Obesity & Centers of Disease Control and Prevention. (2022b). *Childhood obesity facts.* https://www.cdc.gov/obesity/data/childhood.html

Division of Nutrition, Physical Activity, and Obesity & Centers for Disease Control and Prevention. (2022c). *Childhood overweight and obesity.* https://www.cdc.gov/obesity/childhood/

Elder, R. W., Nichols, J. L., Shults, R. A., Sleet, D. A., Barrios, L. C., Compton R., & Task Force on Community Preventive Services. (2005). Effectiveness of school-based programs for reducing drinking and driving and riding with drinking drivers: A systematic review. *American Journal of Preventive Medicine, 28*(5S), 288–304. https://doi.org/10.1016/j.amepre.2005.02.015

Freedman, D. S., Khan, L. K., Dietz, W. H., Srinivasan, S. R., & Berenson, G. S. (2001). Relationship of childhood obesity to coronary heart disease risk factors in adulthood. *Pediatrics, 108*(3), 712–718. https://doi.org/10.1542/peds.108.3.712

Friedlander, S. L., Larkin, E. K., Rosen C. L., Palermo, T. M., & Redline, S. (2003). Decreased quality of life associated with childhood obesity. *Archives of Pediatrics & Adolescent Medicine, 157*, 1206–1211. https://doi.org/10.1001/archpedi.157.12.1206

Fuemmeler, B. F., Lovelady, C. A., Zucker, N. L., & Ostbye, T. (2013). Parental obesity moderates the relationship between childhood appetitive traits and weight. *Obesity, 21*(4): 815–823. https://doi.org/10.1002/oby.20144

Gordon-Larsen, P., Adair, L. S., Nelson, M. C., & Popkin, B. M. (2004). Five-year obesity incidence in the transition period between adolescence and adulthood: The National Longitudinal Study of Adolescent Health. *American Journal of Clinical Nutrition, 80*(3), 569–575. https://doi.org/10.1093/ajcn/80.3.569

Hemmingsson, E. (2018). Early childhood obesity risk factors: Socioeconomic adversity, family dysfunction, offspring distress, and junk food self-medication. *Current Obesity Reports, 7*, 204–209. https://link.springer.com/content/pdf/10.1007/s13679-018-0310-2.pdf

Heron, M. (2021). Deaths: Leading causes for 2019. *National Vital Statistics Reports, 70*(9), 1–114. https://doi.org/10.15620/cdc:107021

Hu, F. B., Li, T. Y., Colditz, G. A., Willet W. C., & Manson, J. E. (2003). Television watching and other sedentary behaviors in relation to risk of obesity and type 2 diabetes. *Journal of American Medical Association, 289*(14), 1785–1791. https://doi.org/10.1001/jama.289.14.1785

Insurance Institute for Highway Safety, Highway Loss Data Institute. (2023a). *Fatality facts 2021: Children.* https://www.iihs.org/topics/fatality-statistics/detail/children

Insurance Institute for Highway Safety, Highway Loss Data Institute. (2023b). *Fatality facts 2021: Teenagers.* https://www.iihs.org/topics/fatality-statistics/detail/teenagers

International Association for the Study of Obesity. (2012). Obesity the global epidemic. *Obesity & Research.* http://www.iaso.org/iotf/obesity/obesitytheglobalepidemic/

International Association for the Study of Obesity. (2014). *About obesity.* http://www.iaso.org/resources/aboutobesity/

Keener, D., Goodman, K., Lowry, A., Zaro, S., & Kettel Khan, L. (2009). *Recommended community strategies and measurements to prevent obesity in the United States: Implementation and measurement guide.* Centers for Disease Control and Prevention.

Li, L., Law, C., Lo Conte, R., & Power, C. (2009). Intergenerational influences on childhood body mass index: The effect of parental body mass index trajectories. *The American Journal of Clinical Nutrition, 89*(2), 551–557. https://doi.org/10.3945/ajcn.2008.26759

McNeely, C., & Crosnoe R. (2008). Social status peer influence, and weight gain in adolescence: Promising directions for addressing the obesity epidemic. *Archives of Pediatrics & Adolescent Medicine, 162*(1), 91–92. https://doi.org/10.1001/archpediatrics.2007.23

Moran, R. (1999). Evaluation and treatment of childhood obesity. *American Academy of Family Physicians, 59*(4), 861–868. https://pubmed.ncbi.nlm.nih.gov/10068710/

Moreno, L. A., & Rodriguez, G. (2007, May). Dietary risk factors for development of childhood obesity. *Current Opinion in Clinical Nutrition and Metabolic Care, 20*(3), 336–341. https://doi.org/10.1097/MCO.0b013e3280a94f59

National Center for Health Statistics & Centers for Disease Control and Prevention. (2010). *Health, United States, 2009: With special feature on medical technology.* National Center for Health Statistics.

National Center for Health Statistics & Centers for Disease Control and Prevention. (2022a). *About the national health and nutrition examination survey.* http://www.cdc.gov/nchs/nhanes/about_nhanes.htm

National Center for Health Statistics & Centers for Disease Control and Prevention. (2022b). *Health, United States, 2020-2021.* https://www.cdc.gov/nchs/data/hus/2020-2021/InjEDVis.pdf

National Center for Injury Prevention and Control & Centers for Disease Control and Prevention. (2020). *Core VIPP summary report.* https://www.cdc.gov/injury/stateprograms/svipp_summary.html

National Center for Injury Prevention and Control & Centers for Disease Control and Prevention. (2022a). *Child passenger safety.* https://www.cdc.gov/transportationsafety/child_passenger_safety/index.html

National Center for Injury Prevention and Control & Centers for Disease Control and Prevention. (2022b). *Core state injury prevention program (Core SIPP).* https://www.cdc.gov/injury/stateprograms/coresipp/index.html

National Center for Injury Prevention and Control & Centers for Disease Control and Prevention. (2022c). *Injury center timeline 1992–2022.* https://www.cdc.gov/injury/about/timeline.html

National Center for Injury Prevention and Control & Center for Disease Control and Prevention. (2022d). *Leading causes of death and injury.* https://www.cdc.gov/injury/wisqars/LeadingCauses.html

National Center for Injury Prevention and Control & Centers for Disease Control and Prevention. (2022e). *Teen drivers and passengers: Get the facts.* https://www.cdc.gov/transportationsafety/teen_drivers/teendrivers_factsheet.html#theproblem

National Center for Injury Prevention and Control & Centers for Disease Control and Prevention. (2022f). *Transportation safety.* https://www.cdc.gov/transportationsafety/

National Center for Injury Prevention and Control & Center for Disease Control and Prevention. (2023). *Injury and violence prevention and control.* http://www.cdc.gov/injury/

Organization for Economic Development and Cooperation. (2011). *Obesity update 2012.* http://www.oecd.org/health/49716427.pdf

Robert Wood Johnson Foundation. (2021). *New data compares latest child obesity rates by age, gender, and race.* https://stateofchildhoodobesity.org/new-data-compares-latest-child-obesity-rates-by-age-gender-and-race/

Robinson, T. N. (1998). Does television cause childhood obesity? *Journal of American Medical Association, 279*(12), 959–960. https://doi.org/10.1001/jama.279.12.959

Serdula, M. K., Ivery, D., Coates, R. J., Freedman, D. S., Williamson, D. F., & Byers, T. (1993). Do obese children become obese adults? A review of the literature. *Preventive Medicine, 22*(2), 167–177. https://doi.org/10.1006/pmed.1993.1014

Spencer, M. R., Hedegaard, H., & Garnett, M. (2021). Motor vehicle traffic death rates, by sex, age group, and road user type: United States, 1999–2019. *NCHS Data Brief No. 400.* https://www.cdc.gov/nchs/data/databriefs/db400-H.pdf

Task Force on Community Preventive Services. (2005). *The guide to community preventive services: What works to promote health.* Oxford University Press.

Task Force on Community Preventive Services. (2018). Motor vehicle injury child safety seats: Laws mandating use. *Guide to community preventive services.* https://www .thecommunityguide.org/findings/motor-vehicle-injury-child-safety-seats-laws -mandating-use.html

Trevino, R. P., Fogt, D. L., Wyatt, T. J., Leal-Vasquez, L., Sosa, E., & Woods, C. (2008). Diabetes risk, low fitness, and energy insufficiency levels among children from poor families. *Journal of the American Dietetic Association, 108*(11), 1846–1853. https://doi .org/10.1016/j.jada.2008.08.009

Whitaker, R. C., Wright, J. A., Pepe, M. S., Seidel, K. D., & Dietz, W. H. (1997). Predicting obesity in young adulthood from childhood and parental obesity. *New England Journal of Medicine, 337*(13), 869–873. https://doi.org/10.1056/NEJM199709253371301

World Health Organization. (2022). *Obesity and overweight.* https://www.who.int/ news-room/fact-sheets/detail/obesity-and-overweight

Xu, J. Q., Murphy, S. L., Kochanek, K. D., & Arias, E. (2021). Deaths: Final data for 2019. *National Vital Statistics Reports, 70*(8). https://www.cdc.gov/nchs/data/nvsr/ nvsr70/nvsr70-08-508.pdf

Appendix 5.1. Community-Based Changes in the Environment

Category 1: Strategies to promote the availability of affordable healthy food and beverages

Strategy 1: Increase availability of healthier food and beverage choices in public service venues

Community Example

- In St. Paul, Minnesota, the "Five a Day Power Plus Program" increased the variety of fruits and vegetables offered in schools by providing an additional fruit item on days baked desserts were served, promoting fruits and vegetables at point-of-purchase, and enhancing the attractiveness of fruits and vegetables. Evaluation of the program found that fruit and vegetable consumption increased significantly among children in the intervention group as compared with a control group.

- The Farm to School Network, which works to bring local produce into schools, improves the health of the children by providing increased access to healthy food. It also promotes living a healthy lifestyle by introducing the students to community gardens, cooking lessons, and field trips to local farms. An added bonus is that the community farmers are able to sell their crops close to home. This program is active across the country, with a program in every state.

Strategy 2: Improve availability of affordable healthier food and beverage choices in public service venues

Community Example

- The New York City Department of Health operates the Health Bucks Program to make fruits and vegetables more affordable to residents who receive food stamps. For every $5 worth of food stamps spent at farmers' markets, individuals receive a $2 Health Bucks coupon that can be redeemed year round at more than 30 farmers markets citywide. In 2007, the City Health Department reported that New Yorkers used more than 40% of the 9,000 Health Bucks distributed in 2006.

Strategy 3: Improve geographic availability of supermarkets in underserved areas

Community Example

- The Philadelphia Food Marketing Task Force investigated the lack of supermarkets in Philadelphia and released 10 recommendations to increase the number of supermarkets in Philadelphia's underserved communities. A new

(continued)

funding initiative was created using public funds to leverage supermarket development. To date, the initiative has committed $67 million in funding for 69 supermarket projects in 27 Pennsylvania counties, creating or preserving 3,900 jobs.

Strategy 4: Provide incentives to food retailers to locate in and/or offer healthier food and beverage choices in underserved areas

Community Example

- The city of Richmond, California, attracted a national discount grocery store to an urban retail center with adjacent affordable housing by offering an attractive incentive package, which included land sold at a reduced cost to the developer; a federal Urban Development Action Grant of $3.5 million for commercial development; a zoning designation that provided tax incentives; assistance in negotiations with state regulatory agencies; improvements to surrounding sidewalks, streetscape, and traffic signals; and concessions on design standards.

Strategy 5: Improve availability of mechanisms for purchasing foods from farms

Community Example

- In 2005, Jefferson Elementary School, in Riverside, California, launched a farm-to-school salad bar program that provides elementary school students access to a daily salad bar stocked with a variety of locally grown produce as an alternative to the standard hot lunch. Two small, locally owned family farms, within 30 miles of the school, sell their produce at an affordable price and make weekly deliveries to the school. Since implementing the farm-to-school salad bar program, the Riverside school district has expanded the program to four additional elementary schools.

Strategy 6: Provide incentives for the production, distribution, and procurement of foods from local farms

Community Example

- The Hartford Food System (HFS) in Connecticut is a nonprofit organization working to create an equitable and sustainable food system that addresses the underlying causes of hunger and poor nutrition facing low-income and elderly residents. In addition to developing innovative projects and initiatives that tackle food cost, access, and nutrition, the organization actively participates in public policy initiatives aimed at increasing production, distribution, and procurement of foods from local farms at the local, state, and federal government levels.

(continued)

Category 2: Strategies to support healthy food and beverage choices

Strategy 7: Restrict availability of less healthy foods and beverages in public service venues

Community Example

- The city of Baldwin Park, California, established nutrition standards for all snack foods and beverages sold in over 30 afterschool programs (including snack offerings in vending machines). The afterschool nutrition standards primarily focus on eliminating less healthy snacks and beverages that exceed recommended fat, calorie, and sugar intake for school-aged children.

Strategy 8: Institute smaller portion size options in public service venues

Community Example

- Although the following example describes a program that targets private restaurants, it may serve as a model for local communities that wish to promote greater access to healthy portion sizes in public service venues.

- The Texas Department of State Health Services developed the *Tex Plate* program to assist Texas restaurants in serving healthier portion sizes to consumers. Participating restaurants receive specialized 9-inch plates that indicate proper portions of key food groups such as vegetables, protein, and whole grains. The program is designed to encourage participating restaurants to increase the vegetable portion of the meal and decrease the entrée and starch portions of the meal.

Strategy 9: Limit advertisements of less healthy foods and beverages

Community Example

- The Mercedes Independent School District in Mercedes, Texas, adopted a comprehensive Student Nutrition/Wellness Plan in 2005 that includes a marketing component. The policy states that schools will promote healthy food choices and will not allow advertising that promotes less nutritious food choices. The plan also defines and prohibits possession of foods of minimal nutritional value at school.

Strategy 10: Discourage consumption of sugar-sweetened beverages

Community Example

- In 2002, the Los Angeles Unified School District adopted the Motion to Promote Healthy Beverage Sales. The motion bans the sale of soft drinks on school campuses; prohibits schools from entering into new or extended sales contracts of unapproved beverages; allows only approved beverages

(continued)

to be sold in vending machines, cafeterias, and student stores; monitors compliance through an audit program; disseminates information on healthy beverage sale options; and develops a new revenue model to make up for anticipated net loss of Associated Student Body monies related to the ban on soft drinks.

Category 3: Strategy to encourage breastfeeding

Strategy 11: Increase support for breastfeeding
Community Example

- In 1998, California passed the Breastfeeding at Work law, which requires all employers to ensure that employees are provided with adequate facilities for breastfeeding or expressing milk. In 2002, the state passed Lactation Accommodation, which expands prior workplace provisions to require adequate break time and space for breastfeeding or milk expression, with a violation penalty of $100.

Category 4: Strategies to encourage physical activity or limit sedentary activity among children and youth

Strategy 12: Require physical education in schools
Community Example

- In 2006, West Virginia enacted Senate Bill 785, which calls for the Department of Education to establish a requirement that every student enrolled in a public school participates in physical education (PE) classes during the school year. The bill also specified participation times for PE classes by grade level. For example, elementary school students are required to participate in at least 30 minutes of PE class 3 days a week, middle school students are required to participate in at least one full period of PE each school day for a semester, and high school students are required to complete no less than one full course credit of PE class prior to graduation.

Strategy 13: Increase the amount of physical activity in physical education programs in schools
Community Example

- Owensboro, Kentucky, overhauled its school-based PE curriculum after a study found that 60% of the Owensboro-area population was obese or overweight. A partnership was formed between the city's hospitals and schools and $750,000 was donated to equip 11 school-based fitness centers with treadmills, stationary bikes, rowing machines, and weightlifting stations.

(continued)

PE teachers were trained using "new PE" techniques, which stress the importance of keeping students physically active for at least 30- to 60-minute increments during class time.

- Equestrian Trails Elementary School, located in Wellington, Florida, received a STARS award from the National Association for Sport and Physical Education in recognition of its outstanding PE program. The PE staff at Equestrian Trails Elementary designed a yearly plan of instruction using physical activity and fitness components as the primary foundation for its curriculum. The curriculum teaches students the basic skills of several movement forms, including team, dual, and individual sports, and dance.

Strategy 14: Increase opportunities for extracurricular physical activity

Community Example

- The city of Eugene, Oregon, and the Bethel School District pooled their resources to purchase and develop a 70-acre parcel of land. The property now includes a 35-acre site for Meadow View School and 35 acres for Bethel Community Park, which includes wetlands, a running path, ball fields, and a skate/community park. Many students can walk through the park to get to school.

- Michelle Obama's "Let's Move" Campaign is the former First Lady's initiative to reduce the rates of childhood obesity. It focuses on giving parents the tools to encourage healthy eating, promoting physical activity for young people, and working to ensure all people have access to healthy, affordable food. This is an example of just one of many very prominent public figures that have brought the issue of childhood obesity to the forefront of the social conversation.

Strategy 15: Reduce screen time in public service venues

Community Example

- In 2006, the New York City Department of Health and Mental Hygiene Board of Health implemented an amendment to the New York City Health Code, which regulates group day care in New York City. The amended article prohibits television, video, and visual recordings for children younger than 2 years of age. In addition, television, video, and visual recordings are limited to 60 minutes per day of educational programming for children 2 years or older.

(continued)

Category 5: Strategies to create safe communities that support physical activity

Strategy 16: Improve access to outdoor recreational facilities
Community Example

- KaBOOM! is a national nonprofit organization that empowers local communities to build playgrounds in neighborhoods that lack play spaces for children. The KaBOOM! process helps residents of local communities bring together the capacity, resources, volunteers, and planning needed to fulfill the vision of a great place to play within walking distance of every child in America. The KaBOOM! Website provides information and resources for community residents to apply for a KaBOOM!-led playground build or to follow detailed steps to build their own playground.

Strategy 17: Enhance infrastructure supporting bicycling
Community Example

- In May 2005, Boulder, Colorado, was awarded Gold status as a Bicycle-Friendly Community by the League of American Bicyclists. The city committed 15% of its annual transportation budget, $3.1 million, toward bicycle enhancement and maintenance activities. More than 95% of Boulder's arterial streets have bicycle facilities and all local and regional buses are equipped with bike racks. In addition, Boulder has created an online bike routing system that provides cyclists a direct and safe bike route to travel within city limits.

Strategy 18: Enhance infrastructure supporting walking
Community Example

- In 2002, Oakland, California, adopted a Pedestrian Master Plan which designates a network of pedestrian facilities and distinguishes segments and intersections in need of particular attention for safety enhancements. The city estimated pedestrian volumes throughout the city based on land use, population, and other network characteristics, and used these estimates in conjunction with crash data, traffic data, and community input to identify and prioritize areas with both safety problems and high pedestrian demand.
- The Walk, Bike, & Roll to School campaign, which encourages children to walk to school through the promotion of safe walking paths, national "Walk-to-School" and "Bike-to-School" days.

(continued)

Strategy 19: Support locating schools within easy walking distance of residential areas

Community Example

- In 2005, the City of Milwaukee began its Neighborhood Schools initiative. As a result of this initiative, the city decided to build six new schools from the ground up and spent millions of dollars revamping and expanding dilapidated schools that were located in and around community neighborhoods. The goals of the initiative were to reduce the number of students being bused to schools around the city and to increase the number of students walking or biking to schools that were centrally located and close to their neighborhoods.

Strategy 20: Improve access to public transportation

Community Example

- Local business owners and residents of the South Park neighborhood of Tucson, Arizona, received funding from the local government and the Federal Transit Administration (FTA) to implement a series of improvements to the existing public transit system. Funds were used to install six new artistic bus shelters, new traffic signals, and additional sidewalk and curb access ramps for public transit users, bicyclers, and pedestrians. As a result of the efforts to revitalize its public transit infrastructure, South Park has experienced renewed pride in its community and helped to rebuild its local economy.

Strategy 21: Zone for mixed-use development

Community Example

- The concept of mixed-use development is the official growth management policy for Eugene, Oregon, which focuses on integrating mixed-use developments within the city's urban growth boundary. The city's regional transportation master plan targets dozens of potential "mixed-use centers" for development into quality neighborhoods that enjoy higher densities, more transportation options, and convenient access to shopping, consumer services, and basic amenities. By combining mixed-use centers with improved transit options, the plan aims to reduce dependence on automobile travel, encourage walking, and reduce the need for costly street improvements.

Strategy 22: Enhance personal safety in areas where persons are or could be physically active

Community Example

- Detroit, Michigan, has one of the highest home foreclosure rates in the country, resulting in a dramatic increase in the number of abandoned buildings and

(continued)

boarded-up homes which attract vandals and petty crime. In response, Urban Farming, an international nonprofit organization, joined forces with the local county government to transform 20 abandoned properties into active fruit and vegetable garden plots that feed the homeless and improve the aesthetic appeal of city neighborhoods. Since establishing the gardens, residents report less vandalism and blight in their community and the local county government donates water to maintain the city gardens on an ongoing basis.

Strategy 23: Enhance traffic safety in areas where persons are or could be physically active

Community Example

- In the mid-1990s, the city of West Palm Beach, Florida, adopted a downtown-wide traffic calming policy to improve street safety for nonmotorized users. The city's main streets were retrofitted with important pedestrian safety measures, including raised intersections, two-way streets, road narrowings and roundabouts to slow traffic, wide sidewalks, tree-lined streets, and shortened pedestrian crossings. As a result of these efforts, city streets are perceived as safe by pedestrians, property values more than doubled in the downtown area, and commercial retail space is 80% occupied.

Category 6: Strategy to encourage communities to organize for change

Strategy 24: Participate in community coalitions or partnerships to address obesity

Community Example

- PedNet Coalition in Columbia, Missouri, is a community coalition that includes 5,000 individuals and 75 businesses, government agencies, and nonprofit organizations. The goal of the coalition is to develop and restore a network of nature trails and urban "pedways" connecting residential subdivisions, worksites, shopping districts, parks, schools, and recreation centers.

Keener, D., Goodman, K., Lowry, A., Zaro, S., & Kettel Khan, L. (2009). *Recommended community strategies and measurements to prevent obesity in the United States: Implementation and measurement guide.* Centers for Disease Control and Prevention.

6 | Public Health System Performance

LEARNING OBJECTIVES

Students will learn . . .

1. What is evidence-based public health and why it is important.

2. That system performance is judged on effectiveness, efficiency, and equity.

3. What are the indicators of public health system performance at the population level.

4. The role of professional organizations in measuring and improving U.S. public health performance.

5. How well the U.S. public health system performs based on various performance measures.

Evaluation of the public health system is increasingly important in this era of accountability and finite budgets. Like the health care system, the public health system's performance is generally evaluated on three criteria: (a) effectiveness, (b) efficiency, and (c) equity (Aday et al., 1993, 2004). Therefore, the overall evaluation of public health performance asks the question: How effective, efficient, and equitable is public health in achieving its mission to prevent disease, injury, disability, and premature death by "assuring conditions in which people can be healthy" (Institute of Medicine [IOM], 1988, p. 1)?

Effectiveness focuses on whether the desired benefits of public health practices—programs, policies, services—are achieved. Efficiency focuses on how the benefits achieved by public health compare to the resources expended to realize them, and whether alternate practices would have achieved greater benefits or the same benefits using fewer resources. "Equity addresses the fairness and effectiveness of policies in minimizing population health disparities" (Aday, 2005, p. 2). The effectiveness, efficiency, and equity criteria are often complementary. Improving effectiveness while holding resources constant increases efficiency, and those increases in efficiency may create opportunities for improved effectiveness and equity. These criteria—effectiveness, efficiency, and equity—provide a basis for evaluating the performance of the public health system, as they do for evaluating the health care system.

A system such as public health can be evaluated at two levels: at the micro-level of discrete programs, policies, and services; and at the macro-level of the system, as a whole. In this chapter, we describe how discrete public health services, programs, and policies are evaluated in evidence-based public health practice. Afterward, we discuss how the performance of the public health system, as a whole, is addressed and assessed.

EVIDENCE-BASED PUBLIC HEALTH PRACTICE

> **KEY IDEA**
>
> The movement to evaluate public health practices, systematically, has resulted in *evidence-based public health (EBPH)*.

EBPH is an effort to demonstrate what works and what does not work in public health practice, based on scientifically valid empirical research. We explicitly seek to base our services, program initiatives, and policies aimed at preventing disease, injury, disability, and premature death in populations on knowledge that has resulted from sound research about the effectiveness, efficiency, and equity of public health practices. Echoing the leading voice for change in public health in the late 20th century—the IOM report, *The Future of Public Health (1988)*—Kohatsu and his colleagues write, "Decisions and policies in public health are frequently driven by crises, political concerns, and public opinion. A number of researchers, however, are proposing a more evidence-based approach to public health, based on the advances of evidence-based medicine" (2004, p. 417).

> The logic of evidence-based practice identifies a cyclic relation between evaluation, evidence, practice, and further evaluation. It is based on the premise that evaluations determine whether anticipated intervention effects occur in practice, and identify unanticipated effects. The reports of such evaluations are a valuable source of evidence to maximize the benefits, and reduce the harms, of public health policy and practice. The evidence can also inform evaluation planning, and thus improve the quality and relevance of new research. (Rychetnik et al., 2004, p. 541)

"Formal discourse on the nature and scope of EBPH (evidence-based public health) originated about two decades ago" (Brownson et al., 2018, p. 3), and while EBPH methods have improved, the concept is well-established. Table 6.1 contains three well-known definitions of EBPH. Taken together, we see that the essence of EBPH is the development of information, using scientific principles,

Table 6.1. Three Definitions of Evidence-Based Public Health

Definition 1[a]	Definition 2[b]	Definition 3[c]
EBPH is the conscientious, explicit, and judicious use of current best evidence in making decisions about the care of communities and populations in the domain of health protection, disease prevention, and health maintenance and improvement (health promotion)	EBPH is the development, implementation, and evaluation of effective programs and policies in public health through application of principles of scientific reasoning, including systematic uses of data and information systems and appropriate use of program-planning models	EBPH is the process of integrating science-based interventions with community preferences to improve the health of populations

EBPH, evidence-based public health.

[a]Jenicek (1997).
[b]Brownson et al. (1999, 2003).
[c]Kohatsu et al. (2004).

Source: Kohatsu, N. D., Robinson, J. G., & Torner, J. C. (2004). Evidence-based public health: An evolving concept. *American Journal of Preventive Medicine, 27*(5), 417–421. https://doi.org/10.1016/s0749-3797(04)00196-5

to inform public health practice so that it is effective, efficient, and equitable. The importance of community preferences is explicitly noted in the more recent definition (Kohatsu et al., 2004), because this issue has considerable bearing on the effectiveness of public health practices, as discussed in Chapter 7 and later in this chapter.

Evidence-Based Public Health Process

EBPH is an activity with direct parallels to evidence-based medicine. The goals and general methods are the same, although some of the specifics differ because of the differences between medicine and public health. As some authors have noted, public health is a broader, more diverse field, and therefore a wider range of scientific approaches is needed to gather information for practice improvement. Kohatsu et al. (2004) have identified differences between evidence-based medicine and EBPH, which are summarized in Table 6.2.

Public health policies, programs, and services target for improvement specific health problems in populations. These include noninfectious diseases such as heart disease, cancer, and stroke; intentional injuries due to such acts as gun violence and suicide; unintentional injuries from motor vehicle crashes, falls, and other calamities; and infectious diseases including foodborne illnesses, tuberculosis, and COVID-19. Public health policies, programs, and services may also attempt to change environments and conditions that cause disease and injury. For example, they might address the origins of hunger and poor nutrition; limited physical activity and recreation; or mental health and violence toward others.

Table 6.2. A Comparison of Evidence-Based Medicine and Evidence-Based Public Health

Step	Evidence-Based Medicine[a]	Evidence-Based Public Health[b]
1. State the scientific question of interest	Convert the need for information (about prevention, diagnosis, prognosis, therapy, causation) into an answerable question	Develop an initial statement of the issue
2. Identify the relevant evidence	Track down the best evidence to answer that question	Search the scientific literature and organize information
3. Identify the relevant evidence	Critically appraise that evidence for its validity (closeness to the truth), impact (size of the effect), and applicability (usefulness in one's clinical practice)	Quantify the issue using sources of existing data
4. Determine what information is relevant to answering the scientific question of interest	Integrate the critical appraisal with one's clinical expertise and with the patient's unique biology, values, and circumstances	Develop and prioritize program options; develop an action plan and implement interventions
5. Determine the best course of action considering the patient or population	Evaluate one's effectiveness and efficiency in executing Steps 1 to 4 and seek ways to improve both for the next time	Evaluate the program or policy

[a]Sackett et al. (2000).
[b]Brownson et al. (1999, 2003).

Source: Kohatsu, N. D., Robinson, J. G., & Torner, J. C. (2004). Evidence-based public health: An evolving concept. *American Journal of Preventive Medicine, 27*(5), 417–421. https://doi.org/10.1016/s0749-3797(04)00196-5

KEY IDEA

Each policy, program, or service can be evaluated on whether it achieved its goals; that is, whether it has been effective. Therefore, measures of effectiveness; that is, measures that indicate whether the desired or intended result was brought about, are population and program specific.

The basic components of any evaluation are *structure, process,* and *outcomes*:

Structure. When assessing a program, service, or policy, structure refers to the resources available for the initiative, including organization and financing; the characteristics of the populations targeted by the initiative; and the physical, social, and economic environments in which the initiative occurs.

Process. Process refers to the implementation of the public health program, service, or policy. "*Process evaluations* focus on the degree to which the program has been implemented as planned and on the quality of the program implementation. *Process evaluations* are known by a variety of terms, such as monitoring evaluations, depending on their focus and characteristics" (Issel, 2009, p. 9).

Outcomes. Outcomes refer to the expected results of implementation. *Outcome evaluations*, often used interchangeably with impact evaluations, focus on whether the goals of the program, service, or policy have been achieved and whether the changes desired can be attributed to the program (Issel, 2009). The outcomes of policies, programs, and services usually consist of *short-term goals*, *longer-term goals*, and *impact*, which is the ultimate purpose of the effort. Often *short-term* goals are changes in knowledge, while *longer-term* goals seek change in the more intractable attitudes and behavior. Impact goals are frequently improvements in health status or utilization of health care or other services.

EBPH Case Study: Intolerance Among High School Students

Bullying and intolerance among students has been associated with severe symptoms of mental health problems, including self-harm and suicidality. "Bullying was shown to have detrimental effects that persist into late adolescence and contribute independently to mental health problems" (Kallmen & Hallgren, 2021, p. 1).

An example of an EBPH program is a project in a local school that used theater to reduce intolerance and bullying among 10th graders. Focus groups with 10th-grade students were conducted to identify their experiences and concerns about intolerance and bullying in their lives. A theater production was developed by a group of young actors using the results of the focus groups to recreate the experiences of students in the school. The theater production contained skits based on the personal experiences of students, increasing the relevance of the production to the audience. The production was presented to all 10th graders during school hours. The *short-term goal* of the program—by the end of the performance—was to increase knowledge about what constitutes intolerance and how intolerance was perceived by both victim and perpetrator. The *longer-term goal*—during the remainder of the school year—was to increase discussions among students about tolerance issues. The desired *impact* of the program was a decrease in the number of incidences of intolerance reported to the high school administration. Questionnaires specific to the program were developed to measure *short- and long-term* attitudes about intolerance and bullying among the students. They were systematically administered to students in a class before the production and in a class 2 months afterward. Records from administration were used to indicate *impact*. There was a decline in reports of bullying to school officials after the program, as well as in the student surveys.

Outcome Measures: Population-Level Morbidity and Mortality

KEY IDEA

Measurement is the key to providing the scientifically sound evidence needed to determine what works and what does not in public health practice.

Population-level measures of morbidity and mortality are often used to assess the *impact* of programs, services, and policies, whether they are implemented at the micro-level of group, community, or organization or the macro-level—counties, regions, cities, states, or nations. Table 6.3 identifies the most widely used of these measures.

Age-Adjusted Mortality Rate and Age-Specific Mortality Rate

Both measures are used to control the effect of age on the results of programs, services, and policies. *Age-adjusted rates* allow comparison of two or more populations at one point in time or comparison of one population at two or more points in time. Age-adjusted rates are calculated (using the direct method) by applying a population's age-specific rates to a standardized age distribution; for example, the age distribution of the year 2000 population. In this way, differences in observed rates that result from age differences in the population are eliminated

Table 6.3. Measures of Mortality and Morbidity

Term	Definition
Prevalence	The number of existing cases of a disease in a population at a given point in time
Incidence	The number of new cases of a disease that occurred in a population during a given time period, often a year
Crude mortality rate	The number of deaths in a population during a given time period, often a year
Age-adjusted mortality rate	The number of deaths in a population during a given time period, often a year, adjusted for the population's age distribution
Age-specific mortality rate	The number of deaths in a specified age-group in a population during a given time period, often a year
Disease-specific mortality rate	The number of deaths from a specified disease in a susceptible population during a given time period, often a year
Infant mortality rate (IMR)	The probability of dying between birth and exactly 1 year of age
Life expectancy	The number of years of life that can be expected on average in a population
Years of potential life lost (YPLL)	The number of years of life lost due to death before the expected age of death in a population during a given time period, often a year
Healthy life expectancy (HALE)	The average number of years that a person at birth can expect to live in full health
Disability-adjusted life years (DALY)	The number of years lost due to illness, disability, or premature death in a population during a given time period, often a year

(Centers for Disease Control and Prevention [CDC], 2022a). An *age-specific mortality rate* is a mortality rate limited to a particular age group. The numerator is the number of deaths in that age group; the denominator is the number of persons in that age group in the population.

Infant Mortality Rate

The United Nations International Children's Emergency Fund's (UNICEF) definition of infant mortality rate (IMR) is the probability of dying between birth and exactly 1 year of age (CDC, Reproductive Health, 2023). This rate is expressed per 1,000 live births per year. IMR is an important measure of population well-being as infant death is associated with poor maternal health, inadequate quality and access to health care, and deficiencies in other life conditions, all of which may be remedied.

Life Expectancy and Years of Potential Life Lost

By using the life expectancy within a population, the time lost to premature death, also called years of potential life lost or life expectancy and **years of potential life lost (YPLL)**, can be calculated. YPLL indicates that death occurred at an age less than what would be expected, and the more premature a death, the greater the loss of life (World Health Organization [WHO], 2019).

> This indicator is a summary measure of premature mortality, providing an explicit way of weighting deaths occurring at younger ages, which may be preventable. The calculation of Potential Years of Life Lost (PYLL) involves summing up deaths occurring at each age and multiplying this with the number of remaining years to live up to a selected age limit (age 75 is used in OECD Health Statistics). In order to assure cross-country and trend comparison, the PYLL are standardised, for each country and each year. The total OECD population in 2010 is taken as the reference population for age standardisation. This indicator is presented as a total and per gender. It is measured in years lost per 100,000 inhabitants (total), per 100,000 men and per 100,000 women, aged 0–69. (Organisation for Economic Cooperation and Development [OECD], 2022a, para. 1)

Healthy Life Expectancy and Disability-Adjusted Life Years

Healthy life expectancy (HALE) and disability-adjusted life years (DALY) are concepts of population health that take into account the quality of life as well as the length of life. They allow the comparison of health status by age and gender within countries and between countries and regions. HALE and DALY are measures used to indicate the Global Burden of Disease.

HALE at birth is defined by WHO as the average number of years that an individual can expect to live in "full health" by taking into account years lived in less than full health due to disease and/or injury (WHO, 2019). HALE is a measure that "combines length and quality of life into a single estimate that indicates years that can be expected in a specified state of health" (Kindig, 1997, p. 45).

> Substantial resources are devoted to reducing the incidence, duration and severity of major diseases that cause morbidity but not mortality and to reducing their impact on people's lives. It is important to capture both fatal and non-fatal health outcomes in a summary measure of average levels of population health. Healthy life expectancy (HALE) at birth adds up expectation of life for different health states, adjusted for severity distribution making it sensitive to changes over time or differences between countries in the severity distribution of health states. (WHO, 2022a, para. 1)

The DALY was first used in 1993 in the World Development Report of the World Bank. The sum of DALYs across the population, or the burden of disease, can be thought of as a measurement of the gap between current health status and an ideal health situation where the entire population lives to an advanced age, free of disease and disability.

> Mortality does not give a complete picture of the burden of disease borne by individuals in different populations. The overall burden of disease is assessed using the disability-adjusted life year (DALY), a time-based measure that combines years of life lost due to premature mortality (YLLs) and years of life lost due to time lived in states of less than full health, or years of healthy life lost due to disability (YLDs). One DALY represents the loss of the equivalent of one year of full health. Using DALYs, the burden of diseases that cause premature death but little disability (such as drowning or measles) can be compared to that of diseases that do not cause death but do cause disability (such as cataract causing blindness). (WHO, 2022b, para. 1)

Benchmarking

Benchmarking as part of a performance improvement methodology was pioneered by Xerox decades ago as part of an approach to improve production costs and later incorporated into performance improvement methodology applicable to any sector including health care (Ettorchi-Tardy et al., 2012). The term benchmark is derived from physical marks representing specifically measured heights through geographic surveys and there are historical markers of high water marks reached by the waves of tsunamis going back centuries (Fackler, 2011). In that vein, performance benchmarks—such as those for public health measures—establish high water marks of performance against which a peer or similar entity may compare their performance. Benchmarks themselves may be based on accepted "gold standards," which represent the best available performance under reasonable conditions (Cardoso et al., 2014; Versi, 1992), peer entities or populations (for whose performance should be comparable), or past performance by the same or similar units.

The last approach is sometimes referred to as internal benchmarking (in financial and accounting functions the term "internal variance analysis" may be more common; Ettorchi-Tardy et al., 2012). The primary benefit of this approach is that the data are typically readily available and avoid practical and legal issues of sharing data across organizations and entities (Ettorchi-Tardy et al., 2012). Additionally, data within the same organization are more likely to be defined and measured the same way (reducing the need for "data normalization").

In many cases internal benchmarking may not be possible for functions or performance areas when they are one-of-one in the entity or jurisdiction or it is believed that other entities have achieved significantly higher performance. In these situations, "peer" or external benchmarks are preferable. For example, IMRs and life expectancy at birth are two common public health measures available for most countries across the world. Countries may set the benchmark for comparison as the best or the best of economic peer countries or a function of the available statistics (e.g., top quartile of countries). What makes these comparisons possible are consistent measure definitions and collection of the underlying data. (One of the original intentions of the *International Classification of Diseases* discussed earlier was to standardize recording and reporting of causes of death to allow such comparisons.) When peers use different definitions (particularly common for financial and cost-related measures given the very different approaches to public health and delivery sector financing used by different countries) data normalization, sometimes substantial, is required. Sometimes this normalization is implicit in a metric such as using infant deaths per 1,000 live births rather than total infant deaths per year. In other cases, data needs to be normalized to a standardized demography prior to comparison and/or inclusion or exclusion of data may be required. For example, while the IMR has been standardized for decades, some countries continued to use slightly different definitions of stillbirth for decades and not all countries' rates have been directly comparable without normalization for all available time periods (Liu et al., 1992).

However, while establishing a benchmark can be a key foundational step as part of a performance improvement effort, it will not by itself result in higher performance. The results of a benchmarking exercise may then be used to highlight gaps in performance and the potential impact from closing those gaps (e.g., lives saved by reaching mortality rates among the best achieved), prioritize areas of focus (e.g., focus current efforts on those areas with the highest potential impact possibly incorporating available resources), and identify higher performers from which to learn (Ettorchi-Tardy et al., 2012). For example, countries may look to similar peer countries who perform better on key mortality statistics or public health departments may look to other public health departments that have achieved lower incidence rates of foodborne illnesses.

EBPH would be applied to the development of new programs and to the evaluation of existing programs that are perceived to need improvement. For example, if a community chose to focus on reducing childhood obesity, public health and community leaders would research programs with similar aims and select and implement one that seemed appropriate for their community. Not finding an existing model to implement, the community would develop a unique program with an evaluation component, which would provide evidence about the effectiveness of the program.

PUBLIC HEALTH SYSTEM PERFORMANCE

How do we evaluate the performance of the system as a whole? The sum of its policies, programs, and services individually? Or macro-level summary measures that assumes the effect of all programs, and so on?

As discussed previously, there are two basic types of evaluation: process and outcomes evaluation. This is true of systems as well as programs, services, and policies. In this section on public health system performance, we turn first to process improvement initiatives.

Accreditation and Credentialing

Desired outcomes result from well-thought-out, well-executed processes. This is true of the public health system, as it is of any other system or initiative. Therefore, the performance of the public health system depends on the:

- Quality and commitment of the workforce;
- Quality of policies, services, and programs in public health organizations at every level—local, state, and federal; and
- Quality of data that are available to assess performance.

There are several initiatives intended to ensure the quality of these three aspects of the public health system. The *quality of the workforce* is addressed by the accreditation of public health programs and schools by the Council on Education for Public Health (CEPH); the core competencies project developed by the Public Health Foundation's (PHF) Council on Linkages Between Academia and Public Health Practice; and the certification of individual public health professionals by the National Board of Public Health Examiners (NBPHE).

The *quality of policies, services, and programs* offered by public health organizations is addressed by the accreditation of state and local public health departments by the **Public Health Accreditation Board (PHAB)**. Data that are needed to assess and improve public health system performance are continually being developed, and some important sources of EBPH are listed under the "Data Sources" section at the end of this chapter. One that we will discuss later is the report card initiative.

The organizations involved in improving public health performance are private, nonprofit entities, supported by members and organizations, chief among them the American Public Health Association (APHA), the Association of Schools and Programs of Public Health (ASPPH), and the Association for Prevention Teaching and Research (APTR). The Association of State and Territorial Health Officials (ASTHO), the National Association of County and City Health Officials (NACCHO), the National Association of Local Boards of Health (NALB), and the National Indian Health Board (NIHB) have also been heavily involved with accreditation of health departments.

Several private foundations have been committed to improving public health performance through these initiatives, including the Robert Wood Johnson Foundation, the American Legacy Foundation, the Foundation to Advance Public Health through Certification, and the Josiah Macy, Jr. Foundation. Each certification—individual, educational program, and public health organization—is voluntary at this time, although **CEPH** accreditation confers many benefits on schools and programs of public health and their graduates.

Council on Education for Public Health

The CEPH is one of the oldest of the initiatives. CEPH is an independent agency recognized by the U.S. Department of Education to accredit schools of public health and certain public health programs offered in settings other than schools of public health. These schools and programs prepare students for entry into careers in public health. The primary professional degree is the Master of Public Health (MPH), but other masters and doctoral degrees are offered as well. The mission is to ensure "quality in public health education and training to achieve excellence in practice, research and service, through collaboration with organizational and community partners" (CEPH, 2022, para. 1).

The Council's focus is the improvement of health through the assurance of professional personnel who are able to identify, prevent, and solve community health problems. The Council's objectives are:

1. To promote quality in public health education through a continuing process of self-evaluation by the schools and programs that seek accreditation;
2. To assure the public that institutions offering graduate instruction in public health have been evaluated and judged to meet standards essential for the conduct of such educational programs;
3. To encourage—through periodic review, consultation, research, publications, and other means—improvements in the quality of education for public health. (CEPH, 2022, para. 6)

As of spring 2023, there were 67 accredited schools of public health, 154 accredited programs in public health, and 27 standalone baccalaureate programs, mostly in the United States (CEPH, 2023).

Council on Linkages Between Academia and Public Health Practice

The Council on Linkages is a collaborative of 24 national organizations that aims to improve public health education and training, practice, and research. It was established in 1992 to implement the recommendations of the Public Health Faculty/Agency Forum to increase the relevance of public health education to the practice of public health. The Council's mission is "to improve the performance of individuals and organizations within public health by fostering, coordinating, and monitoring collaboration among the academic, public health practice, and healthcare communities; promoting public health education and training for health professionals throughout their careers; and developing and advancing innovative strategies to build and strengthen public health infrastructure" (Council on Linkages, 2021, para. 1).

The core competencies developed by the Council on Linkages are organized into eight domains:

- Data analytics and assessment skills,
- Policy development and program-planning skills,
- Communication skills,
- Health equity skills,
- Community partnership skills,
- Public health sciences skills,
- Management and finance skills, and
- Leadership and systems thinking skills.

The core competencies have three tiers, which differentiate the skills needed by entry-level individuals, individuals with management and/or supervisory responsibilities, and senior-level managers and/or leaders of public health organizations. The core competencies are used by educational programs to build their curriculum and by public health organizations to identify their workforce needs (Council on Linkages, 2021).

National Board of Public Health Examiners

The NBPHE was established in 2005 as an independent organization to make certain that students and graduates from CEPH-accredited schools and programs of public health have mastered the knowledge and skills required by contemporary public health. To this end, the NBPHE has administered the Certified in Public Health (CPH) exam each year, beginning in 2009. In addition to developing, administering, and scoring the exam, the NBPHE prepares students to take the exam through study guides and study sessions. The CPH exam is another method of ensuring the quality of the public health workforce.

The goals of credentialing are to:

- Increase recognition of the public health professions,
- Raise the visibility of public health,
- Set standards of knowledge and skills in public health,
- Foster environment of a professional community, and
- Encourage life-long learning (NBPHE, 2022).

To be eligible for the CPH exam, applicants must have a degree from a CEPH-accredited school or program of public health or sufficient work experience in the field (NBPHE, 2022).

Public Health Accreditation Board

The newest accrediting body for public health is the PHAB, whose:

> . . . vision is a high-performing governmental public health system that will make the U.S a healthier nation. All health departments in the U.S. should be accredited. Accreditation is a vehicle to transparency and trust in public health—communities can feel confident that their health departments are providing Foundational Capabilities and meeting national standards for performance and quality. (PHAB, 2022, p. 1)

PHAB's mission is "to advance and transform public health practice by championing performance improvement, strong infrastructure, and innovation. We support health departments in their work to promote the health of the communities they serve through accreditation and recognition, education, technical assistance, and research and evaluation" (PHAB, 2022, p. 2). State and local health departments are the target for this accreditation initiative.

The initiative to accredit local health departments originated with the groundbreaking report, *The Future of Public Health*, which was sponsored by the IOM (1988). The report galvanized public health with a study that had been in the making for 10 years after the IOM assessment that there was a "deplorable lack of reliability, even availability, of an identifiable local component of the public health system in many parts of the country and an unexplainable variability in configuration and performance in the rest of the country" (Tilson, 2008, p. xv). Tilson has written an excellent summary of the history of public health accreditation, part of which is repeated in the following:

> The IOM committee reframed the mission of public health as "fulfilling society's interest in assuring conditions in which people can be healthy." And the committee created a new conceptual framework with which to comprehend the scope of public health's activities as core functions at all government levels: assessment, policy development, and assurance. Into that landmark IOM report a prior thread was woven to strengthen the fabric. *The Model Standards for Community Preventive Health Services* . . . were recognized as providing necessary materials with which to weave this new cloth.
>
> These standards, in turn, had undergone a ten-year development process under the leadership of the Centers for Disease Control and Prevention (CDC). They were initiated at CDC in response to the public health delivery system's failure in the United States to respond adequately or coherently to the substantial challenges in a short-notice nationwide immunization initiative against swine influenza in 1976. For each of the major content areas of public health practice, indicators recognizable and countable in any local community were identified through a consensus process deriving from the same leadership organizations now working together on accreditation. As model standards, the proposal outlined the challenges to the local community using an open-ended,

fill-in-the-blanks approach to modeling: By 19xx, the rate of problem Y will not exceed (or will be reduced to) Z. In association with the *Healthy People 2000* undertaking, an effort at depicting benchmarks, the project developed either national averages or synthetic composite metrics from multiple reporting jurisdictions about each of the objectives in the *Model Standards*, now still part of the *Healthy People* publications. . . . The IOM and many other advocates saw that accreditation could be done in such a way as to recognize local unique situations but still achieve the dual purposes of accountability and continuous process improvement. They based this position on what they observed to be a breakthrough concept, the National Public Health System Performance Standards, which "provide a way to conceptualize the system as the unit of accreditation and, from there, to evaluate the role of the agencies in facilitating the work of the system." (Tilson, 2008, p. xvi)

The current accreditation program administered by PHAB has standards and measures that reflect the changes in public health practice including an emphasis on health equity, data and documentation processes, and updated preparedness requirements based on the COVID-19 pandemic (PHAB, 2022). The National Public Health Performance Standards (NPHPS or the Standards) continue to provide a framework to evaluate the performance and capacity of public health systems and governing bodies. This framework helps to identify areas for system improvement, strengthen state and local partnerships, and ensure that a strong system is in place for providing the 10 essential public health services (CDC, 2022b).

Report Card Initiatives

The report card initiatives can be viewed as outcome evaluations of the public health system as a whole. They collect, organize, and present information about the outcomes that are central to the public health system: population health status, morbidity, and mortality. These indicators are used in macro-level performance evaluations of such areas as cities, counties, regions, states, and nations. We assume the impact of public health care on these rates even though we are not directly measuring exposure to any specific public health service, program, or initiative among the population considered. If, for example, an infectious disease-specific mortality rate is higher in one region than another, we assume that the public health system (and health care system) has not been optimal in the region with the higher mortality rate.

The initiatives discussed here are *Healthy People* and *America's Health Rankings*.

Healthy People

Healthy People, the health-promotion and disease-prevention agenda for the United States, sets health objectives for the nation, monitors progress toward achieving those objectives, and issues regular reports on the results. *Healthy People* has been a highly influential initiative for assessing the health of the nation and, by implication, the performance of the public health system. The *Healthy People* initiative acknowledges that even though the agenda is national, the improvements will come through local actions, which will then affect the state, regional, and national outcomes reports.

The history of *Healthy People* spans three decades (CDC, 2010a, 2010b). The initiative is an outgrowth of *Healthy People: The Surgeon General's Report on Health Promotion and Disease Prevention* (Office of the Assistant Secretary for Health and Surgeon General, 1979), a document presenting quantitative goals to reduce preventable death and injury by 1990. In 1980, the U.S. Public Health Service released a companion report, which contained specific, quantifiable objectives to achieve the *Healthy People* goals. Since then, the U.S. Department of Health and Human Services (DHHS) has updated these national health promotion and disease prevention goals and objectives each decade, beginning with in *Healthy People 2000* (IOM, 1990) and now *Healthy People 2030* (DHHS, 2022).

The goals for each version of *Healthy People* change to reflect changes in the country's health priorities and health realities.

- The goals of the first *Healthy People* initiative were to reduce mortality among four age groups—infants, children, adolescents and young adults, and adults—and increase independence among older adults. There were 15 priority areas and 226 objectives.

- *Healthy People 2000* had three overarching goals: to increase years of healthy life, reduce disparities in health among different population groups, and achieve access to preventive health services. There were 22 priority areas, with 319 supporting objectives.

- *Healthy People 2010* had two overarching goals: to increase quality and years of healthy life and to eliminate health disparities, which served to guide the development of objectives that would be used to measure progress. There were 28 focus areas (changed from priority areas) and 467 objectives.

- *Healthy People 2020*, the initiative just completed, has four goals: to attain longer, healthier, and higher-quality lives; to eliminate health disparities; to create environments both social and physical that promote good health; and to promote healthy lifestyles across all life stages. These goals reflect the state of the United States when initiated, which had an aging population and many health disparities. *Healthy People 2020* contains 42 topic areas with a total of 1,200 objectives. This was by far the most ambitious *Healthy People* initiative at the time of inception, with far more objectives than any years and 13 new topic areas, which included Older Adults and Lesbian, Gay, Bisexual, and Transgender Health.

- *Healthy People 2030* is now developed. It has more topic areas and objectives than previous initiatives, but has identified Leading Health Indicators—a small subset of high-priority *Healthy People 2030* objectives that cover the life span. They address "important factors that impact major causes of death and disease in the United States, and they help organizations, communities, and states across the nation focus their resources and efforts to improve the health and well-being of all people" (DHHS, 2022, para. 1).

The process of selecting priority/focus areas for *Healthy People* has become more participatory over time.

> The process for creating objectives evolved from one that was largely expert-driven with opportunities for feedback from the public (for the 1990 Health Objectives), to one that emphasized public engagement, feedback, and participation throughout the development process (for *Healthy People 2010*). Emphasis on public participation has continued in the two-phased process for developing *Healthy People 2020*. (DHHS, 2013, para. 3)

The CDC's National Center for Health Statistics (NCHS) is responsible for monitoring *Healthy People* objectives using its own and other data sources. As a result, there is a great deal of dependence on the data collected at state and local levels from government and nongovernment organizations. For example, the NCHS made data available for *Healthy People 2010* through DATA2010, an interactive database system accessible through the NCHS website, and the CDC WONDER system. The online *Tracking Healthy People 2010* publication informs that effort. This report includes technical information on general data issues and major data sources, detailed definitions for each objective, and additional resources (DHHS, 2013). These processes continue to be updated for each successive *Healthy People* initiative.

Healthy People has become a strategic management tool for the federal government, states, communities, and many private sector partners.

DID YOU KNOW?

To date, 47 states, the District of Columbia, and Guam have developed their own *Healthy People* plans. Most states have emulated national objectives, but virtually all have tailored them to their specific needs. A 1993 NACCHO [National Association of County and City Health Officials] survey showed that 70% of local health departments use *Healthy People 2000* objectives. Within the federal government, *Healthy People* provides a framework for measuring performance in the Government Performance and Results Act. Success is measured by positive changes in health status or reductions in risk factors, as well as improved provision of services. Progress reviews are conducted periodically on each of the 22 priority areas and on population groups, including women, adolescents, people with disabilities, and racial/ethnic groups. *Healthy People* objectives have been specified by Congress as the metric for measuring the progress of the Indian Health Service, the Maternal and Child Health Block Grant, and the Preventive Health and Health Services Block Grant. Ongoing involvement is ensured through the *Healthy People Consortium*—an alliance of 350 national membership organizations and 300 state health, mental health, substance abuse, and environmental agencies. (*Healthy People*, 2000, 2010)

As *Healthy People* developed, it encountered challenges and criticisms. Criticisms include its printed format that constrains usability; the extensive list of objectives that is hard to manage; a disease-specific approach to organizing objectives that has not encouraged crosscutting collaboration around risk factors; lack of transparency about target-setting methods for specific objectives; and lack of data to assess progress. These criticisms continue to be addressed by the *Healthy People* initiative. The current Leading Health Indicators high-priority objectives attempt to address the concern about large numbers of objectives. There are also more interactive and easily obtained graphics and *Healthy People* data (DHHS, 2022). See **Figure 6.1.**

Several criticisms about *Healthy People* seem inappropriate, including lack of progress or slow progress in achieving objective targets; inadequate guidance on how to achieve the objectives; and lack of guidance to users in setting priorities. As a report card system, it can be argued that the *Healthy People* initiative is not responsible for achieving the targets. Rather, the public health system, as a whole, is accountable for progress toward *Healthy People* objectives.

Table 6.4 contains summary information about the nation's progress toward achieving *Healthy People* objectives through 2010. There was a greater success in achieving 1990 objectives than those in 2000 or 2010 (midcourse)—32%, 21%,

Target Year		Overarching Goals	Topic Areas	Objectives
1990	HEALTHY PEOPLE	**Decrease** mortality: infants-adults **Increase** independence among older adults	15	~200
2000	HEALTHY PEOPLE 2000	**Increase** span of healthy life **Reduce** health disparities **Achieve** access to preventive services for all	22	~300
2010	HEALTHY PEOPLE 2010	**Increase** quality and years of healthy life **Eliminate** health disparities	28	~1,000
2020	Healthy People 2020	**Attain** high-quality, longer lives free of preventable disease **Achieve** health equity, eliminate disparities **Create** social and physical environments that promote good health **Promote** quality of life, healthy development, healthy behaviors across life stages	42	~1,300

Figure 6.1. Evolution of the *Healthy People* Initiative Over the Decades

Source: National Center for Health Statistics. (2022). *Healthy people 2020: An end of decade snapshot.* https://health.gov/sites/default/files/2021-03/21%20HP2020EndofDecadeSnapshot2.pdf

Table 6.4. Most Recent Data on Achievement of Past *Healthy People* Objectives

Most Recent Data Source	Objectives/ Targets	Achieved Target	Toward Target	Regressed From Target	Data Unavailable
1990 Health objectives (*Final review, NCHS, 1992*)	226 objectives, 266 targets[a]	32%	34%	11%	23%
Healthy People 2000[b] (*Final review, NCHS, 2001*)	319	21%	41%	17%	10%
Healthy People 2010[c] (*Final review, NCHS, 2012*)	969	17.5%	17.5%	36%	24%

NCHS, National Center for Health Statistics.
[a]All percentages for the 1990 Health objectives reflect attainment of the 266 measured *targets*.
[b]Percentages for *Healthy People 2000* objectives do not add up to 100% in this table because 11% of objectives (35) that showed mixed progress have been excluded.
[c]Percentages for *Healthy People 2010* objectives do not add up to 100% in this table because 5% of objectives (39) that showed no progress have been excluded.

and 6% achieved, respectively. Also note that 40% of the 2010 objectives could not be assessed because of insufficient tracking data.

This information is available for *Healthy People 2020* in *An End of Decade Snapshot*: https://health.gov/sites/default/files/2021-03/21%20HP2020EndofDecade Snapshot2.pdf. This report details the progress made toward achieving the 985 trackable objectives of *Healthy People 2020*. In sum, about 40% of targets were exceeded or met, 21% showed improvement, 31% showed no change, and 14% were worse at the end of the decade (NCHS, 2022).

Healthy People has raised awareness—as all good report cards do—about the public health problems that we have, the progress that we have made toward solving them, and the problems that remain unsolved, and, therefore, are in need of continued attention and action. *Healthy People* results show, especially, that we have not been able to eliminate health disparities between White and minority populations at the community level (The Secretary's Advisory Committee on National Health Promotion and Disease Prevention Objectives for 2020 & DHHS, 2008). Although health care has been proposed as the solution to health disparities, the ecological orientation of public health tells us that health care alone will not eliminate them. "Health disparities, however, are multidimensional, complicated issues that cannot be addressed through the provision of health care alone. Health disparities are rooted in fundamental social structure inequalities" (Aday, 2005, p. 241).

America's Health Rankings™

America's Health Rankings is a report card initiative that ranks each state on health outcomes and health determinants for the purpose of helping localities, counties, states, and regions make decisions about how to improve population health.

America's Health Rankings is a longstanding platform that builds on the United Health Foundation's work to help draw attention to the cornerstones of public health and better understand the health of various populations. The platform is a demonstration of the United Health Foundation's mission of helping build healthier communities, and reflects UnitedHealth Group's commitment to help people live healthier lives.

As the longest-running state-by-state analysis of our nation's health, the platform provides actionable, data-driven insights that stakeholders can use to effect change either in a state or nationally. The United Health Foundation provides the platform to help policymakers, community leaders and health officials better understand the specific health concerns in their own communities so we can all work together to address health challenges. (America's Health Rankings, 2023, paras. 1 and 2)

The model used by America's Health Rankings is reproduced in **Figure 6.2**.

The model evaluates a historical and comprehensive set of health outcomes, social and economic factors, clinical care, behaviors and physical environmental data to determine national health benchmarks and state rankings.

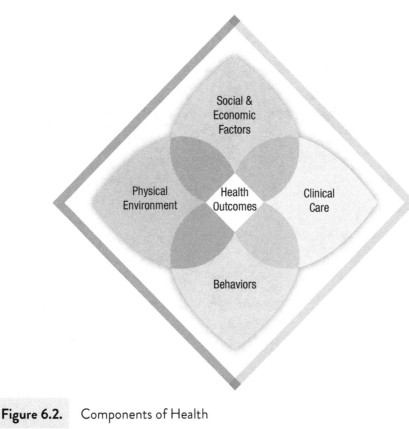

Figure 6.2.   Components of Health

Source: America's Health Rankings. (n.d.). *Introduction.* https://www.americashealthrankings.org/about/methodology/introduction

As an example of their work, **Table 6.5** contains information from America's Health Rankings for 2013. The top three- and bottom three-ranked states on premature death are listed, along with their rankings on other measures including socioeconomic indicators, health behaviors, medical care, and public health funding. There is a general tendency for the states to be similarly ranked on premature death and other indicators. With a few exceptions, the top three are ranked higher than 15 and the bottom three are ranked lower than 35. Public health funding is the least associated with premature death, however.

Table 6.5. Three High- and Three Low-Ranked States on Premature Death, With Selected Health Determinants by County

Selected Counties Ranked on Overall Health	Poor or Fair Health	Adult Obesity	College Degrees	Children in Poverty Parent	Single-Parent Households	Uninsured Adults
Two Highest- and Two Lowest-Ranked Counties on Selected Indicators						
1. Vermont						
Chittenden	8%	19%	45%	8%	9%	12%
Addison	10%	21%	30%	10%	8%	13%
Orange	12%	26%	30%	14%	8%	15%
Essex	17%	25%	15%	21%	9%	16%
3. Massachusetts						
Nantucket	7%	20%	42%	5%	7%	20%
Norfolk	9%	19%	47%	6%	6%	10%
Hampden	15%	26%	24%	25%	12%	12%
Suffolk	17%	21%	37%	28%	11%	15%
5. New Hampshire						
Grafton	10%	23%	34%	10%	8%	14%
Rockingham	10%	23%	36%	6%	7%	10%
Sullivan	12%	27%	25%	12%	10%	13%
Coos	17%	27%	17%	17%	9%	12%
47. Louisiana						
St. Tammany	14%	26%	30%	15%	9%	23%
Lafayette	16%	25%	28%	22%	12%	22%
Madison	21%	33%	13%	49%	16%	14%
East Carroll	20%	34%	14%	56%	18%	12%

(continued)

Table 6.5. Three High- and Three Low-Ranked States on Premature Death, With Selected Health Determinants by County (*continued*)

Selected Counties Ranked on Overall Health	Poor or Fair Health	Adult Obesity	College Degrees	Children in Poverty Parent	Single-Parent Households	Uninsured Adults
48. Alabama						
Shelby	11%	28%	39%	9%	7%	13%
Baldwin	13%	25%	26%	15%	9%	21%
Greene	20%	44%	12%	44%	16%	15%
Lowndes	N/A	40%	12%	43%	15%	15%
50. Mississippi						
DeSoto	16%	32%	20%	11%	11%	20%
Rankin	17%	29%	28%	14%	10%	19%
Tallahatchie	37%	36%	12%	40%	16%	16%
Holmes	25%	42%	12%	51%	22%	13%

N/A, not available.

Source: Population Health Institute at the University of Wisconsin. (2013). *County health rankings.* https://www.countyhealthrankings.org/explore-health-rankings/county-health-rankings -model/health-outcomes/length-of-life/premature-death?keywords=&f%5B0%5D=type%3Astates &f%5B1%5D=type%3Acounties&year=2013

EFFECTIVENESS AND EQUITY OF PUBLIC HEALTH SYSTEM

In the following section, we develop an informal report card for the U.S. public health system by comparing population-level indicators across countries and within subgroups of the United States. Although these indicators are not specific to any one public health program, service, or policy, we assume the overall impact of the public health system on two of the performance criteria—effectiveness and equity—is reflected in these measures.

As an example of how population-level outcomes are used to assess public health performance, consider the case of life expectancy. Life expectancy can be used as an assessment measure in at least two ways. First, we can compare the life expectancy in one society to life expectancy in another. Second, we can compare life expectancies among subgroups within one society. In the first case, life expectancy rates indicate that the United States has a problem with public health effectiveness. In the second case, life expectancy rates indicate that the United States has a problem with equity.

Comparisons With Other Countries

We compare the United States to other member nations in the OECD. The OECD is a forum where the governments of 38 democracies with market-based economies collaborate to develop policy standards to promote sustainable economic growth. For the list of these countries, see **Table 6.6** (WHO, 2019).

Life Expectancy and HALE

First, we consider life expectancy in the United States compared to other nations in the OECD. In 2019, the United States ranked 30 out of 38 countries in life expectancy at birth for males—76.3 years. Switzerland had the highest life expectancy for men at 81.8 years. Only seven countries had a lower life expectancy for men than the United States—Poland, Slovakia, Hungary, Lithuania, Mexico, Latvia, and Estonia. The United States ranked 33 out of 37 countries in life expectancy at birth for females—80.7 years. Japan had the highest life expectancy for women at 86.9 years. Only four countries had a lower life expectancy for women than the United States—Lithuania, Mexico, Latvia, and Hungary.

When we examine healthy life expectancy (HALE) at birth and at 60 years of age a similar story emerges. Americans have, on average, fewer years of healthy life compared to most of countries in the OECD. For example, healthy life expectancy at birth for men is highest in Japan at 72.6 years, while the United States is ranked 33 out of 37 with 65.2 years of healthy life, on average. Only four countries had a lower HALE than the United States—Hungary, Lithuania, Mexico, and Latvia. For women, Japan is also ranked first with 75.5 years of healthy life expected, and the United States is ranked last of the 37 OECD countries with a HALE of 65 years.

Infant and Maternal Mortality

Comparison of the IMR in the United States to the same 38 peer countries also indicates a problem of public health effectiveness and equity in the United States. In 2020, the United States' IMR was 5.4 per 1,000 live births (OECD, 2022b). Although this rate is low, it is among the highest of the 38 peer countries. Only Mexico, Colombia, Turkey, Costa Rica, and Chile had higher IMR rates. Similarly, maternal mortality in the United States was among the highest of the OECD countries at 20.1/100,000 live births in 2019 and 23.8/100,000 live births in 2020. The lowest rates were under 11/100,000 live births. Only 9 of the 38 countries in 2019 and 10 countries in 2020 had maternal mortality rates above 11/100,000 live births (OECD, 2022b).

Comparisons Within the Country

We can also compare groups within the United States to indicate disparities in health and well-being. These include life expectancy, age-adjusted mortality, and IMR. Overall, we find significant differences in these measures within the United States, and we present some key findings for them by age, gender, race, and ethnicity.

Table 6.6. Life Expectancy and Healthy Life Expectancy (HALE) in OECD Countries, 2019 (WHO, 2019)

Country	Life Expectancy at Birth (Years)			Life Expectancy at Age 60 (Years)			Healthy Life Expectancy (HALE) at Birth (Years)			Healthy Life Expectancy (HALE) at Age 60 (Years)		
	Both Sexes	Male	Female	Both Sexes	Male	Female	Both Sexes	Male	Female	Both Sexes	Male	Female
United States	78.5	76.3	80.7	23.1	21.8	24.4	66.1	65.2	67	16.4	15.6	17.1
Australia	83	81.3	84.8	25.6	24.4	26.8	70.9	70.2	71.7	19	18.2	19.7
Austria	81.6	79.4	83.8	24.1	22.4	25.6	70.9	69.9	71.9	18.3	17.2	19.4
Belgium	81.4	79.3	83.5	24	22.3	25.6	70.6	69.8	71.3	18.2	17.2	19.1
Canada	82.2	80.4	84.1	25.2	23.8	26.4	71.3	70.5	72	19	18.2	19.7
Chile	80.7	78.1	83.2	24.3	22.4	25.9	70	69	71.1	18.4	17.3	19.3
Colombia	79.3	76.7	81.9	24	22.5	25.3	69	67.4	70.5	18.1	17.1	18.9
Costa Rica	80.8	78.3	83.4	25	23.6	26.4	70	68.6	71.3	18.7	17.8	19.5
Czechia	79.1	76.3	81.9	22.1	19.9	24	68.8	67	70.6	16.3	14.7	17.8
Denmark	81.3	79.6	83	23.6	22.3	24.9	71	70.7	71.4	18.2	17.6	18.9
Estonia	78.9	74.7	82.6	22.5	19.3	25	69.2	66.4	71.7	17.3	14.8	19.1
Finland	81.6	79.2	84	24.2	22.4	25.8	71	69.9	72	18.5	17.3	19.5

(continued)

Table 6.6. Life Expectancy and Healthy Life Expectancy (HALE) in OECD Countries, 2019 (WHO, 2019) *(continued)*

Country	Life Expectancy at Birth (Years)			Life Expectancy at Age 60 (Years)			Healthy Life Expectancy (HALE) at Birth (Years)			Healthy Life Expectancy (HALE) at Age 60 (Years)		
	Both Sexes	Male	Female	Both Sexes	Male	Female	Both Sexes	Male	Female	Both Sexes	Male	Female
France	82.5	79.8	85.1	25.3	23.3	27.2	72.1	71.1	73.1	19.7	18.5	20.8
Germany	81.7	78.7	84.8	24.4	21.9	26.9	70.9	69.7	72.1	18.5	17	19.9
Greece	81.1	78.6	83.6	23.8	22.1	25.5	70.9	69.9	71.9	18.4	17.3	19.5
Hungary	76.4	73.1	79.6	20.2	17.7	22.3	67.2	65	69.3	15.3	13.4	16.8
Iceland	82.3	80.8	83.9	24.6	23.7	25.5	72	71.7	72.3	19	18.6	19.4
Ireland	81.8	80.2	83.5	24.2	23	25.3	71.1	70.7	71.4	18.6	18	19.2
Israel	82.6	80.8	84.4	24.9	23.6	26	72.4	72	72.7	19.3	18.7	19.9
Italy	83	80.9	84.9	25	23.4	26.5	71.9	71.2	72.6	18.9	17.9	19.8
Japan	84.3	81.5	86.9	26.3	23.9	28.6	74.1	72.6	75.5	20.4	18.8	21.8
Latvia	75.4	70.6	79.8	20.5	17.2	23	66.2	62.9	69.3	15.6	13.2	17.4
Lithuania	76	71.2	80.4	20.9	17.6	23.5	66.7	63.4	69.7	15.9	13.4	17.8
Luxembourg	82.4	80.6	84.2	24.4	22.9	25.8	71.6	71.1	72	18.5	17.7	19.3
Mexico	76	73.1	78.9	21.8	20.5	23.1	65.8	64.3	67.2	16.1	15.3	16.8

(continued)

Netherlands	81.8	80.4	83.1	24.1	23	25.1	71.4	71.3	71.5	18.4	17.9	18.9
New Zealand	82	80.4	83.5	24.8	23.8	25.8	70.2	69.6	70.8	18.6	17.9	19.2
Norway	82.6	81.1	84.1	24.7	23.5	25.8	71.4	71	71.6	18.5	17.8	19.1
Poland	78.3	74.5	81.9	22.1	19.5	24.3	68.7	65.9	71.3	16.8	14.9	18.5
Portugal	81.6	78.6	84.4	24.3	22.1	26.3	71	69.6	72.2	18.6	17.3	19.8
Korea	83.3	80.3	86.1	25.8	23.4	27.9	73.1	71.3	74.7	19.8	18.2	21.2
Slovakia	78.2	74.8	81.4	21.8	19.3	23.9	68.5	66.2	70.8	16.6	14.6	18.2
Slovenia	81.3	78.6	84.1	23.8	21.8	25.6	70.7	69	72.5	17.8	16.4	19.2
Spain	83.2	80.7	85.7	25.4	23.3	27.3	72.1	71.3	72.9	19.2	18	20.3
Sweden	82.4	80.8	84	24.5	23.3	25.6	71.9	71.7	72.1	18.9	18.3	19.4
Switzerland	83.4	81.8	85.1	25.4	24.1	26.6	72.5	72.2	72.8	19.5	18.8	20.2
Turkey	78.6	76.4	80.7	22	20.6	23.2	68.4	67.8	69	16.6	15.8	17.3
United Kingdom	81.4	79.8	83	24.1	23	25.2	70.1	69.6	70.6	18.3	17.6	18.9

Life Expectancy and Age-Adjusted Mortality

Next, we examine life expectancy and age-adjusted mortality among subgroups within the United States. There are significant differences among population subgroups, which have been noted historically (Adler et al., 1993; IOM, 2003; Pappas et al., 1993). First, race and ethnicity are predictors of disparities in life expectancies. **Figure 6.3** displays the life expectancy at birth by Hispanic origin and race in 2019 and 2020. Although there was a decline in life expectancy between 2019 and 2020, the disparity by race and ethnicity remains. The authors write:

> Regardless of Hispanic origin, life expectancy for the black population has consistently been lower than that of the white population but the gap between the two races had generally been narrowing since 1993 when it was 7.1. The gap of 6.0 observed in the first half of 2020 is the largest since 1998. Conversely, the gap between the Hispanic and non-Hispanic white populations decreased by 37% between 2019 and the first half of 2020 (from 3.0 to 1.9 years). This indicates that the Hispanic population lost some of the mortality advantage it has evidenced since 2006 relative to the non-Hispanic white population, despite experiencing generally lower socioeconomic status. (Arias et al., 2021, p. 3)

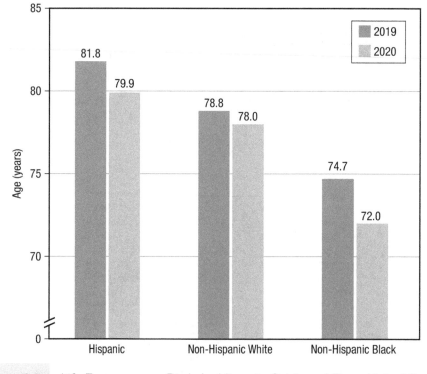

Figure 6.3.   Life Expectancy at Birth, by Hispanic Origin and Race: United States, 2019 and 2020

Source: Arias, E., Tejada-Vera, B., & Ahmad, F. (2021). Provisional life expectancy estimates for January through June 2020. *NVSS Vital Statistics Rapid Release, 10.* https://www.cdc.gov/nchs/data/vsrr/VSRR10-508.pdf

In 2019, the age-adjusted death rate was 715.2 per 100,000 population. However, there was considerable variation by race and ethnicity and sex. (Age adjustment statistically accounts for the fact that life expectancy from birth is shorter for males than for females.) Overall, men have substantially higher death rates than women, and among men in 2019, Black males had the highest rate (1,092.8), followed by White men (868.8) and Hispanic men (633.2). Among women, the highest age-adjusted mortality rate was for Black women with 724.9/100,000, followed by White women at 627.4, and then Hispanic women at 430.7. See **Figure 6.4**. Also note that the death rate increased for all race and ethnic groups in 2020, but especially for Hispanics and Blacks (Murphy et al., 2021). Much of the increase in death was due to COVID-19.

This uneven pattern holds for age-adjusted death rates for selected diseases. In 2019, the rate/100,000 population for diabetes was lowest for Asian Americans at 16.6 and Whites at 19. The age-adjusted mortality rate was highest for Black Americans at 38.2 and American Indians at 41.5. Disparities in age-adjusted death from heart disease also shows disparities, although Whites and Black Americans had the highest levels at 165.8 and 205.7, respectively (Kaiser Family Foundation, 2022). See **Figure 6.5**.

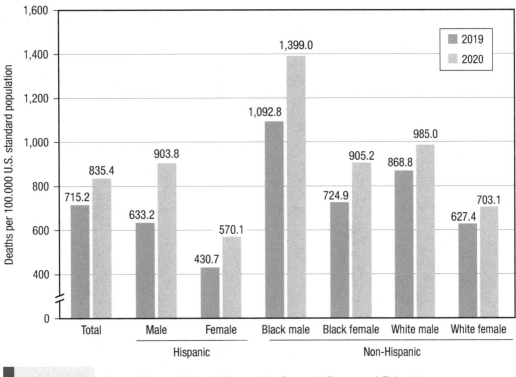

Figure 6.4. Age-Adjusted Death Rates, by Sex and Race and Ethnicity: United States, 2019 and 2020

Source: Murphy, S. L., Kochanek, K. D., Xu, J., & Arias, E. (2021). Mortality in the United States, 2020. *NCHS Data Brief, 427.* https://www.cdc.gov/nchs/products/databriefs/db427.htm#section_2

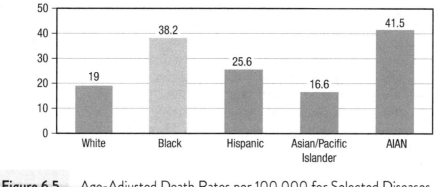

Figure 6.5.   Age-Adjusted Death Rates per 100,000 for Selected Diseases by Race/Ethnicity, 2021

Source: Hill, L., Ndugga, N., & Artiga, S. (2023). *Key data on health and health carte by race and ethnicity.* KFF. https://www.kff.org/report-section/key-facts-on-health-and-health-care-by-race-and-ethnicity-health-status -outcomes-and-behaviors/

Infant Mortality Rate

The subgroup comparison of infant mortality within the United States also indicates problems. The difference in the IMR in the United States between racial and ethnic groups is striking and long-standing. In 2018, the IMR ranged from 3.6 deaths/1,000 births for Asian Americans to 10.8 deaths/1,000 births for Black Americans. The rate for Whites and Hispanic women are very similar—4.6/1,000 births and 4.9/1,000 births, respectively (Kaiser Family Foundation, 2022). See **Figure 6.6**. Note, too, that the Black American IMR has been at least double that for Whites since 1915, when the rate was first recorded as 99.9 per thousand overall (Grove & Hetzel, 1968).

Overall, the statistics on life expectancy, mortality, and infant mortality indicate existing disparities between men and women, as well as between persons of different races and ethnicities. Typically, Blacks and Native Americans have worse scores than Whites and Asians, and persons of Hispanic ethnicity fall

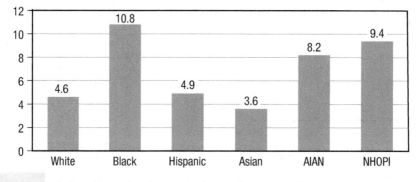

Figure 6.6.   Infant Mortality (per 1,000 Live Births) by Race/Ethnicity, 2018

Source: Hill, L., Ndugga, N., & Artiga, S. (2023). *Key data on health and health carte by race and ethnicity.* KFF. https://www.kff.org/report-section/key-facts-on-health-and-health-care-by-race-and-ethnicity-health-status -outcomes-and-behaviors/

somewhere in between. It is notable, though, that Hispanics have the highest life expectancy of any race or ethnic group. These differences indicate the magnitude and complexity of the work before public health to achieve equity in health status effectively and efficiently. The work will require different emphases for different communities. Health problems will differ and methods will need to be tailored to fit specific community attributes. Health determinants to be considered will include access to education, nutritious food, clean water and air, opportunities for physical activity, adequate housing, safe workplaces, health care, and others.

CHAPTER SUMMARY

Performance of the public health system can be evaluated at the micro-level of programs, policies, and services that are targeted at defined populations, and it can be evaluated at the system level using population health indicators such as IMR, life expectancy, and premature death rate for geographic locales and sub-populations. The criteria for evaluating the public health system, as a whole, as well as its component programs, policies, and services are effectiveness, equity, and efficiency. There is strong evidence from the report card initiatives that the effectiveness and equity of the system are not satisfactory, and, therefore, the efficiency of the system cannot be acceptable either. This is a continuing challenge for public health professionals and organizations in the coming years.

DISCUSSION QUESTIONS

Q: What is EBPH and how does it relate to evidence-based medicine?

Q: What is meant by public health system effectiveness, efficiency, and equity?

Q: How well does the U.S. public health system perform? What measures are you using to evaluate the system?

Q: What organizations collect information on the performance of the U.S. public health system?

Q: Where does the information on performance come from?

Q: What organizations evaluate U.S. public health organizations?

DATA SOURCES

The following websites provide links to scientific studies and published reports that contain guidance for local health departments, health care providers, community leaders, employers, and others to improve the performance of public health programs, services, and policies. Together, these sites provide innumerable examples of what has been tried and how well it worked—EBPH programs, services, and policies.

- Centers for Disease Control and Prevention (CDC)

  The CDC's *Guide to Community Preventive Services* provides a summary of effective community interventions that promote health and prevent disease. The *Guide* is a valuable source of systematic reviews and evidence-based recommendations for public health practice. In addition, the Task Force on Community Preventive Services has developed methods that may be used to evaluate the impact of EBPH interventions. Explore these resources here: https://www.thecommunityguide.org/

- The Cochrane Collaboration

  Cochrane is an international network with headquarters in the U.K. It is a registered not-for-profit organization and does not accept commercial or conflicted funding.

  For 28 years, the Cochrane Collaboration's global network has gathered and summarized peer-reviewed research that can be used to improve public health performance. Topics of the systematic reviews include child health, health and safety at work, infectious disease, tobacco, and drugs and alcohol, among many others. Cochrane's systematic reviews are available from the *Cochrane Library*, which can be found here: https://www.cochranelibrary.com/cdsr/reviews

- ASTHO

  ASTHO has archived information on health initiatives and research that increases the evidence base supporting public health interventions. The site includes *Program Development 3 (PD 3)*, which provides the proportion of a health department's programs that are currently implementing evidence-based intervention. This site can be explored at: https://www.astho.org/globalassets/pdf/accreditation/performance-dashboard-tool/performance-dashboard-tool-pd3.pdf

  In addition, ASTHO contains descriptions of evidence-based projects in every major area of public health practice. For example, ASTHO's Early Brain Development project includes tested policy approaches, such as evidence-based home visiting and maternal depression screening, that can buffer the effects of adverse child experiences and help shape the social environments in which children grow up and build a strong foundation for their health and wellness. Many more topics are found on the ASTHO website: https://www.astho.org/topic/

- NACCHO

  NACCHO's *Model Practices Database* is a searchable database of local health agency practices between 2003 and 2014, graded as model or promising. Applications were required to include an evaluation of the program, policy, or service. This website can be explored at: https://eweb.naccho.org/eweb/DynamicPage.aspx?site=naccho&webcode=mpsearch&OrderBy=progname&dir=%7B?dir==

NACCHO's more recent examples of EBPH are found in four areas—Public Health Preparedness, Community Health, Environmental Health, and Public Health Infrastructure and Systems—at the following website: https://www.naccho.org/programs

- U.S. Preventive Services Task Force

  The U.S. Preventive Services Task Force, an activity of the Agency for Healthcare Research and Quality, develops recommendations on the efficacy of preventive clinical services such as disease screening and health counseling. The recommendations of the Task Force can be searched in the *Electronic Preventive Services Selector ePSS*. Recommendations are grouped into three categories: Recommended; Not Recommended; and Uncertain Recommendations. Start here for your search: https://www.healthit.gov/resource/electronic-preventative-services-selector-epss

To explore how the United States compares to other countries in health and health system performance, the WHO and the OECD obtain and make available this information.

- The Global Health Observatory (WHO) can be found at: https://www.who.int/data/gho
- OECD Health Statistics can be explored here: https://www.oecd.org/els/health-systems/health-data.htm

---

A robust set of instructor resources designed to supplement this text is located at **http://connect.springerpub.com/content/book/978-0-8261-8615-7**. Qualifying instructors may request access by emailing **textbook@springerpub.com**.

REFERENCES

Aday, L. A. (2005). *Reinventing public health: Policies and practices for a healthy nation.* Jossey-Bass.

Aday, L. A., Begley, C. E., Lairson, D. R., & Balkrishnan, R. (2004). *Evaluating the healthcare system: Effectiveness, efficiency, and equity.* Health Administration Press.

Aday, L. A., Begley, C. E., Lairson, D. R., & Slater, C. H. (1993). *Evaluating the medical care system: Effectiveness, efficiency, and equity.* Health Administration Press.

Adler, N. E., Boyce, W. T., Chesney, M. A., Folkman, S., & Syme, S. L. (1993). Socioeconomic inequalities in health: No easy solution. *Journal of the American Medical Association, 269*(24), 3140–3145. https://doi.org/10.1001/jama.1993.03500240084031

America's Health Rankings. (2013). *About the report.* http://www.americashealthrankings.org/

Arias, E., Tejada-Vera, B., & Ahmad, F. (2021). Provisional life expectancy estimates for January through June, 2020. *Vital Statistics Rapid Release, 10.* https://www.cdc.gov/nchs/data/vsrr/VSRR10-508.pdf

Brownson, R. C., Baker, E. A., Deshpande, A. D., & Gillespie, K. N. (2018). *Evidence-based public health* (3rd ed.). Oxford University Press.

Brownson, R. C., Baker, E. A., Leet, T. L., & Gillespie, K. N. (2003). *Evidence-based public health.* Oxford University Press.

Brownson, R. C., Gurney, J. G., & Land, G. H. (1999). Evidence-based decision making in public health. *Journal of Public Health Management and Practice, 5,* 86–97. https://doi.org/10.1097/00124784-199909000-00012

Cardoso, J. R., Pereira, L. M., Iversen, M. D., & Ramos, A. L. (2014). What is gold standard and what is ground truth? *Dental Press Journal of Orthodontics, 19*(5), 27–30. https://doi.org/10.1590/2176-9451.19.5.027-030.ebo

Centers for Disease Control and Prevention. (2010a). *Healthy people 2000.* http://www.cdc.gov/nchs/healthy_people/hp2000.htm

Centers for Disease Control and Prevention. (2010b). *Healthy people 2010.* http://www.cdc.gov/nchs/healthy_people/hp2010.htm

Centers for Disease Control and Prevention. (2022a). *Sources and definitions. Health United States, 2020–2021.* https://www.cdc.gov/nchs/hus/sources-definitions.htm

Centers for Disease Control and Prevention. (2022b). *National Public Health Performance Standards.* https://www.cdc.gov/publichealthgateway/nphps/index.html

Centers for Disease Control and Prevention, Reproductive Health. (2023). *Infant mortality.* https://www.cdc.gov/reproductivehealth/maternalinfanthealth/infantmortality.htm

Council on Education for Public Health. (2022). *About.* https://ceph.org/about/org-info/

Council on Education for Public Health. (2023). *Accreditation statistics.* https://ceph.org/about/org-info/

Council on Linkages Between Academia and Public Health Practice. (2021). *Core competencies for public health professionals.* https://www.phf.org/resourcestools/Documents/Core_Competencies_for_Public_Health_Professionals_2021October.pdf

County Health Rankings. (2013). *About the county program.* http://www.countyhealthrankings.org/about-project

Ettorchi-Tardy, A., Levif, M., & Michel, P. (2012). Benchmarking: A method for continuous quality improvement in health. *Healthcare Policy, 7*(4), e101–e119. https://www.ncbi.nlm.nih.gov/pmc/articles/PMC3359088/

Fackler, M. (2011). Tsunami warnings, written in stone. *The New York Times.* https://www.nytimes.com/2011/04/21/world/asia/21stones.html

Grove, R. D., & Hetzel, A. M. (1968). *Vital statistics rates in the United States: 1940–1960.* U.S. Government Printing Office.

Institute of Medicine. (1990). *Healthy people 2000: Citizens chart the course.* National Academy Press.

Institute of Medicine. (2003). *Unequal treatment: Confronting racial and ethnic disparities in health care.* National Academies Press.

Institute of Medicine & Committee on the Study of the Future of Public Health. (1988). *The future of public health.* National Academies Press.

Issel, L. M. (2009). *Health program planning and evaluation.* Jones and Bartlett.

Jenicek, M. (1997). Epidemiology, evidenced-based medicine, and evidence-based public health. *Journal of Epidemiology, 7*(4), 187–197. https://doi.org/10.2188/jea.7.187

Kaiser Family Foundation. (2022). *Key facts on health and health care by race and ethnicity.* https://www.kff.org/report-section/key-facts-on-health-and-health-care-by-race-and-ethnicity-health-status-outcomes-and-behaviors/

Kallmen, H., & Hallgren, M. (2021). Bullying at school and mental health problems among adolescents: A repeated cross-sectional study. *Child and Adolescent Psychiatry and Mental Health, 15*(74). https://doi.org/10.1186/s13034-021-00425-y

Kindig, D. A. (1997). *Purchasing population health: Paying for results.* University of Michigan Press.

Kohatsu, N. D., Robinson, J. G., & Torner, J. C. (2004). Evidence-based public health: An evolving concept. *American Journal of Preventive Medicine, 27*(5), 417–421. https://doi.org/10.1016/s0749-3797(04)00196-5

Liu, K., Moon, M., Sulvetta, M., & Chawla, J. (1992). International infant mortality rankings: A look behind the numbers. *Health Care Financing Review, 13*(4), 105–118. https://www.ncbi.nlm.nih.gov/pmc/articles/PMC4193257/

Murphy, S. L., Kochanek, K. D., Xu, J., & Arias, E. (2021). Mortality in the United States, 2020. *NCHS Data Brief, 427.* https://www.cdc.gov/nchs/products/databriefs/db427.htm#section_2

National Board of Public Health Examiners. (2022). *CPH: Certified in Public Health.* https://www.nbphe.org/why-get-certified/

National Center for Health Statistics. (1992). *Prevention profile, health, United States, 1991.* Public Health Service.

National Center for Health Statistics. (2001). *Healthy people 2000: Final review.* National Center for Health Statistics.

National Center for Health Statistics. (2012). *Healthy people 2010: Final review.* National Center for Health Statistics.

National Center for Health Statistics. (2022). *Healthy people 2020: An end of decade snapshot.* https://health.gov/sites/default/files/2021-03/21%20HP2020EndofDecadeSnapshot2.pdf

Office of the Assistant Secretary for Health and Surgeon General. (1979). *Healthy people: The surgeon general's report on health promotion and disease prevention.* U.S. Government Printing Office.

Organisation for Economic Cooperation and Development. (2022a). *Potential years of life lost*. https://data.oecd.org/healthstat/potential-years-of-life-lost.htm

Organisation for Economic Cooperation and Development. (2022b). *Health status: Maternal and infant mortality*. OECD.Stat. https://stats.oecd.org/index.aspx?queryid=30116

Pappas, F., Queen, S., Hadden, W., & Fisher, G. (1993). The increasing disparity in mortality between socioeconomic groups in the United States, 1960 and 1986. *New England Journal of Medicine, 329*(2), 103–109. https://doi.org/10.1056/nejm199307083290207

Population Health Institute at the University of Wisconsin. (2013). *County health rankings*. https://www.countyhealthrankings.org/reports/county-health-rankings-reports

Public Health Accreditation Board. (2022). *About*. https://phaboard.org/

Rychetnik, L., Hawe, P., Waters, E., Barratt, A., & Frommer, M. (2004). A glossary for evidence based public health. *Journal of Epidemiology and Community Health, 58*, 538–545. https://doi.org/10.1136/jech.2003.011585

Sackett, D. L., Straus, S. E., Richardson, W. S., Rosenberg, W., & Haynes, R. B. (2000). *Evidence-Based medicine: How to practice and teach EBM*. Churchill Livingstone.

Tilson, H. H. (2008). Public health accreditation: Progress on national accountability. *Annual Review of Public Health, 29*, xv–xxii. https://doi.org/10.1146/annurev.pu.29.031708.100021

The Secretary's Advisory Committee on National Health Promotion and Disease Prevention Objectives for 2020 & U.S. Department of Health & Human Services. (2008). *Phase I report recommendations for the framework and format of healthy people 2020*. https://health.gov/sites/default/files/2021-11/Secretary%27s%20Advisory%20Committee%20Recommendations%20for%20HP2020%20Framework%20and%20Format.pdf

U.S. Department of Health & Human Services. (2000). *Healthy people 2010: Understanding and improving health* (2nd ed.). U.S. Government Printing Office.

U.S. Department of Health & Human Services (2022). *Healthy people 2030*. https://health.gov/healthypeople/objectives-and-data/leading-health-indicators

Versi, E. (1992). "Gold standard" is an appropriate term. *British Medical Journal, 305*, 187. https://doi.org/10.1136/bmj.305.6846.187-b, https://www.ncbi.nlm.nih.gov/pmc/articles/PMC1883235/

World Health Organization. (2019). *Life expectancy and healthy life expectancy data by country*. Global Health Observatory. https://apps.who.int/gho/data/node.main.688

World Health Organization. (2022a). *Healthy life expectancy at birth*. The Global Health Observatory. https://www.who.int/data/gho/indicator-metadata-registry/imr-details/66

World Health Organization. (2022b). *Disability-adjusted life years*. The Global Health Observatory. https://www.who.int/data/gho/indicator-metadata-registry/imr-details/158

7 Building Healthy Communities

LEARNING OBJECTIVES

Students will learn . . .

1. Describe the three major approaches for changing risky behaviors.

2. Describe the differences between the population-based tools of social marketing and community engagement.

3. Describe the five groups of communities.

4. Describe the nine principles of community engagement.

5. Describe the principles of comprehensive worksite wellness programs.

There is incredible power within local communities to build truly healthy communities, and public health organizations need to understand how to tap that power in order to be successful. Since all communities are unique in composition and needs, there is no single model to do that. Rather, healthy communities must be built community by community. Having the tools to facilitate true community engagement is the key to success.

KEY IDEA

Unfortunately, much of what has been done historically in the name of community engagement is actually community coercion (Dwelle & Musumba, 2013).

Many community initiatives start with a single person or organization within the community and blossom as community members and organizations identify with and discuss perceived needs and solutions at the community level. These initiatives often begin with a focus on risky behaviors and how to reduce them. Important community issues may include those around major risk factors like tobacco, diet and exercise, nutrition, alcohol and substance abuse, and the built environment. In addition, there is increasing recognition that the built environment has a major influence on community health. The built environment includes community design and organization that decrease exposure to environmental contaminants, increase access to healthy foods, encourage adequate exercise, decrease the risk of injury, and decrease the risk of violence and crime.

There are three major approaches to changing risky behaviors: policy, influencing individuals or families in a clinic-like setting, and population-based interventions (see **Figure 7.1**).

> Policy developed by local, state and federal governments, businesses, and organizations is an effective tool to encourage healthy behaviors but must be implemented and enforced to be effective. Clinicians are trained in one-on-one counseling, another powerful strategy to encourage the change of risky behaviors. Population-based interventions provide yet another potent behavioral impact and can be divided into two tool subsets; social marketing and community engagement. (Dwelle & Musumba, 2013, p. 35)

Additional elements contributing to building healthy communities are effective local coalitions and community-level integration among policy, clinical, and public health interventions. All of these approaches are important to building healthy communities and must be integrated through collaboration and partnerships.

Population-based expertise lies primarily in the discipline of public health. Increased public health investments, especially in low-resource communities, have been associated with decreased mortality from preventable causes of death,

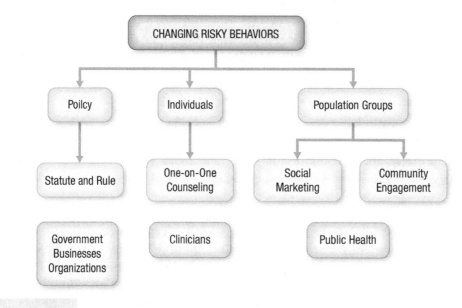

Figure 7.1.   Changing Risky Behaviors Involves Individuals, Groups, and Policy

Source: Dwelle, T. L., & Musumba, A. (2013). *Engagement or coercion: A community engagement toolkit.* Unpublished.

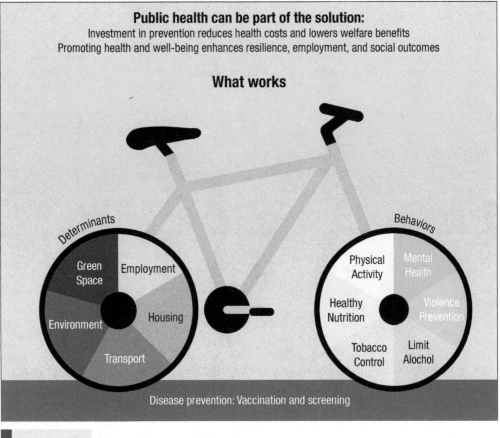

Public health can be part of the solution:
Investment in prevention reduces health costs and lowers welfare benefits
Promoting health and well-being enhances resilience, employment, and social outcomes

What works

Determinants

Green Space
Employment
Environment
Housing
Transport

Behaviors

Physical Activity
Mental Health
Healthy Nutrition
Violence Prevention
Tobacco Control
Limit Alochol

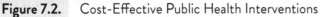

Disease prevention: Vaccination and screening

Figure 7.2. Cost-Effective Public Health Interventions

Source: World Health Organization Regional Office for Europe. (2014). *The case for investing in public health.*
https://www.researchgate.net/publication/277189955_The_case_for_investing_in_public_health

including those associated with infant mortality and deaths due to cardiovascular disease, diabetes, and cancer (Mays & Smith, 2011). For instance, they report that for each 10% increase in local public health spending, mortality rates fell between 1.1% and 6.9%. According to the World Health Organization (WHO), population-based approaches cost five times less than individual interventions, and provide a return on investment (ROI) of $4.00 for every dollar invested (WHO, 2014).These include impacting determinants such as green space, employment, housing and the environment, as well as behaviors including physical activity, alcohol abuse, and nutrition. See **Figure 7.2**: Cost-Effective Public Health Interventions for a visual example.

COMMUNITY ENGAGEMENT

A major role of active, engaged communities throughout history has been to support and encourage the health and well-being of community members. Consistent with WHO's definition of health (1946), health is generally defined by

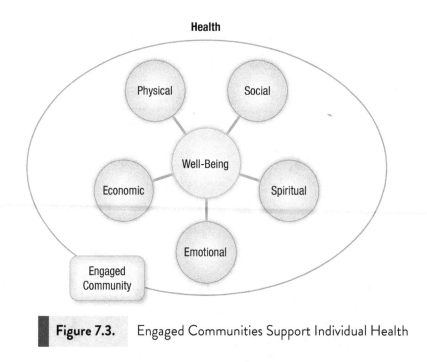

Figure 7.3.   Engaged Communities Support Individual Health

most cultures as much more than absence of disease. It may include the physical, social, economic, emotional, and spiritual well-being of a person and community. Some cultures define health as harmony with one's self, others, the supernatural, and the environment. A community's perception of the world, including its definition of health and wellness, stems from the community's deep cultural beliefs and values—its worldview. Communities will only express interest and invest their time and resources in issues their members feel are important to them—their perceived needs. These community perceptions define the boundaries of community engagement and ownership and are essential for public health professionals working with communities on health issues to understand (see **Figure 7.3**).

KEY IDEA

Building sustainable healthy communities requires community ownership.

It takes exceptional patience and special community engagement skills and competencies to facilitate community ownership of problems and solutions as they move from unhealthy behaviors to health and wellness. This approach is often not supported by the rigid requirements and timelines of grants. The special skills of a community engagement specialist include expertise in facilitating group participatory discussions using concepts like LePSA(S) (**L**earner-centered training which involves three phases: **P**roblem-posing, **S**elf-discovery, and **A**ction; Lennon & Coombs, 1992) or Open Space Facilitation (Owen, 1993), which fosters group ownership.

To a community engagement facilitator, a community is often much more than a geopolitical area. A true community exhibits the following key characteristics: people who know each other by first name and have a sense of shared responsibility for each other. If these characteristics are met, community engagement concepts can often be used to facilitate community ownership of their problems and solutions.

People are generally members of not just one, but multiple communities. These communities impact how members think, act, and believe, often through the influence of horizontal communicators, also known as opinion leaders or champions. These individuals are most often informal rather than formal leaders and due to their community status can exert exceptional impact on the beliefs, values, institutions, and behaviors of community members. A major goal of a public health community engagement facilitator is to find and engage these horizontal communicators in target communities.

Communities that meet the definition of community can be divided into five general categories, including:

- Rural towns and villages,
- Worksites,
- Schools,
- Civic and faith-based groups, and
- Other groups (e.g., Optimists, Rotary, Knights of Columbus, NAACP, and others).

Fundamental community engagement concepts generally apply to engaging all of these and other communities. Yet there are unique concepts that apply to each group and must be mastered by facilitators to truly engage them. Faith-based communities have a strong belief in the supernatural. A facilitator must understand how to encourage using those deep beliefs to change risky behaviors. In the school community, it is essential to understand the worldview and development of children and youth versus adults. In the worksite, a facilitator must appreciate that the business' bottom line is always an essential consideration.

Another major concept of community engagement is realizing that a community does not exist in a vacuum within a target area. Community members are commonly members of multiple communities or subcommunities in that area (e.g., churches, school organizations, worksites). Consistent messages within all the communities to which an individual belongs will usually result in reaching a behavioral threshold more quickly. Therefore, an effective community engagement strategy is to engage as many communities in a target area as possible. Rural target areas can generally use community engagement in all five of these community groups while urban areas are often limited to worksites, faith-based groups, schools, and other organizations.

Community Engagement and Maslow's Hierarchy of Needs

Maslow described a hierarchy of needs that can be further divided into deficiency needs and growth needs (**Figure 7.4**).

Maslow's Hierarchy of Needs

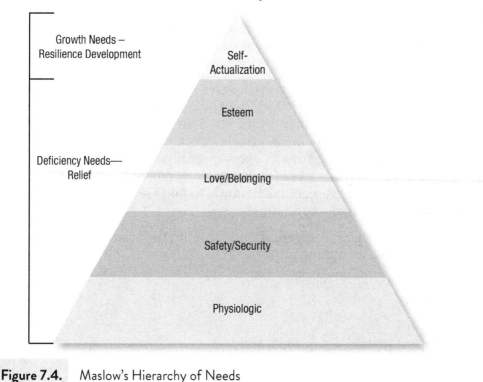

Figure 7.4. Maslow's Hierarchy of Needs

Source: Maslow, A. H. (1954). *Motivation and personality.* Harper.

The deficiency needs include physiologic, safety and security, love and belonging, and esteem, where the growth needs fall into the area of self-actualization. In a way, Maslow's hierarchy of needs defines the scope of the determinants of health. Deficiency needs are generally more temporal in nature, focusing on the now, while growth needs relate to longer-term goals and strategies. Public health and community development primarily relate to longer-range goals, therefore falling into the area of self-actualization. Community deficiency needs must be met to a significant degree to release community energy for self-actualization. Therefore, some early community building interventions may need to address the social determinants around deficiency needs first before being able to facilitate community engagement for longer-range goals. Public health must be willing to collaborate, partner, and strategize with key stakeholders to significantly meet the deficiency needs of communities during the community-building process.

Many organizations attempt to short-circuit this process, resulting in failure. Transitional strategies are often important to allow adequate time for community infrastructure, political, and policy changes. Progressive change is a necessary part of life and public health indicating healthy growth. As childhood growth is often associated with growing pains, public health growth is also associated with discomfort and sometimes even disapproval from colleagues, friends, the public, and politicians. Public health must always seek to improve the well-being of people using good science, but also use wisdom to design reasonable transitional strategies to reach the goal.

Community Engagement and Social Marketing

Behaviors are the result of deeper influences on individuals from their cultures and communities. Behaviors arise from an individual's worldview, that is, their deep beliefs in four areas (Redfield, 1957):

- Self (humanity),
- Nature,
- The supernatural, and
- Time (past, present, and future).

It is from this worldview that we build our belief systems including ideology or philosophy of life and cosmology (where everything comes from). Values, the things we feel are important in life, are developed based on deep beliefs. It's upon these deep beliefs and values that we build our institutions, how we do things, including how we govern ourselves, how we educate our children, how we marry, how we organize and run our businesses, and how we develop our laws. Finally, all of these deeper layers emerge as our behaviors and artifacts. Cultural communications experts strongly suggest that to make permanent changes in the risky behaviors of a society, the underlying beliefs and values that drive those risky behaviors must be changed. This is a major premise of community engagement (see **Figure 7.5**).

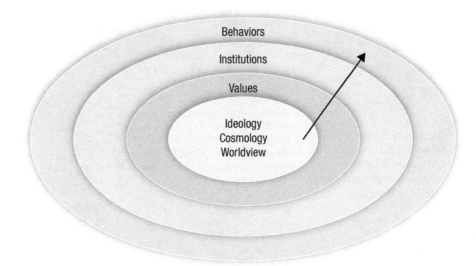

Figure 7.5. Cultural Egg

Source: Hesselgrave, D. (1991). *Communicating christ cross-culturally: An Introduction to missionary communication.* Zondervan Press.

Social marketing has been a major part of health messaging since the 1970s, when Kotler and Zaltman (1971) recognized that tools used to market items could be used to influence health-related behaviors. Social marketing strategy may be described with this statement, "I don't really care what a person thinks, feels, or believes. I just want a change in the target behavior." Effective social marketing relies on convincing presentations of timely and culturally appropriate messages provided through effective message channels. A common problem with social marketing is permanency of change, since the underlying beliefs and values that ultimately drive risky behaviors are not often addressed with these techniques. Social marketing works at the outer behavioral layer of the cultural egg and is particularly useful in one-time behaviors like immunizations and cancer screenings. It commonly utilizes highly trained communication specialists who are often external to a target community.

In contrast, **community engagement** is the facilitation of communities in the process of problem-solving, encouraging communities to own their problems and solutions. Community engagement could be described as changes in the beliefs, feelings and thinking of individuals . . . essential for permanent changes of risky behaviors. Community engagement focuses on the center of the cultural egg, the area of worldview, deep beliefs, and values, and as such changes the forces that drive more permanent risky community behaviors. Community engagement requires specialized skills and patience to move at the pace of the community and utilizes the horizontal communication systems within the community to reach into the area of beliefs and values that drive risky behaviors (see **Figure 7.6**).

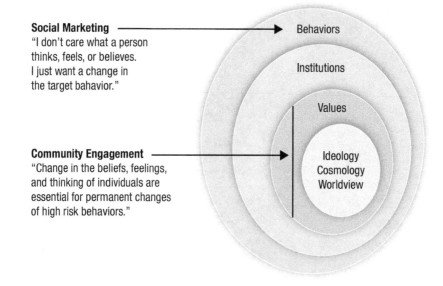

Figure 7.6. Community Engagement, Social Marketing, and the Cultural Egg

Source: Dwelle, T. L., & Musumba, A. (2013). *Engagement or coercion: A community engagement toolkit.* Unpublished.

Principles of Community Engagement

The Centers for Disease Control and Prevention (CDC) identified nine key principles of community engagement (CDC, 2011).

Prepare for Community Engagement

1. "Be clear about the purposes or goals of the engagement effort and the populations and/or communities you want to engage . . .
2. Become knowledgeable about the community's culture, economic conditions, social networks, political and power structures, norms and values, demographic trends, history, and experience with efforts by outside groups to engage it in various programs. Learn about the community's perceptions of those initiating the engagement activities" (CDC, 2011, pp. 46–47).

Develop Relationships in the Community

3. "Go to the community, establish relationships, build trust, work with the formal and informal leadership (horizontal communicators), and seek commitment from community organizations (not structures) and leaders to create processes for mobilizing the community . . .
4. Remember and accept that collective self-determination is the responsibility and right of all people in a community. No external entity should assume it can bestow on a community the power to act in its own self-interest (community engagement versus coercion)" (CDC, 2011, pp. 48–49).

Foundational Beliefs Needed for Successful Community Engagement

5. "Partnering with the community is necessary to create change and improve health.
6. All aspects of community engagement must be recognized, and respect the diversity of the community. Awareness of the various cultures of a community and other factors affecting diversity must be paramount in planning, designing, and implementing approaches to engaging a community.
7. Community engagement can only be sustained by identifying and mobilizing community assets and strengths and by developing the community's capacity and resources to make decisions and take action.
8. Organizations that wish to engage a community as well as individuals seeking to effect change must be prepared to release control of actions or interventions to the community and be flexible enough to meet its changing needs.
9. Community collaboration requires long-term commitment and patience by the engaging organization and its partners." (CDC, 2011, pp. 50–52)

Community Engagement and Religiosity

As an important determinant of worldview and values, religion is an attribute that should be assessed when engaging communities and incorporated into the plan for engagement, if relevant to the community.

Though previous theoretical models have suggested that perceived religious influence on health behavior (e.g., healthy lifestyle as a result of one's religious beliefs) is a main reason why individuals who are religiously involved experience positive health outcomes, there has been surprisingly little research aimed specifically at testing this hypothesis. More broadly, religious involvement might have both positive and negative influences on one's health. (Holt et al., 2014, p. 321)

Examples of the religious impact on health and health behaviors follow.

Religiosity and Dietary Beliefs and Behaviors

Lukwago et al. (2001) conducted a study of African American women from Alabama, St. Louis, and Kansas. They used a scale that they previously developed and validated. Seventy-four percent of the women identified with the Christian faith, 11.8% had no religious group identification, 0.9% were Muslim, 1.7% were Jehovah's Witnesses, and 9.4% were unspecified. The results demonstrated that women who engaged in religious behaviors and/or held strong religious beliefs consumed more fruits and vegetables.

These findings support some association between religious beliefs in African American women in the South and positive dietary habits, particularly regarding fruit and vegetable intake. Another study of White women from the Northwest did not show a similar positive association between religiosity and fruit and vegetable intake, but did show a positive association between religiosity and low-fat dietary behaviors. Observed association between religious beliefs and positive dietary behaviors could suggest an enhanced role for faith-based organizations in health messaging to target communities.

Parent Religiosity and Teen Transition to Sex and Contraception

The 1997 National Longitudinal Survey of Youth obtained information from sexually inexperienced adolescents aged 12 to 14 years, and looked for the association between parent and family religiosity and transition to first sexual experience and contraceptive use at first sex during the teen years. More frequent parental religious attendance and family religious activities were related to later timing of sexual initiation but did not translate into improved contraceptive use (Manlove et al., 2006).

Faith-Based HIV Intervention for African American Women

A large African American church with 25,000 members, 98% of whom were African American, participated in an Emory University study of the effectiveness of two HIV interventions intended to reduce risky behaviors (Wingood et al., 2013). *Sisters Informing Sisters About Topics on AIDS* (SISTA) is a CDC evidence-based, HIV intervention for African American women. *P4 for Women* is a faith-based adaption of SISTA.

A 10-member Church Advisory Board (CAB) was formed, which included the Director of Pastoral Services, the Co-Director of Health Services Ministries, the Director of the College and Singles Ministry, and members of the church's Women's Ministry. CAB members were able to modify the study as desired to avoid risks to participants and perceived undermining of the churches beliefs and values. Participants were randomly assigned to either two 3-hour SISTA or two P4 for Women sessions. HIV testing was provided to all participants. Table 7.1 compares the general content of the SISTA and P4 for Women intervention programs.

Both the SISTA and P4 for Women programs had a statistically significant effect on condom use and other sexual behaviors in the previous 90 days. P4 for Women had a statistically significant impact on the number of weeks participants were abstinent and on all measures of religious social capital. P4 for Women was more acceptable to participants than SISTA.

Table 7.1. Content for Sisters Informing Sisters About Topics on AIDS (SISTA) and P4 for Women

Discussion/Activities Session Content	SISTA	P4 for Women
Session 1: Ethnic and Gender Pride	The joys and challenges of being an African American woman	The values of being an African American Christian woman
	Role models and how they positively influence our lives	The role Christianity has played in the African American community
	Reviewing HIV risk-reduction strategies	Promoting sexual abstinence and safer sex
	Personal values clarification	Enhancing norms supportive of sexual abstinence
Session 2: Enhancing Coping and Skills	Enhancing norms supportive of HIV risk reduction	Exploring the use of religious coping (i.e., participation in church ministries and religious activities, talking to peers and leaders within the church) to remain sexually abstinent
	Building sexual negotiation, condom use, and partner selection skills	Building sexual negotiation, condom use, and partner selection skills
	Exploring risk levels involved in behaviors	Encouraging HIV and STI testing

STI, sexually transmitted infection.

Notes: SISTA is a CDC evidence-based, HIV intervention for African American women. P4 for Women is a faith-based adaption of SISTA.

TACTICS FOR BUILDING HEALTHY COMMUNITIES

Integrating Primary Care and Public Health

The goal of public health integration with primary care is to provide primary population-based prevention services to prevent risk factors associated with disease and death. Secondary and tertiary prevention services are the main mission of clinical institutions. The Institute of Medicine (IOM) in 2012 strongly suggested that enhanced integration of public health and primary care with more true collaboration and partnerships is essential to building healthy individuals and communities in the future. The IOM expert committee on integration identified a continuum of integration for primary care and public health from isolation to merger (Figure 7.7).

Current integration of public health and primary care primarily rests in mutual awareness and cooperation with less true collaboration or partnership. Integration requires a commitment to an ongoing process and continual dialogue that should lead to greater collaboration, partnerships, and even merging of public health and primary care (IOM, 2012). Public health is well positioned to lead and facilitate that dialogue. The IOM additionally identified essential principles for successful integration, including:

- A shared goal of population health improvement;
- Community engagement in defining and addressing population health needs;
- Aligned leadership that bridges disciplines, programs, and jurisdictions to reduce fragmentation and foster continuity;
- Clarifies roles and ensures accountability, develops and supports appropriate incentives;
- Has the capacity to manage change;
- Sustainability, the key to which is the establishment of a shared infrastructure;
- Building for enduring value and impact; and
- The sharing and collaborative use of data and analysis. (IOM, 2012, pp. 5–6)

The ongoing process and dialogue should lead to greater collaboration, partnerships, and even merging of public health and primary care programs.

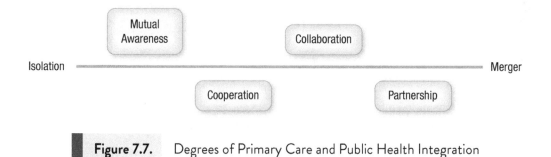

Figure 7.7.   Degrees of Primary Care and Public Health Integration

Comprehensive worksite wellness by integrating best practices of primary prevention with clinical interventions of chronic disease management, case management, call-a-nurse services, and onsite clinics represents "low-hanging fruit" for sustainable integration of public health and primary care at the community level. Other examples of sustainable integration include public–private partnerships for community-based chronic disease management, case management with clinical services provided by private clinics, and home visitation by public health nursing.

Utilizing Community Health Workers

Community health workers (CHWs) are usually respected members of the community they serve. As such, they are culturally aware and have established relationships with community members. These attributes of community respect, cultural awareness, and established relationships are crucial to community engagement initiatives since many community members may be disengaged from and even skeptical of health systems and professional health workers.

Persons in poor households often do not seek health care outside the home, due to costs of clinic and hospital visits, lack of health insurance, other access issues like transportation, personal beliefs, and occasionally the misperception of the skills, attitudes, politics, and agendas of professional health personnel. CHWs tend to stay in their communities unlike many other health professionals who, even if they originate from a rural community, tend to seek employment in other areas, particularly urban settings, that offer higher salaries and more opportunities for advancement. As a result, CHWs can be key to providing home visits—a vital function for most CHW programs worldwide. Moreover, CHWs are almost always welcomed, due to their being part of the community.

In the United States, community health workers (CHWs) help us meet our national *Healthy People* goals by conducting community-level activities and interventions that promote health and prevent diseases and disability. CHWs are trusted, respected members of the community who serve as a bridge between their community members and professionals in the field of health and human services. They provide an important service by establishing and improving relationships between these professionals and members of the community. As community health educators and role models, CHWs promote, encourage, and support positive, healthful self-management behaviors among their peers. As community advocates, CHWs help people get the services and follow-up care they need. CHWs serve as patient and community advocates, as "coaches" for disease management, and as patient "navigators," guiding patients through the health care system. They also strengthen their community's understanding and acceptance of medical care. The recognition of their successes has led to recommendations that CHWs be included as members of health care teams to help eliminate racial and ethnic disparities in health care. (CDC, 2022, para. 1)

CHWs work either for pay or as volunteers in association with the local public health and/or health care systems in both urban and rural environments. CHWs are part of the community they serve, and therefore, share ethnicity, culture, language, socioeconomic status, and life experiences with other community members. Since CHWs typically reside in the community they serve, they have the unique ability to provide information where it is needed most. They can reach community residents where they live, eat, play, work, and worship. CHWs are frontline agents of change, helping to reduce health disparities in underserved communities. Table 7.2 lists the most common health problems

Table 7.2. Health Problems Addressed and Services Provided by Percent of Respondents

	Paid Only	Volunteer Only	Paid and Volunteer	Total
Health problems (N = 620)				
Cancer	22.0	38.2	36.5	26.8
Cardiovascular disease	22.0	38.2	32.9	25.8
Child health	43.4	26.5	36.5	40.6
Diabetes	32.9	55.9	46.1	37.7
Heart disease	19.6	38.2	28.7	23.1
High blood pressure	27.9	44.1	37.1	31.3
HIV/AIDS	35.8	17.6	52.1	39.2
Immunizations	39.6	23.5	32.9	36.9
Infant health	40.3	20.6	35.3	37.9
Nutrition	46.8	55.9	47.9	47.6
Obesity	31.0	32.4	38.3	33.1
Physical activity	27.2	38.2	29.3	28.4
Pregnancy, prenatal care	43.7	20.6	38.3	41.0
Sexual behavior	31.0	17.6	44.3	33.9
Women's health	44.9	29.4	52.1	46.0
Services (N = 596)				
Assist in accessing medical services/programs	85.0	85.3	82.7	84.4
Assist in accessing nonmedical services/programs	71.5	67.6	72.8	71.6

(continued)

Table 7.2. Health Problems Addressed and Services Provided by Percent of Respondents (*continued*)

	Paid Only	Volunteer Only	Paid and Volunteer	Total
Build community capacity	30.8	38.2	44.4	34.9
Build individual capacity	33.8	52.9	48.1	38.8
Case management	46.3	32.4	44.4	45.0
Community advocacy	50.0	52.9	60.5	53.0
Counsel	29.8	20.6	34.6	30.5
Cultural mediation	17.8	29.4	16.0	18.0
Interpretation	33.5	35.3	33.3	33.6
Mentor	18.8	11.8	27.2	20.6
Patient navigation	16.0	29.4	19.8	17.8
Provide culturally appropriate health promotion/education	81.3	79.4	83.3	81.7
Provide direct services	37.8	14.7	41.4	37.4
Risk identification	39.8	17.6	48.8	40.9
Social support	43.3	52.9	50.6	45.8
Translation	36.5	26.5	35.2	35.6
Transportation	35.8	20.6	38.3	35.6
Other	10.3	5.9	12.3	10.6

Note: Multiple responses were permitted.

Sources: Department of Health and Human Services, Health Resource and Services Administration, & Bureau of Health Professions. (2007). *Community health worker national workforce study*. https://bhw.hrsa.gov/sites/default/files/bureau-health-workforce/data-research/community-health-workforce.pdf

faced and services provided by CHWs with the most common service being culturally appropriate health education and service access assistance (Health Resources and Services Administration, 2007).

Evidence of Community Health Workers' Effectiveness

Some of the recognized outcomes of CHW services include improved access to health care services, increases in community member health and screening, better understanding between community members and health care, public health and social service systems, enhanced communication between community members and health providers, increased use of health care services, improved adherence to health recommendations, and reduced need for emergency and specialty services.

The Association of State and Territorial Health Officials (ASTHO) presents the results of many, many studies that have examined the effectiveness of CHWs. This is an important issue for communities and states as they evaluate whether to utilize CHWs. Existing studies on CHWs focus on assessing their effectiveness in improving health outcomes, reducing health care costs, and bridging the gap in health disparities. Research has demonstrated effectiveness across multiple settings and health issues. For example, a systematic review on the effects of CHW interventions to improve chronic disease management and care among vulnerable populations found CHWs to be more effective when compared with alternatives and more cost-effective for certain health conditions, particularly in underserved communities (ASTHO, 2023). Studies on ROI also have found CHWs financially desirable. For example, a health plan in Nevada hired three CHWs to work with an average of 37 patients each day for 30 to 60 days. The average medical costs for the patients decreased from $1,223 pre-intervention to $983 post-intervention (ASTHO, 2023).

Community Health Worker Certification

CHWs are increasingly recognized for their powerful potential to improve health care and population health. CHWs can help reduce costs and improve care, key goals of most governmental health care priorities. For this reason, many states in the United States are promoting and formalizing the CHW's role within state health care systems through certification.

There is great state variability regarding approaches to a certification process for CHWs. As with other health professionals, some sort of licensure and certification credential for CHWs will be necessary for them to bill and receive payment for services provided. Some states have established a board or workgroup to make recommendations for CHW certification and training. In several states, private nonprofit organizations that support the concept of CHWs provide CHW certification that typically includes classroom training on core competencies, a practicum or internship experience, and an evaluation of skills and knowledge. Development of national standards for CHWs' scope of practice, training, certification, licensure, reimbursement, and oversight is needed in the United States.

An example of CHW training is the *Community Health Worker Training Resource for Preventing Heart Disease and Stroke* developed and published by the CDC (2022). It is an evidence-based, plain-language training resource and reference for CHWs, as well as a curriculum that health educators, nurses, and other instructors can use to train CHWs. It includes 15 chapters that show how CHWs can help individuals prevent or manage heart disease, stroke, high blood pressure and cholesterol, diabetes, depression and stress, and other conditions. This training material also includes sections on working with children and teens and helping individuals talk to their doctor and take medicines properly.

The recognition of CHW successes has led to recommendations that they be included as members of health care teams to help eliminate racial, ethnic, and geographic disparities in health care (CDC, 2022). CHWs can conduct community-level activities and interventions that promote health and prevent diseases and disability, serve as a bridge or liaison between community members and other health professionals, and impact community health and wellness significantly. Development of national standards for CHWs scope of practice, training, certification, licensure, reimbursement, and oversight are needed in the United States.

COMPREHENSIVE WORKSITE WELLNESS: THE ENGAGED WORKPLACE

Worksites provide an excellent opportunity for public health to promote health. Poor health is bad for business, and employers have an incentive to support worksite wellness programs. Poor health impacts the bottom line of every business in several ways, including:

- Medical care,
- Pharmaceuticals (medications),
- Absenteeism—employees absent from work due to poor health, and
- Presenteeism—employees at work but not performing to their potential due to poor health.

Current costs of poor employee health are substantial. As of 2023, the cost to employers was estimated to be $530 billion every year due to absences and lost or reduced productivity. This includes:

- $198 billion due to reduced productivity from unmanaged or poorly managed chronic health conditions;
- $178 billion for the cost of wages and benefits for absences due to illness, workers' compensation, and Family and Medical Leave (FMLA) expenses;
- $82 billion for the cost of missed revenues, hiring temporary workers, and overtime; and
- $73 billion for workers' compensation payments and related costs (Johns Hopkins Medicine, 2023).

Earlier studies confirming the high cost of poor employee health abound. They include the 2013 Public Health Institute report on the costs to employers of poor employee health. At that time, it was estimated that $153 billion was lost to businesses each year due to absenteeism from workers who were overweight or obese or had chronic health conditions. Overweight and obese workers missed an additional 450 million work days each year (Public Health Institute, 2013).

Loeppke and colleagues (2009) demonstrated that 35% of business health care costs were associated with presenteeism, 33% with absenteeism, 24% with medical costs, and 8% with medications. Another study by Burton and colleagues (2005) looked at the productivity loss of individuals with a variety of risk factors (e.g., smoking, obesity, inadequate exercise, inadequate diet, stress) and found a baseline loss of 14.7% for employees having 0 to 2 risk factors. Productivity loss dramatically increased, with the number of risks approaching 83%

above baseline, with five or more risk factors (see **Figure 7.8**). It is highly desirable to identify and reduce risk factors in employees. Risk factor reduction is primary prevention—the major mission of public health.

A big question for business is whether worksite wellness actually works. The answer is yes, if done appropriately. For example, Chapman conducted a meta-analysis of 56 peer-reviewed articles on worksite wellness. A qualifying worksite wellness program had to have at least three of the following programs:

- Smoking prevention and cessation,
- Physical fitness,
- Stress management,
- Medical self-care,
- High blood pressure control,
- Cholesterol reduction,
- Cardiovascular disease prevention,
- Prenatal care,
- Seat belt use,
- Back injury prevention,
- Back pain prevention,
- Weight management, and
- Nutrition education.

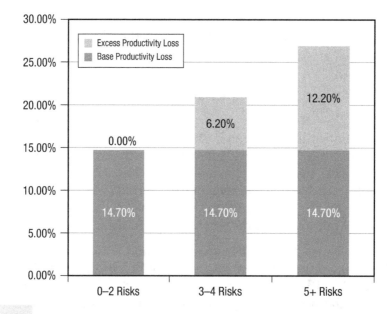

Figure 7.8. Employee Risk Behavior Increases Productivity Loss

Source: Burton, W. N., Chen, C. Y., Conti, D. J., Schultz, A. B., Pransky, G., & Edington, D. W. (2005). The association of health risks with on-the-job productivity. *Journal of Occupational and Environmental Medicine, 47*(8), 769–777. https://doi.org/10.1097/01.jom.0000169088.03301.e4

In qualifying worksites, absenteeism decreased by 26%, health care costs decreased by 26.1%, and workers' compensation costs decreased by 32% with a benefit/cost ratio of 5.81/1. Even with relatively few interventions, worksite wellness, if done appropriately, significantly impacts the bottom line of businesses (Chapman, 2005).

Seven Steps to Successful Worksite Wellness Programs

Seven steps to successful worksite wellness programs have been identified by the Wellness Council of America (2022), and include:

1. Obtain support of management,
2. Create a wellness team,
3. Collect meaningful data,
4. Create an operating plan,
5. Choose appropriate interventions,
6. Create a supportive environment, and
7. Evaluate and modify.

Obtain Support of Management

Upper- and middle-level management support is absolutely essential, without which the program will fail. A worksite wellness program must help meet the mission of the business. Management must understand the benefits of a wellness program for both the employees and the organization, in order to commit sufficient support.

Develop a Wellness Team

A team needs to be developed—a worksite wellness committee—that represents all key groups in the business, including the healthy and less healthy. For instance, reach out and include those who exercise and those who do not, those with disabilities and those without, average and overweight employees, as well as smokers and nonsmokers. This team ideally must design and run the program if employee ownership is desired. This is key to true community engagement in the workplace.

Collect Meaningful Data

Collection of data is important to driving the successful wellness initiative. What is not measured is generally not addressed. Furthermore, the data provide benchmarks that indicate whether the initiative is successful. Important data include:

- Health risk assessments—gives specific individual data and aggregate data for the program;
- Health screenings—for example, lipid profiles, blood pressure, blood sugar, body composition, and so forth;

- Medical claims data—workers' compensation, disability claims, pharmaceutical costs, and so forth;
- Absenteeism records from human resources data;
- Perceived needs—manager and employee interest surveys;
- Environmental assessments; and
- Cultural assessments.

Create an Operating Plan

An operating plan should answer the vision, mission, goals, and objectives of the workplace. Vision is essentially where a workplace wants to be in the future. Mission is what we need to do and why we need to accomplish the vision. Goals and objectives are the detailed steps needed to accomplish the mission. Mission, vision, goals, and objectives set the framework for effective reporting and evaluation.

Choose Appropriate Interventions

The program interventions chosen should flow naturally from the data and align with the goals and objectives of the initiative, as well as the goals of management and employees. Programs should be personalized to health issues and the employees' perceived needs and designed with an appropriate mix of awareness, education/motivation, and interventions to meet those needs. Employees will participate in what they feel is important (ownership). Designing a specific worksite wellness program for a business is a major role for the worksite wellness team.

Create a Supportive Environment

A supportive environment provides employees with encouragement, opportunity, and rewards. Your workplace should celebrate and reward health achievements and have a management team that models healthy behavior. A supportive environment helps retain employees and establishes policies that encourage healthy choices in areas including physical activity, tobacco use, nutrition, ergonomics, alcohol/substance abuse, mental health, seat belt safety, and other safety and emergency procedures. A supportive environment needs to consider employee benefits, including:

- Health insurance,
- Life insurance,
- Sick leave/well days off,
- Vacation,
- Flex time,
- Work at home/telecommuting,
- Family leave,
- Health promotion programs, and
- Employee assistance.

Evaluate and Modify

Evaluation is essential. It is a key to program success and helps adjust program activities as they progress. A facilitator should avoid wasting time on a worksite wellness program not committed to a significant evaluation plan. Regularly assess the program to determine what is working and what is not. Then make changes accordingly. Look to your employees for feedback on possible changes and adjustments. In addition, while it's valuable to evaluate the ROI through lower claims and insurance costs, the greatest savings may be in fewer absences, greater employee retention, and higher productivity. Top elements to measure include:

- Participation;
- Satisfaction;
- Improvements in knowledge, attitudes, and behaviors;
- Biometrics;
- Risk factors;
- Physical environment/corporate culture;
- Productivity; and
- ROI.

An effective comprehensive worksite wellness program will be optimally effective if it strategically combines population-based interventions (wellness behavior change) using social marketing and community engagement techniques, along with appropriate clinical interventions (chronic disease management, case management, call-a-nurse, and onsite clinical services) provided by midlevel practitioners. This is a sustainable integration of public health and primary care models that will significantly impact the fiscal bottom line of businesses (see **Figure 7.9**).

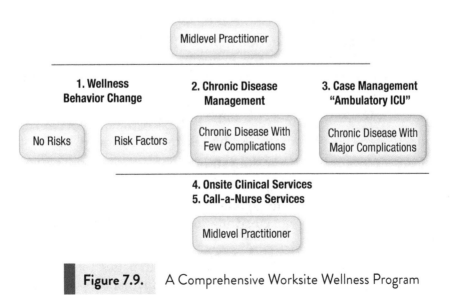

Figure 7.9.   A Comprehensive Worksite Wellness Program

Case Study: Johnson & Johnson Worksite Wellness Program

Many corporations, particularly large ones, provide worksite wellness programs, and a substantial number of private firms in the United States develop and deliver them for these corporations. What are the origins of worksite wellness programs? In the interest of conveying historical context, the Johnson & Johnson Company is the subject of this case study. Johnson & Johnson has been in the forefront of worksite wellness since the 1970s, and it is still a model for programs today.

In 1978, Johnson & Johnson created a wellness program—Live for Life® (LFL)—with a mission to:

- Encourage employees to become the healthiest in the world, and
- Implement on-site programs and services to reduce the cost of health care for the company (Isaac & Flynn, 2001).

LFL provided employees and their families with resources and opportunities to lead healthier lifestyles—a comprehensive program of health screens, life-style improvement programs, and worksite changes to support healthier lifestyles. Key program features included:

- Focus on prevention and education,
- Health benefits links,
- Targeted health interventions, and
- Cost-effective health care delivery.

Health resources provided to participants included:

- Online action planning guides,
- Access to call-a-nurse services,
- Access to health coaches, and
- Access to case management services for high-risk patients.

LFL underwent a rigorous evaluation in its earliest years (Bly et al., 1986). Over the 5-year period 1979 to 1983, the experience of two groups of Johnson & Johnson employees exposed to LFL was compared with that of a control group. The three groups were:

- Group 1—5,192 people from sites with LFL operating for more than 30 months,
- Group 2—3,259 people from sites with LFL operating for 18 to 30 months, and
- Group 3—2,955 people from Johnson & Johnson companies with no LFL program.

To account for baseline differences, analyses of covariance produced adjusted means for inpatient hospital costs, admissions, hospital days, outpatient costs, and other health costs.

Data were reported for all employees working at the sites for the entire study period, whether or not they participated in specific aspects of LFL. The LFL program was based on a "total immersion" hypothesis that constant reinforcing messages would change behavior; that is, the environment would provide the impetus to change independent of formal program participation.

The findings of the evaluation were promising. In summary, all groups experienced increases over time, but the costs and utilization in the non-LFL group (Group 3) began to exceed those of the LFL groups (Groups 1 and 2) in 1982.

The authors found:

- "The hospital costs for the LFL groups doubled over a 5-year period, while costs in the non-LFL group increased fourfold. . . .

- An average savings of $2,450,079 per year in 1979 dollars was obtained or a total of $980,316 for the study period. . . .

- Mean annual inpatient cost increases were $43 and $42 for two Live for Life groups versus $76 for the non-Live for Life group. Live for Life groups also had lower rates of increase in hospital days and admissions. No significant differences were found for outpatient or other health care costs." (Bly et al., 1986, pp. 3235 and 3239)

Johnson & Johnson continued to expand and improve worksite wellness after its initial efforts in the 1970s. Many evaluations followed and were used to modify the company's wellness programs. Today Johnson & Johnson remains a foremost example of the kind of success that can be obtained when company leadership fully supports health promotion for employees.

CHAPTER SUMMARY

In this chapter, we advocate that public health engage communities in the work of improving the health of members. If done well, community engagement is an effective strategy for achieving public health goals in all kinds of communities including rural towns and villages, worksites, schools, civic and faith-based groups, and others. Worksite wellness programs have been especially successful models for engagement. Community engagement is distinguished from social marketing and other non-engaged approaches to impacting the health attitudes, behaviors, and beliefs that result in poor health. Some tactics for community engagement are described including integrating primary care and public health, as well as employing CHWs to facilitate health improvement efforts.

DISCUSSION QUESTIONS

Q: What are the three major approaches for changing risky behaviors?

Q: What situations are most effectively addressed with social marketing?

Q: What situations are most effectively addressed with community engagement?

Q: What are the nine principles of community engagement?

Q: How can CHWs improve community engagement efforts?

Q: Explain how the worksite can be a venue for the integration of public health and primary care.

DATA SOURCES

County Health Rankings & Roadmaps (CHR&R) is an indispensable source of health data for community health improvement efforts. An initiative of the University of Wisconsin Population Health Institute, CHR&R contains health-related data at the county, zip code, and state levels that can be used to compare communities or states and assess trends in health. "The Rankings are unique in their ability to measure the health of nearly every county in all 50 states, and are complemented by guidance, tools, and resources designed to accelerate community learning and action. CHR&R is known for effectively translating and communicating complex data and evidence-informed policy into accessible models, reports, and products that deepen the understanding of what makes communities healthy and inspires and supports improvement efforts" (CHR&R, 2022, para. 1). Begin your exploration of community health at these sites:

- For the measures, data sources, and years collected by CHR&R:

  https://www.countyhealthrankings.org/explore-health-rankings/county-health-rankings-measures
- For health rankings at county, state, or zip code levels:

  https://www.countyhealthrankings.org/explore-health-rankings
- For examples of what works in community health improvement:

  https://www.countyhealthrankings.org/take-action-to-improve-health/what-works-for-health

---

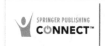 **SPRINGER PUBLISHING** **CONNECT™** A robust set of instructor resources designed to supplement this text is located at **http://connect.springerpub.com/content/book/978-0-8261-8615-7.** Qualifying instructors may request access by emailing **textbook@springerpub.com.**

REFERENCES

Association of State and Territorial Health Officials. (2023). *Community health workers.* https://www.astho.org/topic/population-health-prevention/healthcare-access/community-health-workers/

Bly, J. L., Jones, R. C., & Richardson, J. E. (1986). Impact of worksite health promotion on health care costs and utilization: Evaluation of Johnson & Johnson's Live for Life® program. *Journal of the American Medical Association, 256,* 3235–3240. https://doi.org/10.1001/jama.256.23.3235

Burton, W. N., Chen, C. Y., Conti, D. J., Schultz, A. B., Pransky, G., & Edington, D. W. (2005). The association of health risks with on-the-job productivity. *Journal of Occupational and Environmental Medicine, 47*(8), 769–777. https://doi.org/10.1097/01.jom.0000169088.03301.e4

Centers for Disease Control and Prevention & Clinical and Translational Science Awards Consortium. (2011). *Principles of community engagement* (2nd ed., No. 11-7782). National Institutes of Health.

Centers for Disease Control and Prevention & Division for Heart Disease and Stroke Prevention. (2022). *A community health worker training resource for preventing heart disease and stroke.* https://www.cdc.gov/dhdsp/programs/spha/chw_training/

Chapman, L. S. (2005). Meta-evaluation of worksite health promotion economic return studies: 2005 update. *American Journal of Health Promotion, 19*(6), 1–11. http://dx.doi.org/10.4278/0890-1171-19.4.TAHP-1

County Health Rankings & Roadmaps. (2022). *About us.* https://www.countyhealthrankings.org/about-us

Dwelle, T. L., & Musumba, A. (2013). *Engagement or coercion: A community engagement toolkit.* Unpublished.

Holt, C. L., Clark, E. M., & Roth, D. L. (2014). Positive and negative religious beliefs explaining the religion-health connection among African Americans. *International Journal for the Psychology of Religion, 24*(4), 311–331. https://doi.org/10.1080/10508619.2013.828993

Institute of Medicine. (2012). *Primary care and public health: Exploring integration to improve population health.* National Academies Press.

Isaac, F., & Flynn, P. (2001). Johnson & Johnson live for life® program: Now and then. *American Journal of Health Promotion, 15*(5), 365–367. https://www.researchgate.net/publication/11842975

Johns Hopkins Medicine. (2023). *The cost of employees' poor health.* https://www.johnshopkinssolutions.com/wp-content/uploads/2019/01/Johns_Hopkins_HealthyWorks_Cost_of_Employee_Health_Infographic.pdf

Kotler, P., & Zaltman, G. (1971). Social marketing: An approach to planned social change. *Journal of Marketing, 35*, 3–12. https://doi.org/10.1177/002224297103500302

Lennon, J. L., & Coombs, D. W. (1992). An application of the LePSA methodology for health education in leprosy. *Leprosy Review, 63*(2), 145–150. https://doi.org/10.5935/0305-7518.19920019

Loeppke, R., Taitel, M., Hautte, V., Parry, T., Kessler, R. C., & Jinnett, K. (2009). Health and productivity as a business strategy: A multiemployer study. *Journal of Occupational and Environmental Medicine, 51*(4), 411–428. https://doi.org/10.1097/jom.0b013e3181a39180

Lukwago, S. N., Kreuter, M. W., Bucholtz, D. C., Holt, C. L., & Clark, E. M. (2001). Development and validation of brief scales to measure collectivism, religiosity, racial pride, and time orientation in urban African American Women. *Family and Community Health, 24*(3), 63–71. https://doi.org/10.1097/00003727-200110000-00008

Manlove, J. S., Terry-Humen, E., Ikramullah, E. N., & Moore, K. A. (2006). The role of parent religiosity in teens' transitions to sex and contraception. *Journal of Adolescent Health, 39*(4), 578–587. https://doi.org/10.1016/j.jadohealth.2006.03.008

Mays, G. P., & Smith, S. A. (2011). Evidence links increases in public health spending to declines in preventable deaths. *Health Affairs, 30*(8), 1585–1593. https://doi .org/10.1377/hlthaff.2011.0196

Owen, H. (1993). *A brief user's guide to open space technology.* https://openspaceworld .org/wp2/hho/papers/brief-users-guide-open-space-technology/

Public Health Institute. (2013). *Prevention means business.* http://www.phi.org/uploads/ application/files/0a4evwb07m9clv9crv74ch2anirhfg23xixw3xpc47flvhdyfw.pdf

Redfield, R. (1957). *The primitive world and its transformations.* Cornell University Press.

U.S. Department of Health and Human Services, Health Resources and Services Administration & Bureau of Health Professions. (2007). *Community health worker national workforce study.* https://bhw.hrsa.gov/sites/default/files/bureau-health-workforce/ data-research/community-health-workforce.pdf

Wellness Council of America. (2022) *About us.* https://www.welcoa.org/page/3/ ?s=7+steps&c=site

Wingood, G. M., Robinson, L. R., Braxton, N. D., Er, D. L., Conner, A. C., Renfro, T. L., Rubtsova, A. A., Hardin, J. W., & Diclemente, R. J. (2013). Comparative effectiveness of a faith-based HIV intervention for African American women: Importance of enhancing religious social capital. *American Journal of Public Health, 103,* 2226–2233. https:// doi.org/10.2105/AJPH.2013.301386

World Health Organization. (1946, June 19–22). *Preamble to the constitution of the World Health Organization (signed on July 22, 1946, by the representatives of 61 states [official records of the World Health Organization, no. 2, p. 100] and entered into force on April 7, 1948)* [Conference session]. International Health Conference, New York, NY.

World Health Organization Regional Office for Europe. (2014). *The case for investing in public health.* https://www.researchgate.net/publication/277189955_The_case_for_ investing_in_public_health

8   Public Health Leadership

LEARNING OBJECTIVES

Students will learn . . .

1. The difference between technical and adaptive leadership and the situations associated with each of those sets of skills.

2. The roles of beliefs and values in adaptive change.

3. The attributes of an adaptive leader.

4. The role of community engagement in effecting adaptive change.

5. The importance of scientific training for public health leaders.

6. The importance of two practical skill sets for public health leaders—advocacy and lobbying—as well as disaster and incident management.

Sound leadership is essential for the well-being of any organization, including public health organizations. This is especially true in periods of upheaval such as we are experiencing now. Today, the public health system in the United States faces major challenges to its ability to meet the health and wellness needs of the nation. Effective responses to these challenges will require exceptional leadership.

The following phrases have been used to describe leadership:

- The art of mobilizing others to struggle for shared aspirations (Farber, 2009, p. 5);
- Organizing people around a common goal (Farber, 2009, p. 5);
- Sticking your neck out when it's the right thing to do (Farber, 2009, p. 5);
- Living dangerously, often exceeding authority, and withstanding criticism (Heifetz & Linsky, 2002, p. 2);
- Usually lonely;
- A process of social influence in which one person can enlist the aid and support of others in the accomplishment of a common task (Chemers, 1997);
- Love, edge (energy), audacity, and proof (LEAP; Farber, 2009, p. 19);

- Leadership is like an extreme sport that involves taking risks (Farber, 2009, p. 19);
- Committed, continually improving leadership skills, outward focused, serving others, interdependent (Assemblies of God, personal communication, March 10, 2013);
- Somebody whom people follow: somebody who guides or directs others (Kirkpatrick & Locke, 1991; Richards & Engle, 1986);
- More committed to achieving key goals versus advancement; and
- Demonstrating situational perception and action, power, vision and values, charisma, and intelligence.

The focus of this discussion will be *adaptive leadership*.

LEADERSHIP SPOTLIGHT: STEPHANIE JAY

Stephanie Jay, MPH, is a member of the Turtle Mountain Band of Chippewa Indians whose reservation is located on the border between North Dakota and Canada and has approximately 14,500 members. In 2020, Stephanie became concerned about the impact the COVID-19 pandemic would have on tribal members, given the lack of tribal health resources and historic trends in morbidity and mortality from disease and other health problems among American Indians. With approval from the Tribal Chairman and Tribal Council, Stephanie began to develop a COVID-19 response program and a tribal public health infrastructure, which would provide culturally appropriate programs and services to improve the physical, emotional, and spiritual health of tribal members, instead of relying so heavily on external public health departments.

North Dakota state statute did not allow recognition of any tribal public health departments, although the Turtle Mountain tribe was already federally recognized as the reservation's public health authority through implementation of Public Law 93-638 under which "the employees and administrative control of an otherwise federal program (e.g., the Indian Health Service) are transferred to the tribal government via a 638 contract." However, Stephanie, along with other tribal leaders, decided that with or without state recognition, as a sovereign nation, the tribe would proceed with development of the *Turtle Mountain Public Health Department* and become the first tribal public health department in North Dakota.

With a public health consultant hired in 2021 and her two-person staff, Stephanie developed a Turtle Mountain COVID-19 response program and a *Turtle Mountain Public Health Strategic Plan*, which would initiate a basic public health infrastructure on the reservation. She organized a COVID-19 coalition that included K–12 and tribal college leaders, as well as state, county, and Indian Health Service personnel. The coalition met weekly to review COVID-19 epidemiology reports and discuss and plan for multidisciplinary, collaborative public health interventions. With her staff, Stephanie implemented the tribal COVID-19 response program consisting of:

- Recruiting and training tribal members for a contact tracing program,
- Developing a robust school and community COVID-19 testing program,
- Developing tribal isolation and quarantine protocols,
- Implementing a COVID-19 public information program,
- Developing and coordinating a home quarantine support program,
- Developing and implementing a COVID-19 wastewater surveillance system,
- Obtaining a mobile public health unit, and
- Collaborating with the Indian Health Service clinic and the county local public health department to immunize tribal members with COVID-19 vaccines.

As part of the *Turtle Mountain Public Health Strategic Plan*, the Centers for Disease Control and Prevention (CDC) Foundation was contacted and provided resources to recruit and fund five additional public health positions including an epidemiologist, senior public health advisor, administrative support specialist, environmental health coordinator, and communications specialist. These personnel were in place by January 2022, after which the Tribal Council officially established the *Turtle Mountain Public Health Department*. A community health assessment was completed in 2022 to guide the efforts of the department.

Stephanie's work exemplifies adaptive and technical leadership skills. In the end, her efforts to build a public health department during a pandemic and organize a response to COVID-19 at Turtle Mountain were highly successful. The actual pandemic death rate among tribal members was 2.8/1,000—less than the North Dakota rate at 2.9/1,000 and the United States rate at 3.1/1,000. Indeed, at 6.09/1,000 to 6.51/1,000, the death rate from COVID-19 at Turtle Mountain was far lower than the expected rate for a high-risk, Native American population. This story underscores the significant impact a tribal public health program under an effective public health leader can have on the health and wellness of tribal members. Further, it is a testament to community engagement and the core values of tribal communities to own their problems and solutions. Turtle Mountain and Stephanie Jay can serve as examples for other communities—native and non-native.

ADAPTIVE LEADERSHIP

Many of the phrases and traits mentioned earlier begin to capture the definition of leader. Leaders may have both technical and adaptive leadership skills. Many executives are good managers (technical leadership) and yet have an additional set of skills to guide organizations through perilous and confusing times (adaptive leadership). Knowing when and where to use these various leadership skills requires knowledge of the differences and appropriate judgment to use them effectively. Certain individuals may have many personal qualities that propel them into leadership positions, yet they can enhance their leadership skills, both technical and adaptive, through experiential learning, appropriate training, and mentorship opportunities.

Adaptive leaders often possess the following attributes:

- Technical and adaptive leadership skills matched to organizational needs;
- Deeply committed to the organization's beliefs and values;
- Leadership by example;
- Take appropriate risks;
- Willing to commit time and energy to reach the vision, mission, and goals of the organization;
- Committed to outcomes versus advancement;
- Able to manage fear;
- Appropriately audacious;
- Delegate authority and responsibility;
- Tolerate hostility;
- Excellent judgment;
- A history of stable leadership beliefs and values; and
- Accept casualties.

Technical Versus Adaptive Leadership

Responses to organizational challenges often fall into either the technical (management) or adaptive categories, or both. Technical responses generally result in no significant loss to individuals. The "know how" and procedures are already in place, and many times the solution is fairly obvious to an experienced manager. The leader can orchestrate the "technical fix" with relatively little risk. Technical solutions to problems are relatively comfortable since they do not require changes in the deeply ingrained cultural beliefs and values of the organization. Technical problems tend to be problems of individuals or small groups versus the organization as a whole. In contrast, adaptive responses cause significant losses that are associated with the changes required in the beliefs, values, habits, or current ways of doing business within the organization.

Adaptive problems are often considered crises, though the crises may be acute or chronic. The adaptive solution to such problems is not readily apparent and will likely be determined by ideas and recommendations coming from the organizational community, not the technical leader. A technical leader can throw all the technical ideas they can construct at an adaptive problem, and the problem still persists. Adaptive change requires that the organizational community assume ownership of the problem and resultant solution. This is the realm of community engagement (see Chapter 7). The role of the adaptive leader in this process is not to provide their solutions (technical) to fix the problem, but to facilitate the organizational community to own their adaptive problem and solutions (true community engagement) no matter how painful the process.

At the beginning of an adaptive process, organizational members fail to see how things will be better, yet they clearly perceive the losses they are being asked to endure; a break from tradition. This loss commonly results in significant resistance to the whole adaptive process and often resistance to the adaptive leader. Adaptive change often requires a change in the organization's deep beliefs and values, and to abandon these is tantamount to disloyalty to self and those who are deeply committed to those beliefs and values—often people who have committed their lives to the organization and are deeply respected.

However, if leadership caves to organizational pressure to maintain the status quo in an adaptive situation, which often seems to be a reasonable, short-term, easy way out solution, the adaptive problem persists and the organization's future may be in jeopardy. Thus, adaptive situations are the territory of adaptive leaders. These persons are created to change their world. They are not necessarily easy people to work with since they are passionate, energetic, creative, unafraid to challenge tradition, and willing to take risks that frighten managers (technical leaders). Solutions to adaptive problems are risky and uncomfortable. Posing them may result in a leader being ignored or even fired. Adaptive leadership is not commonly a position that people relish, but is desperately needed to solve critical, complex problems.

In many of these complex situations there are both technical and adaptive elements to the solution and the leader must adeptly navigate the organization to appropriate technical and adaptive "fixes." Effective leaders must have skills to handle both these situations (technical and adaptive) for the organization's health and well-being.

Leadership and Culture

Behaviors are the result of deep cultural influences, as represented in the cultural egg (see **Figure 7.5**). Behaviors start in the center with worldview or deep beliefs—concepts of self, nature, the supernatural, and time (past, present, and future). It is upon these deep beliefs that cultures and communities build their values (things they feel are important). These values inform cultural and community institutions like marriage, education, law, governance—and the way communities, organizations, and businesses operate. Finally, all of these deeper layers ultimately emerge as behaviors. This area of behavior is what public health seeks to impact in order to improve the health of a community.

Technical solutions arise from the institutional level of the cultural egg (see **Figure 8.1**). However, adaptive solutions generally operate using the deep beliefs and values of the organization, but require adjustments at the institutional and behavioral levels. Thus, even though there is change in the way things are done

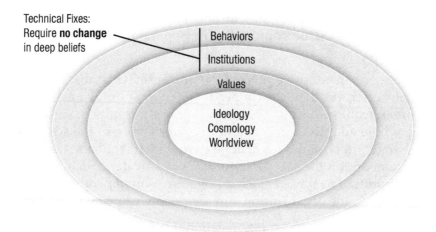

Figure 8.1.   Technical Leadership Solutions

Source: Hesselgrave, D. (1991). *Communicating christ cross-culturally: An introduction to missionary communication.* Zondervan Press.

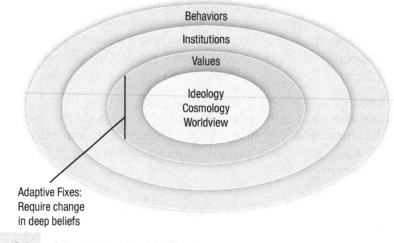
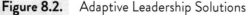

Figure 8.2.   Adaptive Leadership Solutions

Source: Hesselgrave, D. (1991). *Communicating christ cross-culturally: An introduction to missionary communication.* Zondervan Press.

in the organization, there is also substantial organizational comfort in knowing the worldview, deep beliefs, and values are still intact.

Adaptive leadership solutions almost always require changes in the deep beliefs and values of an organization, the very core of the cultural egg. In other words, the very heart and soul of the organization must be changed (**Figure 8.2**).

Organizations and their members do not like to change their deep beliefs and values since they sincerely believe that the way they think, feel, and believe is "right," and anyone who disagrees is obviously wrong. Therefore they often vigorously resist those changes when suggested.

Leadership by Example

Humans learn through three mechanisms: experience, teaching, and imitation (Hall, 1973). Learning by experience is based on trial and error, making mistakes and corrections. Even though this method is a common way to learn, it can be dangerous and even fatal. A person may learn from personal experience that smoking actually causes cancer after 20 years of smoking cigarettes. Even though that experience can be valuable as an example of the dire consequences of risky behavior for others, their personal learning may be too late to prevent the disease. With that example in mind, public health often tries to avoid the trial-and-error method of learning.

A teacher uses a variety of methods to convince or persuade students to learn. Teaching is most effective when reinforcing, as opposed to contradicting, what is being learned through other mechanisms, particularly that through imitation. Hall contends that a great part of culture, including beliefs and values, is learned through imitation, and suggests that if we want to introduce changes, particularly in basic beliefs of a culture, we must introduce or at least strongly reinforce using the imitation model.

An effective adaptive leader must take personal responsibility for their actions. They must not only embody the beliefs and values of the organization but also practically "practice what is preached" through their behaviors.

> A leader lives under a microscope. I'm not saying it's fair or just, but people watch everything a leader does. Everything. They watch the body language and facial expressions; they listen to the tone of voice; they observe the decisions the leader makes; they listen to the leader's questions and how they're asked. Therefore, the most powerful tool a leader has is himself or herself. (Farber, 2009, p. 22)

Leaders are being watched, and many people in the organization will imitate leaders they respect. It is an awesome responsibility to be a leader by example. It is not just about accomplishing the organization's vision, mission, and goals. During the day-to-day leadership process, leaders are actually training by example the next generation of leaders—part of succession planning for the organization. It has been suggested that leaders should:

> Do what you love in the service of people who love what you do. There are three parts (to this statement): "Do what you love." Make sure that your heart's in your work, and that you're bringing yourself fully and gratefully into everything you do. If you're not connected to your own work, you can't expect to inspire others in theirs. "In the service of people" will keep you true, honest, and ethical at the very least. If you're doing what you love, you'll make yourself happy. But extreme leadership is not only about you: It's about your impact on others. "Who love what you do" doesn't mean that you find people who love you and then serve them: It means it's your responsibility to give everyone you serve something to love about you and what you're doing. (Farber, 2009, p. 60)

Attributes of Adaptive Leaders

Beliefs and Values

Adaptive leaders are commonly more committed to outcomes than personal advancement. They want to change the world through what they do. Adaptive leaders are not those that bolt at the first opportunity for a better-paying job or at the first sign of organizational problems. To the adaptive leader, a challenging problem is an incredible stimulus to seek a solution, a blast of heightened awareness and interest, an adrenaline boost to the system. Adaptive leaders often run toward problems instead of away from them. This is what they were created for. They find supreme satisfaction in working through difficult challenges. It is who they are. This trait defines them. Yet there is one caveat: This enhanced commitment often stems from the close alignment of the leader's personal beliefs and values with those of the organization. It would be difficult for leaders to accept risks that could ultimately cost them a job or credibility if they did not deeply believe in the concepts behind the risks. Therefore, before taking a position, a leader should sincerely ask, "How do my beliefs and values align with the organization?" realizing that the answer to that question is the base to their level of commitment and ultimately their leadership performance in that organization. This alignment of beliefs and values, vision and mission, is much more important than salary or position for an adaptive leader who wants to change the world.

Vision

"Leadership qualities begin with a unique vision—the ability to see the broader social dimensions of what otherwise might be viewed as problems specific to certain individuals or communities" (DeBuono et al., 2007, p. 204). Can long-term vision be acquired, or are people born with it? These authors submit that vision can be acquired. It is not simply a sensory gift of perception, but an ability influenced by a leader's beliefs and values and worldview—the glasses through which they see and ultimately interpret the world around them.

Farber (2009) differentiates a bland vision statement from a vision that reflects deeply held values and beliefs and has the ability to motivate others to share that vision:

> Every business book you pick up will tell you that you need to have a vision statement, so any company that's done its required reading will have one. A vision statement doesn't generate energy, love does, great ideas do, principles and values do. A vision statement that comes from a workshop exercise is usually about as energizing and memorable as a saltine cracker.
>
> Vision from the heart is—by definition—an expression of love . . . and not only is that more energizing, it is energy. It's juice . . . Martin Luther King's "I have a dream" speech was juice for a generation. He didn't have to hand out 250,000 laminated cards at the Lincoln Memorial on that hot August day in 1963. Watch the tape: It was pure energy.

Juice. Life itself. This illustrates the love and edge (energy) of the LEAP acronym. (Farber, 2009, p. 71)

The adaptive leader will attempt to connect the "hearts of an organization" and bring everyone into the effort to change the organization and solve adaptive problems. They seek to show the bonds that bind members of the organization and then to motivate them to bring about change together. This ability distinguishes the adaptive leader from the purely technical. Farber argues that the adaptive leader achieves this goal by revealing themselves as a human being with strong values, goals, and beliefs.

> So, instead of reciting a vision statement, feel the intent of that statement, reflect on the ideals that it represents, and take it all into your own heart. Then at every opportunity—whether you're talking one-on-one or standing in front of a crowd—you say, in essence, "This is who I am, this is what I believe. This is what I think we can do together if we put our hearts into it. Look how magnificent our future can be. Please join me and let's help each other make this happen." Then you can burn the document (the vision statement) because, in effect, you've become the vision. . . Energy. . . Generated straight from the heart. (Farber, 2009, pp. 71–72)

KEY IDEA

When the beliefs and values of the organization and leader closely align, leaders are positioned to be successful adaptive leaders in their organizations.

Risk Taking

An adaptive leader must be willing to take risks but will only do that if their beliefs and values say, "It's worth it."

> It's very easy to say (that taking risks is important), but in business, especially, [this is] very hard to do. The irony is, risk is a natural part of the human experience, and we accept it in many areas of our lives without realizing it. But a lot of businesspeople who call themselves leaders want things to be easy and painless. They're either kidding themselves or lying. (Farber, 2009, p. 15)

Organizations commonly face serious challenges that threaten the whole enterprise. They need capable, committed adaptive leaders willing to tackle these situations, taking necessary risks, for the survival and growth of the organization. However, risk comes with fear. Farber argues that this is a natural response, but necessary to bring about change:

> . . . we've been conditioned to believe that fear is bad. And, yeah, fear can save your life or keep you from doing something stupid, but

avoiding it can also keep you from doing something great, from learning something new, and from growing as a human being. Fear is a natural part of growth, and since growth, change, and evolution are all on the extreme leader's agenda, fear comes with the territory. (Farber, 2009, pp. 21–22)

So risk and fear are associated with growth, which is what leaders want to do: grow in their ability to lead. It is like growing pains in adolescence. The pain is an indicator of growth: tendons and muscles being stretched by rapidly growing bones, to the point of discomfort. Analogously, taking risks and their associated fears are indicators of leadership growth. No fear, little growth. That is not necessarily a comforting thought, but should be encouraging for an adaptive leader in the midst of the challenges of bringing change: Though dangerous and frightening, this is the substance of growth.

KEY IDEA

"(Adaptive) leadership is always substantive and rarely fashionable. . . . It is intensely personal and intrinsically scary, and it requires us to live the ideas we espouse—in irrefutable ways—every day of our lives, up to and beyond the point of fear." (Farber, 2009, p. 19)

Audacity

Audacity is one of the leadership qualities of the acronym LEAP (love, edge, audacity, and proofs). Audacity can be synonymous with courage, but in another sense with impudence, temerity, and brazenness. Audacity described by impudence, temerity, and brazenness is often driven by ego and meant to draw attention to the leader where audacity based on heart is courageous; that is, it is the kind of audacity that will change the world (Farber, 2009).

Case Study: Audacity and Courage

Tim Wiedrich, the Emergency Preparedness and Response (EPR) Director for the North Dakota Department of Health, received notice of a new federal legal ruling that certain key EPR resources, including key personnel, could only be used for planning and not response. This meant that during an actual emergency the people who designed and knew the most about the EPR systems in the state would need to be either sent home or detailed to other planning activities while others were called in to run the actual response. This did not make sense and was contrary to the whole idea of the cooperative agreements first initiated in 2002. The whole point of EPR funding was to create a system that could "respond" to a variety of disasters (all hazards), including terrorist attacks like 9/11, floods, hurricanes, tornados, train derailments, and so forth:

(continued)

Case Study: Audacity and Courage (*continued*)

not just plan, plan, plan. Tim was courageous enough to kick back against the ruling, spending a number of hours debating, discussing, and persisting in his demands for an appropriate change in this policy not only for North Dakota but the nation. He was committed to changing his world. He stood up for what he believed was right. Sometimes this seemed very lonely, with few of his EPR colleagues standing with him on this issue with federal leaders. Working with others in the department and the Association of State and Territorial Health Officials through numerous discussions with federal colleagues, the policy was changed. Tim's courage to respond and dogged persistence were based on his beliefs and values (his heart) regarding the whole purpose of the nation's EPR system. Leaders can't be courageous or audacious about issues they don't deeply believe in. It's just not worth the risk if the leader's heart is not in it.

Delegation
Leaders are often confronted with a plethora of technical, adaptive, and complex, mixed problems with only so much time to invest in solutions. "The adaptive process takes an extraordinary level of presence, time and artful communication, but it may also take more time and trust than you have" (Heifetz & Linsky, 2002, p. 52). A reasonable option in a time crunch is to appropriately delegate, if possible, the technical problems to other competent staff, thus freeing an adaptive leader to focus on the adaptive challenge.

Judgment and Compromise
The intent of any general is to win wars, not just a single battle. Sometimes, the loss of a battle in one situation may actually strategically position an army to win a war. Adaptive leaders in extreme situations often encounter this. Ideological polarization may paralyze movement toward real solutions. An extreme leader must see the big picture, how to get from point A to point B, even if it means strategically compromising with opponents on certain issues to get there. This compromising may be interpreted as "caving in"—a sign of weakness by some, even those in the leader's camp. The difficult task of the adaptive leader in these scenarios is to somehow facilitate the organization, if possible, to own their adaptive problems and identify optimal solutions to reach the goal, even though it may entail humbling compromise. Sometimes the adaptive leader must make that decision alone.

"The success of extreme leaders often lies in the capacity to deliver news and raise difficult questions in a way that people can absorb, prodding them to take up the message rather than ignore it or kill the messenger . . . Adaptive leadership is an art" (Heifetz & Linsky, 2002, pp. 12–20).

As in art, there is a strong element of judgment in adaptive leadership, in sometimes going beyond one's authority, compromising, and in disturbing people in the organization and yet surviving. Survival in these situations takes exceptional judgment; that is, knowing how far one can push the envelope of disturbing people and not be eliminated in the process.

Case Study: Judgment and Compromise
In 2005, a bill was introduced to eliminate smoking in all public places in North Dakota. It was clear that the bill in that form would not pass the legislature, so a compromise was reached exempting bars. Many public health folks were not pleased with any compromise. Yet passage of that compromise bill protected at least 30,000 workers in the state from second-hand smoke. An initiated measure in 2012 completed the work by eliminating smoking in all public places. Many leaders felt the compromise in 2005 was a necessary step to achieve the long-term goal, despite the criticism they received.

Casualties
Adaptive leaders prefer not to think about casualties since this is always uncomfortable and painful—a situation they want to avoid. They want everyone to agree and work together to make adaptive changes. They realize that there will be conflict and challenges, but hope that by using good facilitation techniques everyone will eventually understand and come along as one big happy family. Unfortunately, this generally is not true. Adaptive change will leave casualties. Sometimes these casualties are close friends: "people who simply will not or cannot go along" (Heifetz & Linsky, 2002, pp. 98–99) with the proposed change. They will need to go. If a leader is committed to making an adaptive change, they must be willing to accept those casualties. This is not easy for leadership but is an all-too-frequent reality for adaptive leaders.

PUBLIC HEALTH AND POLICY AND ADVOCACY

An important role for public health leaders concerns policy and **advocacy**, which entail leading the community efforts to develop policies to improve health and advocating for them.

The definition of advocacy is to actively promote a cause or principle involving actions that will lead to a goal (Center for Community Health and Development [CCHD], 2023). Much public health advocacy revolves around policy issues involving government organizations, businesses, schools, and other large institutions. Avner (2002) lists several reasons for advocacy, including:

- People working together make a difference in changing laws and policies.
- Advocacy is a democratic tradition.
- Advocacy helps societies find real solutions.
- Policy makers need the input of advocates to make good policy decisions.
- Advocacy gives organizations and the public a voice.

Advocacy is often part of community initiatives (CCHD, 2023). The community engagement principle of facilitating communities to own their advocacy process is important since communities will only invest their resources and time in advocacy issues they feel are important. A community or organization should assess its capacity, enthusiasm, commitment, and patience to engage in an advocacy effort. Avner (2002) suggests seven questions to answer regarding a community's or organization's advocacy capacity:

- Who are the organizational champions for this advocacy effort?
- How deep is the organization's commitment to these advocacy efforts?
- Do we as a group appropriately understand the legislative process and structure?
- What are we prepared to do now?
- What resources are available to support this effort?
- Are we ready for media work?
- Do we know the lobbying rules and laws that apply to this effort?

An important pre-advocacy step is to gather and analyze information including public health and health care data, community needs and political environmental assessments, stakeholder strategic plans, and how allies and opponents invest and utilize resources. This analysis should provide the information needed to develop an advocacy strategic plan. An advocacy strategy should include how to engage with opponents, as well as proponents, and influence their beliefs and values. Opponent relationships may result in helpful compromises. Advocacy needs are always greater than the advocacy capacity of stakeholders, and therefore, advocacy goals must be carefully prioritized.

Advocacy can be confrontational or nonconfrontational. Both types of advocacies are useful but must be employed wisely (CCHD, 2023). Nonconfrontational advocacy is subtle, requires time and patience, and often takes place behind the scenes. It depends on persuasion skills, strength of relationships, and may involve compromise. Activism is commonly synonymous with confrontational advocacy and is generally visible and "in your face,"—associated with forcing results by use of political, media, and legal pressures to accomplish a policy goal. Activism can cause opponent entrenchment and loss of relationships, thus having a negative impact on future collaboration opportunities. In choosing an advocacy strategy, keep in mind the end goal: winning a policy war not just a battle.

An advocacy champion must clearly and convincingly present a vision of the proposed advocacy work to others. Nothing will happen without a champion initiating and leading the effort. Leadership support of a community or organization must be obtained. A planning team of five or six people is then organized to complete preplanning work and develop and implement an advocacy strategic and operational plan. Avner (2002) suggests answering six questions when developing an advocacy policy plan:

- What are the issues?
- What is already being done to address these issues?
- Where are the issues decided and debated (e.g., legislative bodies, administrative branches, courts)?
- What policies need to be changed?
- Should our group be proactive or reactive?
- Will this be a one-time or long-term effort?

There are generally three arenas of policy influence (Avner, 2002): legislative bodies, executive or administrative branches, and courts. The most common route to influence public policy is through advocacy of legislative members. The executive or administrative branches can occasionally influence policy through executive action or orders and is often an easier option. Complex issues are usually settled through court litigation. Lobbying is a special form of advocacy (CCHD, 2023) and is of two types: direct and grassroots. Direct lobbying efforts try to influence elected and appointed officials to adopt a group's position. Grassroots lobbying relies on educating, mobilizing, and activating the public to persuade those officials to support a position.

Planning groups can be categorized as high or low performance based on five basic attributes or principles of strategic effectiveness.

1. There is no relation between the time spent in planning and implementation. If an organization spends excessive time in planning, they get stuck in the planning loop and never progress to implementation. In those situations, the whole plan becomes "to plan." Strategic effectiveness is related to an organization's ability to set reasonable, not perfect, goals and consistently achieve them, which translates into formulating a "good enough" plan. It usually takes no more than a few hours of appropriately facilitated strategic planning and discussion to find a "good enough" plan in most organizations.

2. Once a "good enough" plan is identified, high-performance groups moved quickly to implementation.

3. Both high and low performance groups regularly evaluated their progress, but low performance groups tended to embellish their results, also called "result inflation." High-performance groups were brutally honest with their evaluation data.

4. High-performance groups made real-time adjustments to their strategic plans.

5. High-performance groups focused on results, where low performance groups focused on activities. The low performance groups often said, "We are working hard; therefore, we must be doing well." Working hard doesn't always translate into desired results. Advocacy issues vary greatly, often based on current events, local issues of interest, and politics.

PUBLIC HEALTH AND DISASTERS

Another important role for public health leaders concerns disasters—preparing for them and leading the disaster response. These are essential skills since disasters will likely be more frequent in the future due to:

- Human vulnerability associated with increased poverty and social inequality;
- Urbanization causing concentration of higher risk population groups;
- Environmental degradation and changes like climate change; and
- Rapid population growth.

These factors affect the United States and other developed countries, as well as the developing world. However, countries like the United States are better buffered from the effects of disasters because of the following advantages:

- Greater ability to forecast natural events,
- Greater enforcement of strict codes for fire and seismic construction,
- Existence of high functioning communications networks,
- More extensive emergency medical service systems,
- Contingency planning, and
- Redundancy of services and systems.

Disasters can be divided into two major categories, natural and man-made. Some disasters occur suddenly, like earthquakes, tsunamis, tornadoes, floods, hurricanes, volcanoes, landslides, and many infectious disease outbreaks. Some evolve slowly, over time, like droughts, famine, environmental degradation, and toxic substance exposure. Human-generated disasters include:

- War, which usually results in refugees and their associated challenges;
- Technological disasters, such as those associated with system failures that expose populations to hazardous chemicals or radiation;
- Transportation disasters, such as train collisions and overturns;
- Material shortage disasters, such as those associated with famine due to poor farming practices; and
- Desertification and deforestation.

The disaster cycle can be divided into four phases (see **Figure 8.3**).

- The inter-disaster phase is a time for public health to facilitate communities in the community engagement process, including developing community-level strategic disaster plans.
- The early sub-phase of the emergency and relief phase relates to services like emergency medical response, trauma care, search and rescue, establishment of emergency communications, relocation of vulnerable individuals, and removal of the dead. The late sub-phase of the emergency and relief phase relates to the provision of primary medical care and public health disaster interventions and services.

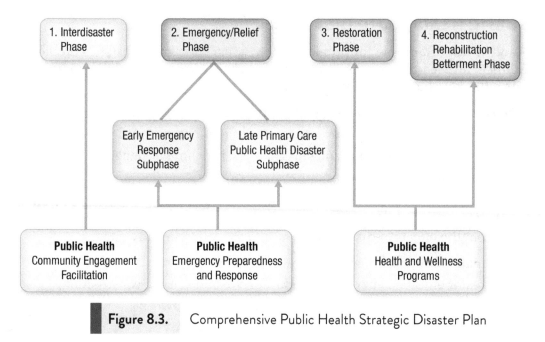

Figure 8.3. Comprehensive Public Health Strategic Disaster Plan

- The restoration phase is when normal services are restored.
- The reconstruction, rehabilitation, and betterment phase is when community development takes place. Traditional state and local public health programs that improve overall health and wellness of community members should be intimately involved with communities during the restoration and reconstruction, rehabilitation, and betterment phases.

Public health is involved throughout the disaster cycle, but in different capacities. The inter-disaster phase is the time for public health to facilitate community engagement, fostering, and enriching community ownership of their problems and solutions. During the emergency relief phase, public health emergency preparedness and response programs function. Incident command is an essential tool used in this phase. During the restoration and reconstruction, rehabilitation, and betterment phases, state and local public health programs—like community health, immunization, regulatory programs, population-based prevention programs—coordinate and collaborate with communities to improve the overall health wellness of all members.

Public health should develop a comprehensive public health strategic disaster plan, including local and state public health, that includes the emergency and relief phase, led by the emergency preparedness and response program, and also covers community engagement strategic planning during the inter-disaster phase. The latter may include strategic planning to support rural grocery stores to ensure adequate local food supplies for a prolonged natural disaster like blizzards, or plans to ensure that individuals on chronic medications have at least a 2-week supply on hand, and so forth.

The public health portion of the late sub-phase of the emergency and relief phase (one) includes:

- Water supplies,
- Disposing of human excreta and solid wastes,
- Food safety,
- Shelter,
- Personal hygiene needs,
- Vector control,
- Surveillance activities,
- Disease control, and
- Facilitating the strategic transition to community ownership and restoration.

DID YOU KNOW?

Potable water is generally the most important public health response in the late portion of the emergency and relief phase. During the Rwanda crisis in Africa, over 50,000 people died in refugee camps in Zaire during the first weeks of July, 1994 due to cholera. The crude mortality rate reached 28–41/10,000 per day. The source of the epidemic was contamination of water sources. The epidemic resolved with appropriate water treatment in the camps.

The early and late subphases of the emergency/relief phase overlap, similar to the general overlap of the relief and development phases previously discussed. Ideally, there should be a steady, seamless, smooth strategic transition from early to late sub-phases (**Figure 8.4**). This needs to be discussed and strategized through the Incident Command process of the public health emergency preparedness and response program linked with other local and state incident command processes responding to the disaster. Public health leadership should ensure that strategic transition discussions are considered at the intra- and inter-agency levels (Noji, 1997, 2000).

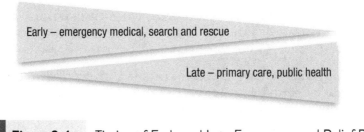

Figure 8.4.   Timing of Early and Late Emergency and Relief Phases

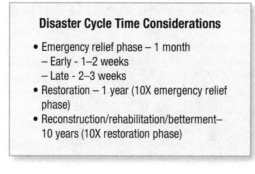

Figure 8.5. Disaster Cycle Time Considerations

Source: Colten, C. E., Kates, R. W., & Laska, S. B. (2008). Community resilience: Lessons from New Orleans and Hurricane Katrina. *Community and Regional Resilience Initiative Report*, 3.

Generally, the emergency and relief phase of most disasters lasts about 1 month (**Figure 8.5**): 1 to 2 weeks in the early sub-phase and 2 to 3 weeks in the late sub-phase. The restoration phase generally lasts 10 times longer than the emergency and relief phase, or about 10 to 12 months. The reconstruction, rehabilitation, and betterment phase lasts approximately ten times the duration of the restoration phase, or approximately 10 years. Major disasters are not short-term events but last for years, long after the cameras and short-term response teams have gone home. The restoration and reconstruction, rehabilitation and betterment phases often require more resources, flexibility, and creativity than the emergency and relief phase. These latter phases are the time for engaged communities to do what they do best, in their own unique ways. This is the area of community resilience. Facilitating communities to truly engage in the inter-disaster phase will dramatically help enhance community resilience when disasters strike (Maguire & Cartwright, 2008).

KEY IDEA

Disaster response is the time for a previously engaged community to do its work, and not the best time for a facilitator to engage a community. The best time to engage the community is in the inter-disaster phase.

Incident Management

Application of incident management principles is essential for effective public health response to major health threats and fundamental information needed by public health leaders.

> Public health emergencies are often complex, protracted, and can overwhelm public health systems typically staffed and equipped for routine operations. . . . Applying the concepts of emergency management, including the use of Emergency Operation Centers (EOCs) and Incident Management Systems (IMS) can help national and subnational public health systems protect populations impacted by a public health threat. (Bryant et al., 2018, p. 1)

The **Incident Management System (IMS)** is a comprehensive, national approach applicable at all jurisdictional levels and across disciplines (Federal Emergency Management Agency, Emergency Management Institute, 2022; U.S. Department of Health and Human Services, Office of the Assistant Secretary for Preparedness and Response, 2012). It improves coordination and cooperation among all response organizations, both private and public. The IMS provides a tool for organizations to respond to any type of incident regardless of size, location, or complexity, and standardizes incident management processes, protocols, and procedures for use by all responders. IMS features include:

- Common terminology to reduce confusion;
- Organizational resources and facilities;
- Manageable span of control;
- Use of position titles;
- Reliance on an Incident Action Plan that answers Who, What, When, Where;
- Management by objectives;
- Integrated communications and interoperability; and
- Accountability for check-in, initial briefings, record keeping, and demobilization.

The incident command organizational structure consists of Incident Command, which could be a single Incident Commander or a Unified Command. All incident command personnel report to and receive assignments from Incident Command. Other components of the incident command structure may include the Command Staff: Liaison, Public Information Officer (PIO), and Safety Officer. The Command Staff oversees the general staff that is usually organized in four sections: Logistics, Planning, Financing, and Operations. See Figure 8.6. Based on the incident, an Information and Intelligence section may also be activated. The Incident Commander activates only the functions and positions that are necessary to meet the specific incident response goals, with each activated element having a person in charge. Line of authority is key and must be maintained.

DID YOU KNOW?

The Incident Commander:

- Provides overall leadership for incident response.
- Delegates authority to others.
- Takes general direction from agency administrators or officials.
- Is responsible for all activities and functions until delegated and assigned to staff.
- Assesses need for staff.
- Establishes incident objectives.
- Directs staff to develop the incident action plan.
- Approves all information released by the public information officer.

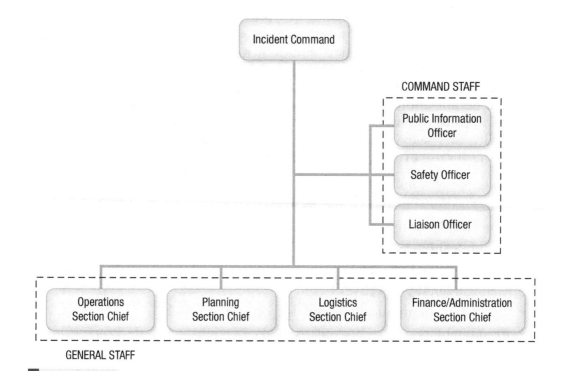

Figure 8.6.   Standard Incident Command System Organizational Structure at FEMA

Source: Federal Emergency Management Agency. (2018). *IS-0100.c: An introduction to the incident command system, ICS 100.* https://training.fema.gov/emiweb/is/is100c/english/student%20manual/is0100c_sm.pdf

Incidents are categorized by five types based on complexity, with Type 5 incidents the least complex and Type 1 the most complex. Incident objectives are established based on the following order of priority:

1. Life saving,
2. Incident stabilization, and
3. Property preservation.

DID YOU KNOW?

The 10 Myths and Facts About Disasters

Myth #1: Foreign medical volunteers with any kind of clinical background are needed. **Fact:** The local population almost always provides for its own immediate health needs. Only medical personnel with skills that are not available in the affected country may be needed.

Myth #2: Any kind of international assistance is needed immediately. **Fact:** A hasty response, not based on an impartial evaluation, contributes to the chaos. Most

(continued)

needs are met by the victims themselves and their government and local agencies, not by foreign aid workers.

Myth #3: Epidemics and plagues are inevitable after every disaster. **Fact:** Epidemics seldom occur after a disaster, and dead bodies do not lead to catastrophic outbreaks of infectious diseases. Improving sanitary conditions and educating the public on hygienic measures are the best means of preventing disease.

Myth #4: Disasters bring out the worst in people (e.g., looting, rioting). **Fact:** While there are isolated cases of antisocial behavior, which tend to be highlighted by the media, most people respond positively and generously.

Myth #5: The affected population is too shocked and helpless to take responsibility for its own survival. **Fact:** Many people find new strength and resiliency during an emergency.

Myth #6: Disasters are random killers. **Fact:** Disasters strike the most vulnerable groups hardest (i.e., minorities and the poor, especially women, children, and the elderly).

Myth #7: Locating disaster victims in temporary settlements is the best solution to the housing problem. **Fact:** This is the least desirable option. The preferred strategy is to purchase construction materials and rebuild.

Myth #8: Food aid is always required for the victims of natural disasters. **Fact:** Massive food aid is not usually required; natural disasters only rarely cause loss of crops.

Myth #9: Clothing is always needed by disaster victims. **Fact:** Clothing is almost never needed; it is usually culturally inappropriate, and although it is accepted by disaster victims it is almost never worn.

Myth #10: Things return to normal within a few weeks. **Fact:** Disasters have enduring effects and major economic consequences. International interest tends to wane just as needs and shortages become more pressing.

Source: Jacob, B., Mawson, A. R., Payton, M., & Guignard, J. C. (2008). Disaster mythology and fact: Hurricane Katrina and social attachment. *Public Health Reports, 123*(5), 555–566. https://doi.org/10.1177/003335490812300505

PUBLIC HEALTH AND SCIENCE

Public health is said to be the *science* of protecting and improving the health of people and their communities (CDC Foundation, 2023), but what is science? Science is the *systematic effort* of acquiring knowledge about the world—physical, behavioral, and social. Scientific knowledge is obtained through unbiased *observation* and *experimentation* and testing hypotheses with the evidence acquired. As Heilbron writes about the development of modern science:

> . . . modern science is a discovery as well as an invention. It was a discovery that nature generally acts regularly enough to be described by laws and even by mathematics; and required invention to devise the techniques, abstractions, apparatus, and organization for exhibiting the regularities and securing their law-like descriptions. (Heilbron, 2003, p. vii)

A sound foundation in science is essential for public health leaders because science is fundamental to effective public health policy and practice.

- Through scientific inquiry, we have learned how to prevent, control, and treat all sorts of health problems—from infectious diseases to heart disease to diabetes to injuries.
- Scientific inquiry has led to our understanding of the conditions required to promote good health—including provision of clean water and food supplies, as well as safe housing and workplaces.
- Scientific investigations have demonstrated the importance of social support, adequate nutrition, and physical activity.
- Application of the scientific method have helped us select the most effective policies and practices to achieve our goals.

Our values determine our goals, but science reveals how to achieve them. If there is a public health problem, solutions are revealed in scientific findings. For example, we may ask:

- How can an infectious disease agent be identified and treated?
- How can teens be prevented from driving under the influence of alcohol?
- How can eating habits among children be improved?

Solutions to public health problems find answers in scientific investigations that have been conducted or studies that must be undertaken.

Thus, public health practice requires professionals from all STEM disciplines, including statisticians, biologists, epidemiologists, informaticians, data scientists, microbiologists, and economists, as well as the liberal arts and the humanities (CDC, 2021). As a result, public health leaders must maintain currency in scientific findings and methods. This attribute is essential when guiding consideration and selection of best practices to solve problems, and then advocating for them. It also follows that leaders must be excellent science communicators. The importance of science communication has been a hard lesson learned from the COVID-19 pandemic. As Francis Collins—former Director of the National Institutes of Health and Current Science Advisor to President Biden—said regretfully:

> I underestimated the degree to which vaccine hesitancy was always going to be resistant to evidence, and I wish we had initiated more intense research on the basis of this kind of decision making and what interventions might actually work. Clearly lecturing people has not done a lot of good. (Luscombe, 2022, para. 6)

Very importantly, leaders advocating for science-based policy solutions must ensure that they communicate the non-static nature of science. Continual scientific inquiry results in new discoveries, that may change previous findings. This is the strength of science, and that must be understood by the general public. As Carl Sagan wrote:

Science is an ongoing process. It never ends. There is no single ultimate truth to be achieved, after which all the scientists can retire. (Sagan, 1980)

CHAPTER SUMMARY

Public health leaders, as in any field, may have technical or adaptive leadership skills, or both. Many executives are good managers (technical leadership) and yet have an additional set of skills to guide organizations through times of change and challenge (adaptive leadership). Knowing when and where to use these different leadership skills requires knowledge of their differences and appropriate judgment to use them effectively. People seeking leadership positions can enhance their leadership skills, both technical and adaptive, through experiential learning, appropriate training, and mentorship opportunities. Training in disaster management or advocacy and lobbying—two skills that are essential for public health leaders—can be learned in these ways. A sound foundation in science and scientific methods are also essential attributes for successful leaders.

DISCUSSION QUESTIONS

Q: Define the difference between management and adaptive leadership.

Q: What are the core cultural forces driving the way people do things, including their institutions and personal behaviors?

Q: How can a leader present vision passionately to their organization?

Q: What are the five major steps to changing organizational culture?

Q: Explain the role of horizontal communicators in the community engagement process.

Q: Explain the importance of advocacy to public health leaders.

Q: What is the role of public health leaders in disaster response and management?

Q: Why is a sound foundation in science essential for public health leaders?

DATA SOURCES

For the new public health professional, there are many training documents available to assist in developing leadership skills. Here are some of them:

Advocacy and Lobbying

Avner, M. (2002). *The lobbying and advocacy handbook for non-profit organizations: Shaping public policy at the state and local level.* Amherst Wilder Foundation.

Center for Community Health and Development. (2023). *Overview: Getting an advocacy campaign off the ground.* The Community Tool Box at the University of Kansas. https://ctb.ku.edu/en/table-of-contents/advocacy/advocacy-principles/overview/main

Emergency Management System and Incident Management

Bryant, J. L., Sosin, D. M., Wiedrich, T. W., & Redd, S. C. (2018). Emergency operations centers and incident management structure. *The CDC field epidemiology manual.* https://www.cdc.gov/eis/field-epi-manual/chapters/EOC-Incident-Management.html

Federal Emergency Management Agency & Emergency Management Institute. (2022). *IS-0100.c: An introduction to the incident command system, ICS 100 (student manual).* https://training.fema.gov/emiweb/is/is100c/english/student%20manual/is0100c_sm.pdf

U.S. Department of Health and Human Services & Office of the Assistant Secretary for Preparedness and Response. (2012). *Incident command system primer for public health and medical professionals.* https://www.phe.gov/Preparedness/planning/mscc/handbook/Pages/appendixb.aspx

---

REFERENCES

Avner, M. (2002). *The lobbying and advocacy handbook for non-profit organizations: shaping public policy at the state and local level.* Amherst Wilder Foundation.

Bryant, J. L., Sosin, D. M., Wiedrich, T. W., & Redd, S. C. (2018). Emergency operations centers and incident management structure. *The CDC field epidemiology manual.* https://www.cdc.gov/eis/field-epi-manual/chapters/EOC-Incident-Management.html

Center for Community Health and Development. (2023). *Overview: Getting an advocacy campaign off the ground.* The Community Tool Box at the University of Kansas. https://ctb.ku.edu/en/table-of-contents/advocacy/advocacy-principles/overview/main

Centers for Disease Control and Prevention. (2021). *Public health in STEM education.* https://www.cdc.gov/stem/education/stem_in_public_health.html

Centers for Disease Control and Prevention Foundation. (2023). *What is public health?* https://www.cdcfoundation.org/What-Public-Health

Chemers, M. M. (1997). *An integrative theory of leadership.* Lawrence Erlbaum Associates.

Colten, C. E., Kates, R. W., & Laska, S. B. (2008). Community resilience: Lessons from New Orleans and Hurricane Katrina. *Community and Regional Resilience Initiative (CARRI) Report 3.* https://biotech.law.lsu.edu/climate/docs/a2008.03.pdf

DeBuono, B., Gonzalez, A. R., & Rosenbaum, S. (2007). *Moments in leadership: Case studies in public health policy and practice.* Pfizer.

Farber, S. (2009). *The radical leap: A personal lesson in extreme leadership.* Dearborn Trade Publishing.

Federal Emergency Management Agency, Emergency Management Institute. (2022). *IS-0100.c: An introduction to the Incident Command System, ICS 100 (student manual)*. https://training.fema.gov/emiweb/is/is100c/english/student%20manual/is0100c_sm.pdf

Hall, E. T. (1973). *The silent language*. Anchor Books.

Heifetz, R. A., & Linsky, M. (2002). *Leadership on the line*. Harvard Business School Press.

Heilbron, J. L. (2003). *The Oxford companion to the history of modern science*. Oxford University Press.

Jacob, B., Mawson, A. R., Payton, M., & Guignard, J. C. (2008). Disaster mythology and fact: Hurricane Katrina and social attachment. *Public Health Reports, 123*(5), 555–566. https://doi.org/10.1177/003335490812300505

Kirkpatrick, S. A., & Locke, E. A. (1991). Leadership: Do traits matter? *Academy of Management Perspectives, 5*(2), 48–60. https://doi.org/10.5465/ame.1991.4274679

Luscombe, B. (2022, February 4). NIH director Francis Collins is leaving with a warning for some politicians. *Time Magazine*. https://time.com/6141545/nih-director-francis-collins-exit-interview/

Maguire, B., & Cartwright, S. (2008). *Assessing a community's capacity to manage change: A resilience approach to social assessment*. Australian Government, Bureau of Rural Services.

National Institutes of Health. (2011). *Principles of community engagement* (2nd ed.). National Institutes of Health.

Noji, E. K. (1997). *The public health consequences of disasters*. Oxford University Press.

Noji, E. K. (2000). The public health consequences of disasters. *Prehospital Disaster Medicine, 15*(4), 147–57.

Richards, D., & Engle, S. (1986). After the vision: Suggestions to corporate visionaries and vision champions. In J. D. Adams (Ed.), *Transforming leadership* (pp. 199–214). Miles River Press.

Sagan, C. (1980). *Cosmos*. Random House.

U.S. Department of Health and Human Services & Office of the Assistant Secretary for Preparedness and Response. (2012). *Incident command system primer for public health and medical professionals*. https://www.phe.gov/Preparedness/planning/mscc/handbook/Pages/appendixb.aspx

9 Public Health Practice and COVID-19: A Case Study

LEARNING OBJECTIVES

Students will learn . . .

1. Characteristics of COVID-19 and its variants.

2. Health impacts of COVID-19.

3. Phases of the public health response to COVID-19 in the United States.

4. Successes and complications during the COVID-19 response.

5. Lessons learned to improve future responses to a pandemic.

> "Learn from the mistakes of others. You can't live long enough to make them all yourself."
>
> —Eleanor Roosevelt

The story of the COVID-19 pandemic of 2020 is essential reading for new public health professionals. Every aspect of public health was involved in the response to COVID-19, which drew upon expertise in infectious disease control, policy development and evaluation, health monitoring, data collection and analysis, and communication with the public. From the first appearance of the disease to endemicity, it illustrates the full range infectious disease principles and methods of control, the need for accurate and timely information, the role of public health leadership, and the importance of community support and trust. Telling the story of public health during COVID-19 identifies successes and missteps, as well as strengths to be celebrated and weaknesses to be fixed. It is particularly instructive as an example of the application of public health principles and practices to a real-life problem that will undoubtedly be faced by public health professionals in the future.

Chapter 9 tells the story from the emergence of COVID-19 in the United States in January 2020 through the fall of 2022. The chapter describes the infectious disease—COVID-19 caused by severe acute respiratory syndrome coronavirus 2 (SARS-CoV-2)—and its impact on morbidity and mortality, including at-risk populations. Then, it identifies the pandemic phases of COVID-19 in the United States with their associated public health goals. Finally, the chapter discusses the difficulties of implementing a public health response to COVID-19—including the difficulties of communicating scientific information and political polarization, which complicated an already difficult job, and for which, in some important ways, public health was unprepared.

KEY IDEA

Understanding the problems that developed in controlling COVID-19 and possible solutions to them is of utmost importance to the future of public health in America and the response of public health to the next pandemic.

The goal would be to prevent the outcome illustrated in the following cartoon (**Figure 9.1**):

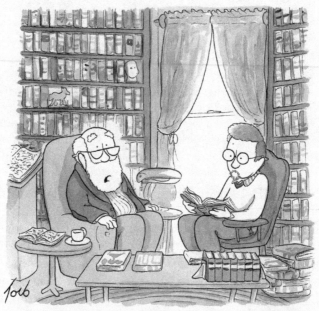

"Those who don't study history are doomed to repeat it.
Yet those who *do* study history are doomed to stand by
helplessly while everyone else repeats it."

Figure 9.1.   Repeating History Political Cartoon

Source: Toro, T. (2012). Those who don't study history. *Litro.*

INTRODUCTION TO THE COVID-19 PANDEMIC

A pandemic is, simultaneously, a public health challenge, a health care challenge, an economic challenge, and a political challenge. Even if the pandemic is caused by a known disease agent with an effective treatment and vaccine, a public health response requires enormous expenditures of resources for:

- Identifying populations at risk;
- Testing to determine infectivity and disease incidence;
- Providing health care and treatment of persons with the disease;
- Implementing public health methods to stem the spread of disease such as public information campaigns, contact tracing, quarantine and isolation protocols and programs; and
- If available, vaccinating the population at risk.

The problem for public health is far greater if the infectious disease agent is unknown and, therefore, the nature of the threat is undetermined when it first appears. What is unknown and must become known includes:

- How fatal is the disease?
- How does it spread and how easily?
- What are its human health effects?
- How can it be treated effectively?
- Who is most at risk of contracting it?
- Can a vaccine be developed?

The COVID-19 pandemic required public health to meet all of these challenges and to implement appropriate control and prevention strategies. In addition, the pandemic occurred in a time of tremendous political polarization in the United States. It began during President Donald Trump's administration and, after the first year, President Joseph Biden's administration assumed leadership. The country's political division increased the challenge of controlling the COVID-19 pandemic for public health. Thus, the story of COVID-19 illustrates the importance of the social and political environment on public health in general, and control of pandemics in particular.

CHARACTERISTICS OF THE DISEASE AND ITS HEALTH IMPACTS

The SARS-CoV-2 Virus

The disease COVID-19 is caused by the SARS-CoV-2 virus, which is a coronavirus. Coronaviruses are a large family of viruses that cause diseases in mammals and birds. Symptoms of coronavirus infection vary from species to species. Chickens often have upper respiratory symptoms, and cows and pigs often have diarrhea. In humans, the disease manifests generally as a respiratory infection. Coronaviruses are enveloped viruses with a single stranded RNA genome and nucleocapsid. The name "coronavirus" is derived from the Latin word corona, meaning "crown" or "halo," which refers to the characteristic appearance of a crown around the virus when viewed by electron microscopy.

Human coronaviruses were first discovered in the 1960s and consisted of seven strains when the COVID-19 outbreak occurred. Four of these strains, OC43, HKU1, NL63 also known as the New Haven coronavirus, and 229E circulate globally, producing common cold-like symptoms. Three coronavirus strains were associated with more severe disease including severe acute respiratory syndrome coronavirus (SARS-CoV or SARS) described in 2003, the Middle East respiratory syndrome coronavirus (MERS-CoV or MERS), associated with occasional outbreaks since 2012, and the SARS-CoV-2 also known as COVID-19. A COVID-19 outbreak was first reported in Wuhan, China, in December 2019. The COVID-19 virus has a 70% genetic similarity to the 2003 SARS virus and is thought to originate from bats since the virus has a 96% genetic similarity to bat coronaviruses.

COVID-19 Variants, Transmissibility, and Severity

Variants are mutations of the original virus. "Viruses constantly change through mutation, and new variants of a virus are expected to occur. Sometimes new variants emerge and disappear. Other times, new variants persist" (Centers for Disease Control and Prevention [CDC], 2021a). Many coronavirus variants and subvariants emerged during the COVID-19 pandemic. The CDC estimated that COVID-19 acquired about one new genetic mutation every 2 weeks. Many of these variants included mutations that affect the "spike protein" on the virus surface. Spike proteins facilitate viral attachment and infection of host cells. Variant spike protein mutations can result in enhanced attachment of COVID-19 to human cells, increasing transmissibility of the virus.

Table 9.1 lists the COVID-19 Variants of Concern as of August 2021. A Variant of Concern is one "for which there is evidence of an increase in transmissibility, more severe disease (for example, increased hospitalizations or deaths), significant reduction in neutralization by antibodies generated during previous infection or vaccination, reduced effectiveness of treatments or vaccines, or diagnostic detection failures" (National Center for Immunization and Respiratory Diseases [NCIRD], 2022d, para. 17). There is only one more designation higher—Variants of High Consequence, but no variants were in this category during the pandemic period described.

The incubation period is the time between exposure of a susceptible person to, and development of, the infection. The incubation period for COVID-19 is 2 to 14 days with a median of 5 days. COVID-19 transmission, or the contagious period, occurs early in the course of the illness, generally from 1 to 2 days prior to

Table 9.1. COVID-19 Variants of Concern, August, 2021

WHO Label	Pango Lineage[a]	Date of Designation to Variant of Concern
Alpha	B.1.1.7 and Q lineages	December 29, 2020
Beta	B.1.351 and descendant lineages	December 29, 2020
Gamma	P.1 and descendant lineages	December 29, 2020
Delta	B.1.617.2 and AY lineages	June 15, 2021
Epsilon	B.1.427 B.1.429	March 19, 2021
Omicron	B.1.1.529, BA.1, BA.1.1, BA.2, BA.3, BA.4, and BA.5 1	August, 2021

WHO, World Health Organization.

[a]Phylogenetic Assignment of Named Global Outbreak (Pango) Lineages Software developed by Aine O'Toole and colleagues at the Andrew Rambaut Laboratory to classify SARS-CoV-2 lineages.*Source*: National Center for Immunization and Respiratory Diseases, Division of Viral Diseases & Centers for Disease Control and Prevention. (2022d). *SARS-CoV-2 variant classifications and definitions.* https://www.cdc.gov/coronavirus/2019-ncov/variants/variant-classifications.html#anchor_1632150752495

2 to 3 days after symptom onset. For some infected individuals, particularly those who have severe disease or are immunocompromised, the duration of viral shedding and ability to transmit the infection to others can be longer. COVID-19 is not only transmissible to others before symptom onset, but can also occur in asymptomatic individuals (25% to 40% of those infected), which enhances transmission and may help explain why COVID-19 spread so rapidly across the globe (Du et al., 2020; Lauer et al., 2020; Lipsitch et al., 2003; Nishiura et al., 2020). Up to 25% to 40% of infected individuals will be asymptomatic but still able to transmit the infection to others.

The mortality rate worldwide of COVID-19 in early 2020 ranged from 2.1% to 4.2% of individuals with confirmed infection. In contrast, the mortality rate of SARS in 2003 was approximately 10%. MERS mortality has been as high as 30%. Though the COVID-19 virus has a lower case fatality rate (CFR) than outbreaks of the SARS and MERS coronaviruses, its high transmissibility and unique ability to transmit the virus before the infected person develops symptoms enhance transmission and result in large numbers of infected individuals, including those who may eventually develop severe disease or die. It is estimated that about 80% of documented COVID-19 infections during the period described came from exposure to those with undocumented infections due to the virus's high transmissibility (Hu et al., 2020). The CFR of COVID-19 is estimated at five to 20 times higher than typical seasonal influenza (note that as data continue to be collected, treatment protocols improve, and variants emerge, an exact comparison is challenging; Faust & del Rio, 2020; Maragakis, 2020; Piroth et al., 2020).

The range of severity for COVID-19 is broad. While many people may be asymptotic, a Chinese study of COVID-19 early in the pandemic showed a distribution of severity of symptoms across 44,000 patients as:

- Mild to moderate: 81%
- Severe: 14%
- Critical: 5%

The outcomes in the United States through May 2020 were similar with 14% hospitalized, 2% overall at the critical care/ICU level, and 5% dying (Stokes et al., 2020).

COVID-19 Impact on Health

Mortality and Morbidity

As of early September 2022, the number of COVID-19 cases in the United States was 94,973,074, and there were 1,044,461 deaths since the first death on February 29, 2020. January 13, 2021 saw the most deaths in a single day—4,082. After that, there were several peaks in death—one in September 2021 and one in February 2022—but none as high as in January 2021. The trajectory in deaths was downward, with 461 deaths on September 8, 2022 (CDC, 2022d). See **Figure 9.2**.

While most patients who developed COVID-19 symptoms had mild-to-moderate symptoms and did not require hospitalization, the proportion who required hospital care was significant when compared to well-known infectious diseases

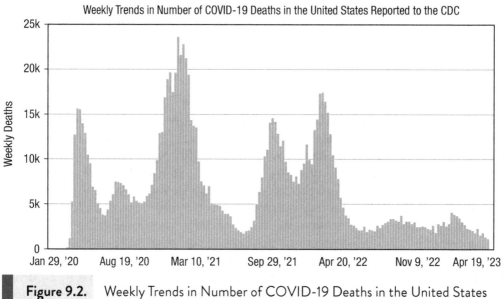

Figure 9.2.   Weekly Trends in Number of COVID-19 Deaths in the United States Reported to the Centers for Disease Control and Prevention

Source: Centers for Disease Control and Prevention. (n.d.). *Trends in United States COVID-19 hospitalizations, deaths, emergency department (ED) visits, and test positivity by geographic area.* https://covid.cdc.gov/covid-data-tracker/#trends_weeklydeaths_select_00

such as influenza ("the flu"), which has an estimated hospitalization rate about 10 times less than COVID-19 (CDC, 2021b). There were 5,272,570 hospital admissions for COVID-19 in total between August 1, 2021 and September 7, 2022. There were four peaks in hospitalizations between August 1, 2021 and September 7, 2022. The highest was on January 15, 2022 with 21,525 admissions (7-day moving average). There were 15,597 on January 1, 2021 and 12,284 on August 27, 2021. On September 7, the 7-day moving average for hospital admissions was 4,559 (CDC, 2022c). See **Figure 9.3**.

The most common complications from severe COVID-19 included pneumonia, hypoxemic respiratory failure/ARDS, sepsis and septic shock, cardiomyopathy and arrhythmia, and acute kidney injury. Additionally, prolonged hospitalization from COVID-19 lead to its own complications including secondary infections, gastrointestinal bleeding, and polyneuropathy/myopathy (CDC, 2021c).

Likelihood of death from COVID-19 varied by age, sex, and race/ethnicity. However, the trajectory was much the same for each group, with five rather large bumps in deaths rates throughout the period from March 1, 2020 through September 10, 2022, and a very small bump in July 2022. The dramatic increases indicated by the "bumps" in death rates would follow an outbreak of COVID-19.

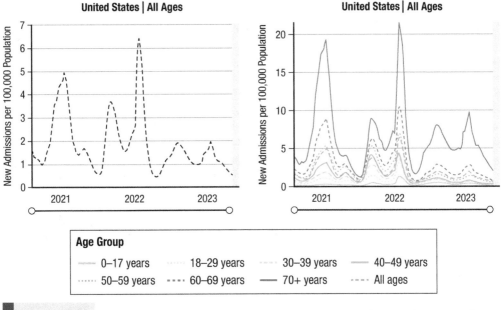

New Hospital Admissions of Patients With Confirmed COVID-19, United States
Aug 01, 2020 - Apr 23, 2023

Figure 9.3.   New Admissions of Patients with Confirmed COVID-19 per 100,000 Population, United States

Source: Centers for Disease Control and Prevention. (n.d.). *COVID data tracker.* https://covid.cdc.gov/covid-data-tracker/#new-hospital-admissions

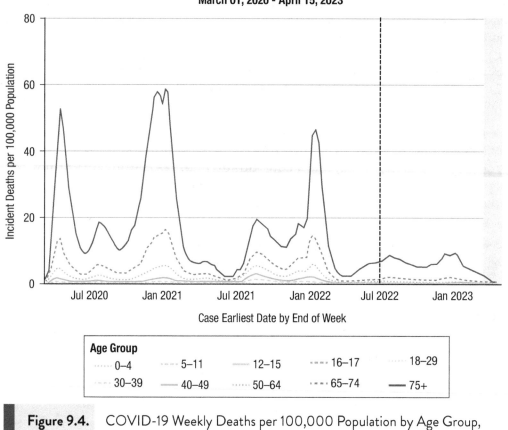

Figure 9.4. COVID-19 Weekly Deaths per 100,000 Population by Age Group, United States

Source: Centers for Disease Control and Prevention. (n.d.). *COVID-19 weekly cases and deaths per 100,000 population by age, race/ethnicity, and sex.* https://covid.cdc.gov/covid-data-tracker/#demographicsovertime

Age was the most influential demographic characteristic predicting death from COVID-19. Throughout the pandemic, persons 50 years and older were substantially more likely to die than younger people. Moreover, as age increased, likelihood of death increased, with people 75 years and older the most likely to die (CDC, 2022b). See **Figure 9.4.**

In addition to older people, those at greatest risk of severe COVID-19 disease and death were individuals with underlying medical conditions. Some of those conditions are listed in the following (NCIRD, 2022e):

- Asthma;
- Cancer;
- Cerebrovascular disease;
- Chronic kidney disease;
- Certain chronic lung diseases;
- Certain chronic liver diseases;

- Cystic fibrosis;
- Diabetes mellitus, type 1 and type 2;
- Heart conditions (such as heart failure, coronary artery disease, or cardio-myopathies); and
- HIV (human immunodeficiency virus).

Race and ethnicity also affected likelihood of death from COVID-19. American Indians/Alaska Natives had markedly higher death rates throughout the pandemic than persons in other groups, except in early 2020 when Blacks had the highest rate. Since June 2022, all ethnic/racial groups have had about the same death rate (CDC, 2022b). See **Figure 9.5**. Men were slightly more likely to die than women, but the trajectory was essentially the same for both sexes (CDC, 2022b). See **Figure 9.6**.

Persistent symptoms noticed in many individuals after COVID-19 infection have been labeled as long-COVID-19. Long-COVID-19 was more common in persons over 65 years old, but was observed in both hospitalized and outpatient cases (Logue et al., 2021). Long-COVID-19 symptoms and signs include fatigue,

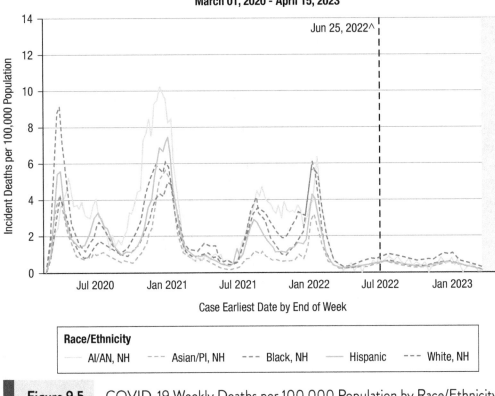

Figure 9.5. COVID-19 Weekly Deaths per 100,000 Population by Race/Ethnicity, United States

AI, American Indians; AN, Alaska Natives; PI, Pacific Islanders; NH, non-Hispanic.

Source: Centers for Disease Control and Prevention. (n.d.). *COVID-19 weekly cases and deaths per 100,000 population by age, race/ethnicity, and sex.* https://covid.cdc.gov/covid-data-tracker/#demographicsovertime

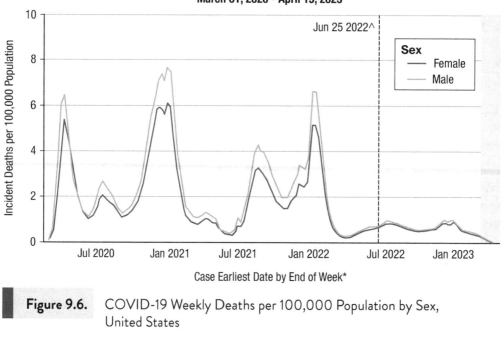

Figure 9.6. COVID-19 Weekly Deaths per 100,000 Population by Sex, United States

Source: Centers for Disease Control and Prevention. (n.d.). *COVID-19 weekly cases and deaths per 100,000 population by age, race/ethnicity, and sex.* https://covid.cdc.gov/covid-data-tracker/#demographicsovertime

weakness, sleep disorders, anxiety, depression, shortness of breath, loss of taste and smell, CT scan abnormalities of the chest, and abnormal lung gas exchange (Editor, *The Lancet*, 2021); brain shrinkage in areas responsible for taste, smell, emotion, and memory processing and storage (Douaud et al., 2021); and neuropsychiatric abnormalities. Neuropsychiatric abnormalities include patterns of brain executive function loss, a frontal lobe syndrome, and memory processing issues and have been more frequently observed in patients hospitalized with COVID-19. Twelve percent of individuals with long-COVID-19 were not able to return to work 12 months after their COVID-19 infection (Editor, *The Lancet*, 2021). Several studies demonstrated an association with new onset diabetes mellitus in children and adults that appeared up to a year after the infection (Gottesman et al., 2022; Rezel-Potts et al., 2021).

Mental Health

Mental health was negatively impacted by the COVID-19 pandemic for many people who shifted from working in offices to working from home. For example, researchers who conducted a study of those working from home in the fall of 2020 found that the majority reported declines in both general and workplace well-being, especially related to increased job demands and home-life difficulties. Only about 22% reported improved well-being (Campbell & Gavett, 2021). See **Figure 9.7**.

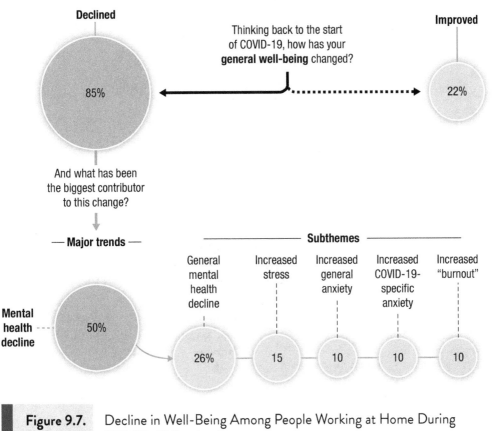

Figure 9.7.   Decline in Well-Being Among People Working at Home During COVID-19 Pandemic

Source: Campbell, M., & Gavett, G. (2021). What COVID-19 has done to our well-being, in 12 charts. *Harvard Business Review.* https://hbr.org/2021/02/what-covid-19-has-done-to-our-well-being-in-12-charts

A survey by the Kaiser Family Foundation asked survey respondents about the impact of COVID-19 on their mental and physical health and the mental health of their children. Over 40% reported negative impacts on both. Other issues that were negatively affected by the pandemic were children's education, relationships with family members, and financial and employment situations. See **Figure 9.8.**

The mental health of health care workers was particularly affected by COVID-19. Hospitalizations from COVID-19 overwhelmed the health care system throughout the pandemic, especially in the beginning when personal protective equipment (PPE) was in short supply and COVID-19-specific treatments were not yet developed. During the pandemic, a relatively high prevalence of anxiety (24.94%), depression (24.83%), and sleep disorders (44.03%) was reported in meta-analyses investigating the mental health of health care workers (Marvaldi et al., 2021; Sahebi et al., 2021). Because of the perceived stigma associated with mental illness and the fear of an impact on their careers, health care workers tend

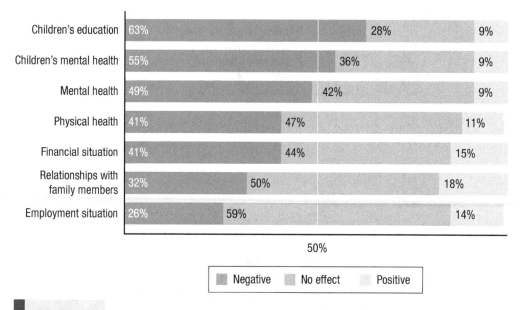

Figure 9.8.   The Impact of the COVID-19 Pandemic on Mental and Physical Health

Source: Sparks, G., Hamel, L., Kirzinger, A., Montero, A., & Brodie, M. (2022). *KFF COVID-19 vaccine monitor: Views on the pandemic at two years.* Kaiser Family Foundation. https://www.kff.org/mental-health/poll-finding/kff-covid-19-vaccine-monitor-pandemic-two-years/

to hide their anxiety and stress (Brower, 2021). Thus, during COVID-19, health care workers struggled with burnout. Moreover, health care workers were three times more likely than the general public to contract COVID-19. And an extensive study by *The Guardian* and *Kaiser Health News* found that 3,607 health care workers in the United States died from COVID-19 during the first year of the pandemic (Spencer & Jewett, 2021).

PHASES OF THE COVID-19 PANDEMIC IN AMERICA

The COVID-19 pandemic can be divided into three phases:

Phase 1: Prevaccine—January 2020 to December 2020

Phase 2: Vaccine Availability and Mass Vaccination—January 2021 to April 2021

Phase 3: COVID-19 Becomes Endemic—May 2021 to Fall 2022

During each phase, public health had goals for control and prevention of COVID-19, as well as achievements and failures, which are described in the following.

Phase 1: Prevaccine (January 2020 to December 2020)

Without a COVID-19 vaccine or proven therapeutics, public health had four primary goals during Phase 1:

Goal 1: Reduce Transmission of COVID-19

Goal 2: Provide Medical Care for the Severely Ill

Goal 3: Develop a COVID-19 Vaccine

Goal 4: Develop COVID-19 Therapies and Diagnostic Tests

Goal 1: Reduce Transmission of COVID-19

In the prevaccine period, the only tools available to prevent transmission of COVID-19 were the long-established public health measures—essentially, placing physical barriers between people, quarantining the infected and those exposed to the virus (isolation), and social distancing. Social distancing resulted in closing schools and offices and having people work or study from home; and prohibiting large gatherings such as concerts, sporting events, and church services. Voluntary interventions were augmented by mandatory interventions in several states and communities and included local, interstate, and international travel bans, closing borders, mandatory testing, and beach closures. Testing was essential to identify persons who needed care, to separate them from others (isolation), and to follow up with contact tracing. Some contact tracing was done early on in the pandemic before the number of cases exploded.

DID YOU KNOW?

Transmission of COVID-19 is primarily by respiratory droplets and aerosols. Respiratory droplets are larger than aerosols, contain large numbers of viral particles, and tend to drop out of the air relatively quickly. The transmission of large droplets from infected individuals could be reduced using a variety of masks. Aerosols are smaller particles that contain fewer viral particles but remain suspended in the air for a longer period and are not as easily removed by masks as the larger droplets are. The COVID-19 virus was detectable in aerosols for up to 3 hours.

Control of transmission was complicated by the difficulty of identifying cases. Infected persons could be symptomatic or asymptomatic. If asymptomatic, individuals continued their normal activities and, unfortunately, spread the virus to others. Even if symptomatic, however, COVID-19 symptoms are not unique. They include fever, chills, cough, shortness of breath or difficulty breathing, fatigue, muscle or body aches, headache, new loss of taste and/or smell, sore throat, congestion, runny nose, nausea, vomiting, and diarrhea, mimicking several other infectious diseases. Thus, even symptomatic COVID-19-infected individuals might not seek care or testing and be identified as having COVID-19. This type of information led to recommending N-95 masks versus cloth masks, which many individuals wore during the initial stages of the pandemic, as well as recommendations to social distance, which helped to decrease transmission of COVID-19 via droplets and aerosols. Wearing a face mask was not recommended as an alternative to social distancing measures, however. See Table 9.2.

Table 9.2. Prevaccine Social Distancing Guidance

1. Stay home and don't go to work if you feel sick

2. Wash your hands regularly with soap and water for 20 seconds

3. Avoid touching your nose, eyes, and mouth

4. Cover coughs and sneezes

5. If someone in the household has COVID-19, keep the entire household at home

6. High risk individuals should stay away from other people

7. Work from home when possible

8. Avoid social gatherings

9. Avoid eating or drinking in bars, restaurants, and food courts

10. Avoid discretionary travel, shopping trips, and social visits

11. Maintain at least a 6-foot distance between people

12. Use a mask when in public

Reducing transmission to the most vulnerable was an early priority during the pandemic. Individuals 60 years and older and those with underlying medical conditions were most likely to develop severe disease and need hospitalization and intensive care. Masking and social distancing guided much social interaction between older and younger people, particularly in long-term care facilities, and between people with underlying health problems. The toll on social relations was high and could include "visiting" relatives in nursing homes at a window, rather than in a room, or conversing with family members only via telephone or virtually.

Resistance to public health control measures began to build during the Prevaccine Phase of the COVID-19 pandemic. Partially as a result of resistance, transmission in the general population varied greatly across the country.

Goal 2: Provide Medical Care for the Severely Ill

During initial pandemic surges, a major goal was to assure adequate medical care for the moderately and severely ill. Due to the marked number of patients needing hospital care, there was an urgent need to protect the hospitals' and clinics' capacities to care for the ill—not only those with COVID-19, but also to continue to provide care for individuals with other medical conditions. The plan to prevent hospital overload was called "flattening the curve" and consisted of plans to decrease public transmission and to develop a hospital mitigation and triage plan (NCIRD, 2021). Hospital mitigation plans altered hospital processes including:

- Rescheduling elective surgeries;
- Shifting select inpatient diagnostic and surgical procedures to outpatient settings, when feasible;
- Limiting or prohibiting visitors to COVID-19 patients;
- Identifying additional space to care for patients including emergency departments and other atypical patient care areas;
- Cohorting hospital staff to a specific COVID-19 space or ward within the institution; and
- Developing new quarantine and isolation plans (NCIRD, 2021).

Another priority was protecting hospital staff with PPE to prevent illness when caring for COVID-19 patients. PPE was in short supply in the early years of the pandemic:

> In protests covered by the news media, healthcare workers compared themselves to firefighters putting out fires without water and soldiers going into combat with cardboard body armor. Medical professionals have called for federal government action to mobilize and distribute adequate supplies of protective equipment, especially gloves, medical masks, goggles or face shields, gowns, and N95 respirators. N95 respirators, which have demonstrated efficacy in reducing respiratory infections among healthcare workers, have been in particularly short supply. (Cohen & Rodgers, 2020, para. 1)

As previously mentioned, health care workers were three times more likely than the general public to contract COVID-19. The causes identified were widespread shortages of masks and other PPE, lack of COVID-19 testing, inconsistent guidance about masking, and lax workplace safety practices (Spencer & Jewett, 2021).

Goal 3: Develop a COVID-19 Vaccine

While the public health and health care systems were responding to the COVID-19 outbreak during 2020, scientists and pharmaceutical companies across the world dedicated themselves to developing a vaccine. In the United States, this effort was supported by a public–private partnership begun under President Donald Trump's administration and named "Operation Warp Speed." One safety concern often expressed as the vaccines were being developed was the perceived "newness" of mRNA vaccine technology.

KEY IDEA

However, the COVID-19 mRNA vaccine technology evolved over decades from research on lipid nanoparticles in the 1980s, the development of techniques to synthesize mRNA for injection into cells in the 2000s, and the 2012 study of MERS-CoV and the potential use of spike proteins in vaccines.

Therefore, there was much existing science to build upon. The COVID-19 vaccine effort was built on the work of generations of vaccine scientists throughout the country and the world—resulting in safe and effective vaccines.

DID YOU KNOW?

The United States has an exceptional multilayered system to monitor the safety of medications and vaccines. This system includes both pre- and post-licensure processes and programs including the safety and efficacy studies of the three phases of clinical trials, the vaccine adverse events reporting system (VAERS), the clinical immunization safety assessment (CISA) project, the vaccine safety datalink (VSD), post-licensure rapid immunization safety monitoring (PRISM) system, and V-safe.

The VSD program is an important active safety monitoring tool developed by the CDC approximately 30 years ago, and covers 12 million people linked through nine participating managed care organizations. Data analyzed includes vaccinations, hospital and outpatient information, and laboratory data. VSD utilizes Rapid Cycle Analysis (RCA), which was developed by the VSD program to monitor pre-specified vaccine related safety outcomes in near real-time. RCA commonly utilizes either self-controlled or current/historical study designs with appropriate control groups, data quality, and adjustment for confounding factors. Every week, RCA compares rates of pre-specified outcomes in pre-specified time windows. Ninety percent of initial adverse events signals turn out to be spurious by RCA. In the history of all licensed vaccines in the United States, no serious side effects have ever been found after 6 weeks. All currently available COVID-19 vaccines have now been studied for over 6 to 12 months. Even with that being said, the vaccine safety monitoring systems mentioned will continue to monitor these COVID-19 vaccines along with all other vaccines for safety. There is no end point for vaccine safety monitoring.

Goal 4: Develop COVID-19 Therapies and Diagnostic Tests

During the first phase of the pandemic, scientists in government, private industry, and academia were also devoting themselves to developing diagnostic tests as well as therapies for persons ill with COVID-19. Similar to efforts to develop a COVID-19 vaccine, these efforts also proved successful, and they were implemented as they emerged beginning in 2020.

Testing was essential for an effective response to the pandemic. If tests were widely available, they could identify persons infected and prevent them from infecting others through isolation and contact tracing. Viral tests look for a current infection with SARS-CoV-2, the virus that causes COVID-19. Antibodies are created by the immune system after infection and indicate past infection by the COVID-19 virus. Antibody (serology) tests were used by public health epidemiologists to determine how many people in a defined population or community were previously infected with COVID-19 (prevalence of a disease). Viral tests indicated current infection by the COVID-19 virus (incidence of a disease; CDC, 2023).

DID YOU KNOW?

There are two types of viral tests—nucleic acid amplification tests (NAATs) and antigen tests. NAATs detect viral genetic material and are usually performed in a laboratory. They are the most accurate tests for detecting infection in persons with and without symptoms. Antigen tests are less accurate than NAATs, but they are rapid and can produce results in 15 to 30 minutes. Antigen tests can be used serially to provide more sensitive results. Home or self-tests are generally antigen tests (NCIRD, 2022c). Both NAATs and antigen tests rarely cause false-positive results, and therefore, a positive from either a NAATs or antigen test was treated as a true positive.

In addition to needing diagnostic tests for COVID-19, therapies were necessary to preserve the life of persons who had developed the disease. In the United States and worldwide, a great deal of effort was expended by scientists to develop effective COVID-19 therapies. However, the introduction of these therapies occurred later in the pandemic—not during the prevaccine period. For example, Pfizer's Paxlovid for treatment of mild-to-moderate COVID-19 in adults and pediatric patients was approved in December 2021. It was the first treatment in the form of a pill (FDA, 2021). Other effective COVID-19 therapies—including antiviral medications and monoclonal antibodies—were also developed later in the pandemic.

However and not surprisingly, especially at the outset of the pandemic, there was controversy over the protocols for testing and providing therapeutics. Which tests or therapeutics should be given, to whom, by whom, and how often? There were also issues with supply and adequate access to testing and effective therapeutics. These issues were major concerns that occupied scientists and public health and health care professionals throughout the pandemic. As examples of controversy and uncertainty, see Binnicker (2020) and Pettengill and McAdam (2020) on testing issues.

Phase 1 Summary

The goals of the prevaccine Phase 1—reduce COVID-19 transmission, provide medical care for the severely ill, and develop a COVID-19 vaccine and effective therapies and diagnostic tests—were met with costs.

- Transmission of the COVID-19 virus was certainly decreased, but the cost in reduced social interaction and weakened social ties was high, especially for the young and old. The mental health consequences in loneliness and isolation were substantial.

- Medical care was provided to those with COVID-19 at a substantial cost to health care workers. They were overburdened by huge caseloads, shortage of personal protection against the virus, fearful of transmitting the virus to family members, and working without proven therapeutics and diagnostics. In this early period, the high death rate among hospitalized patients with COVID-19 was exhausting and demoralizing.
- The development of COVID-19 vaccines, diagnostic tests, and therapeutics for the sick was begun successfully in Phase 1 (**Box 9.1**). These medical advancements represent a success story for the scientific community as well as public health, because they were built on extensive prior research in other, but related, areas. The foundation of existing science—built over decades—allowed the rapid development of the tools needed to control the COVID-19 pandemic and save lives through vaccines, tests, and therapies.

Box 9.1. Highlight: A Source of Pride

Dr. Francis Collins, former National Institutes of Health (NIH) Director and White House Science Advisor at the time, described the tremendous scientific effort around COVID-19: "During 2020, 2021, as the COVID pandemic was raging and spreading across the world, I don't think I ever felt a greater sense of the unanimity of the scientific community to come together, to come up with strategies to battle this worst pandemic in more than a century. Many of us were working 100 hours a week. I certainly was, trying to make sure that no stone was unturned to come up with vaccines and therapeutics and diagnostic tests that might save the lives that we were losing every day. And it felt that way, like every day I've got to make the right decision, or it's going to be potentially the cost of somebody's life." (Cooney, 2022, para 4)

Phase 2: Vaccine Availability and Mass Vaccination (January 2021 to May 2021)

With an effective COVID-19 vaccine ready for adults, public health had two primary goals during Phase 2:

Goal 1: Make Vaccines Available to the Adult Population

Goal 2: Develop Herd Immunity

Goal 1: Make Vaccines Available to the Adult Population

In December 2020, three COVID-19 vaccines for adults received approval from the U.S. Food and Drug Administration (FDA), and vaccinations were available in the United States beginning in January 2021. The approved vaccines included two mRNA vaccines (Pfizer and Moderna) and one adenovirus vector vaccine (Johnson & Johnson).

Once the vaccines were approved for use in the United States, two tremendous logistical efforts were undertaken: (a) produce enough vaccine for administration to millions of eligible adults, and (b) create vaccination sites that could be accessed easily by most adults. The effort to create easily accessible vaccination sites required extensive cooperation throughout the country to ensure that everyone received the same access to vaccinations. The vaccination effort was a "whole-of-society" endeavor that included states, localities, and public and private partners. It was the largest free vaccination program in America's history with 90,000 vaccination locations and the ability to administer more than 125,000 shots a day. Over 9,000 federal personnel supported the vaccination effort, including over 5,000 active-duty troops. The effort included "employers who offered paid time off for their employees; child care providers who offered drop-in services for caregivers to get vaccinated; public transit authorities and ride-sharing companies that provided free rides to vaccination sites; churches, civic organizations, barbershops, and beauty salons, who opened their doors to be trusted spaces for vaccinations; and the families who made vaccination a family affair" (The White House, 2022, p. 8).

Soon after his inauguration in January 2021, President Joseph Biden set a goal to achieve 100 million vaccinations in his first 100 days in office. That number was exceeded by May 2021, with 200 million COVID-19 vaccinations administered (Naylor, 2021). The public health vaccination effort between January and May 2021 was highly successful because of the broad coalition—both private and public—supporting it, including the White House and Congress. Indeed, this achievement would not have been possible without the societal-level cooperation that spanned the smallest communities and the highest levels of leadership.

Goal 2: Develop Herd Immunity

A goal of the COVID-19 vaccination effort was not only prevention of COVID-19 in individuals, but attaining **herd immunity**. Herd immunity occurs when enough people in a community or population are immune to a specific disease to reduce or eliminate transmission among those who are still susceptible. When the community immunity threshold is reached, the infection rate drops because the disease agent is unable to find enough susceptible persons to perpetuate its life cycle. The community immunity threshold may be achieved through vaccination, infection that imparts immunity, or both.

DID YOU KNOW?

To calculate community immunity (CI), scientists first determine the reproduction number ($R0$) for an infectious organism. The $R0$ describes the average number of people that a single person with an infection like COVID-19 will usually infect if those people aren't already immune. The higher the $R0$, the more people need to be immune to reach the CI threshold. The $R0$ for the original COVID-19 virus was between 2 and 3. This means that one person generally would infect two or three other susceptible people. One formula for the CI threshold in percent is CI = $[(R0 - 1)/R0] \times 100$.

(continued)

Using this formula, the lower COVID-19 CI threshold percent, using an $R0$ of 2 would be 50%. The high COVID-19 threshold percent using an $R0$ of 3 would be 67%. So, if the CI threshold, which may include those having natural immunity from infection and those vaccinated, is greater than 50% to 67%, there should be a decline in transmission for that COVID-19 strain in that community. COVID-19 variants that have higher $R0$ values result in a higher community or herd immunity threshold. The $R0$ for omicron variants may range from 8 to 16 with a community threshold range of 88% to 91%.

Unfortunately, herd immunity was not achieved by the mass vaccination efforts of early 2021. Becoming vaccinated was mostly voluntary, and rapid uptake of vaccinations occurred at first. However, vaccination-seeking waned beginning in late spring 2021 with only about 53% of Americans fully vaccinated by May 31—approximately 5 months after vaccinations became available (Our World in Data, 2022a). After that, vaccination rates rose steadily, but slowly. By August 2022, about 15 months after vaccines were first available in the United States, 68% of Americans were fully vaccinated—only 15% more than in May 2021 (Our World in Data, 2022b)—and not enough to provide herd immunity.

KEY IDEA

The major cause for declining vaccination rates was vaccination hesitancy or even resistance based on misinformation and the resultant mistrust of vaccines.

In time, epidemiologists demonstrated that vaccination reduced the likelihood of severe disease, hospitalization, and death among people exposed to the COVID-19 virus. Studies showed that post-hospitalization fatality rates, post-COVID-19 neuropsychiatric problems, and long COVID-19 symptoms were also positively impacted by vaccination (Becker et al., 2021; Douaud et al., 2021). Once the vaccination effort began, almost all hospitalizations occurred among unvaccinated individuals (CDC, 2022a). See **Figure 9.9**. However, many people outside the public health community were unmoved by these findings, choosing instead to believe the misinformation that vaccination was harmful and/or unnecessary.

Phase 2 Summary

The goals of Phase 2—to make vaccines widely available and develop herd immunity—were partially met.

- The COVID-19 vaccination effort was highly successful. By and large, adults throughout the country who wished to be vaccinated were able to access vaccination sites. Public health planning addressed the barriers to obtaining the vaccine including knowledge about vaccine safety, cost, location of sites,

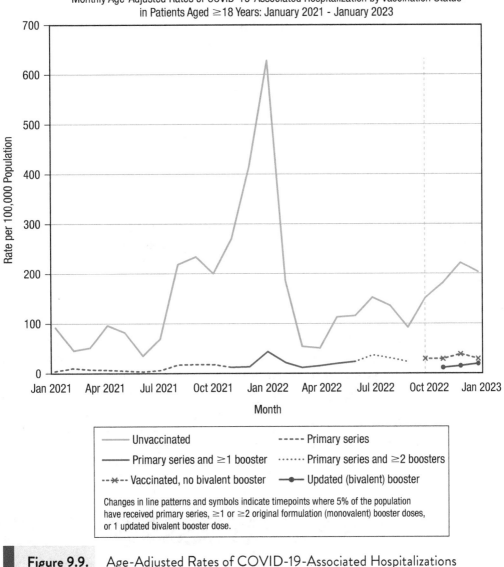

Figure 9.9.   Age-Adjusted Rates of COVID-19-Associated Hospitalizations by Vaccine Status in Adults Aged 18 Years or Older

Source: Centers for Disease Control and Prevention. (n.d.). *COVID-19 update for the United States.* https://www.cdc.gov/coronavirus/2019-ncov/covid-data/covid-net/hospitalizations-by-vaccination-status-report.pdf

and hours of operation. Shots were free or low cost. Vaccination sites were placed in community, not just health care, settings. Hours of operation were extensive. The massive COVID-19 vaccination effort in early 2021 exemplified public health practice at its most successful.

- However, reaching herd immunity was unsuccessful, because the rate of vaccination declined after May 2021. The substantial unvaccinated population provided opportunity for the virus to continue replicating and eventually to form variants—keeping COVID-19 alive.

Phase 3: COVID-19 Becomes Endemic (June 2021 to Fall 2022)

With the mixed results of mass vaccination and the continued transmission of the COVID-19 virus, public health had three primary goals during Phase 3:

Goal 1: Respond to New Variants of COVID-19

Goal 2: Increase Availability of Testing and Therapeutics

Goal 3: Prepare for COVID-19 Endemicity

Goal 1: Respond to New Variants of COVID-19

"Throughout the pandemic, the United States has experienced waves of different variants of SARS-CoV-2, the virus that causes COVID-19. SARS-CoV-2 is constantly changing, and new variants of the virus are expected to occur" (NCIRD, 2022b). The rise of COVID-19 variants—which differed in transmissibility and severity from the original virus—required new vaccines as the effectiveness of the earlier vaccines declined. Booster shots were developed for the vaccinated.

Alpha was the first variant to emerge, early in 2021. It was followed by the delta variant, which became the most common circulating COVID-19 variant worldwide in the summer of 2021. The delta variant was first described in India and shown to be approximately 40% to 60% more transmissible compared to the highly transmissible alpha variant. In addition, vaccination, particularly after the first dose of the Pfizer mRNA vaccine, was 70% less effective in preventing hospitalization. However, hospitalization efficacy increased to approximately 95% after the second dose, similar to the efficacy against the alpha variant. This result emphasized the importance of receiving the two-dose primary series of mRNA vaccines to provide protection from infection, hospitalization, and death with the delta variant.

DID YOU KNOW?

In late 2021 and throughout early 2022, the omicron variant became the predominant variant circulating in the United States. The omicron variant B.1.1.529, or BA.1, and the omicron subvariant BA.2 were much more transmissible than the delta variant. This resulted in about a 70-fold increase of viral particles in various respiratory secretions. The increased transmissibility caused spikes in cases globally. The BA.2 subvariant has been called the "stealth omicron" because certain genetic laboratory tests could not identify the genetic structural differences between BA.2 and BA.1. BA.2 presented with similar clinical symptoms to BA.1. Prior infection with BA.1 provided protection against infection with BA.2. Viral mutations of the omicron variant (BA.1) and "stealth" subvariant (BA.2) resulted in a significant loss of neutralizing antibody protection after a previous COVID-19 infection with other COVID-19 variants or even after vaccination—resulting in increased reinfection rates. Booster doses dramatically increased neutralizing antibody protection against infection and severe disease due to omicron.

New variants continued to emerge throughout Phase 3. Mitigation and vaccination strategies were adapted as variants emerged with increased transmissibility and decreased response to the primary series of mRNA COVID-19 vaccines. Booster shots were developed and made available to the vaccinated, while those who had not been vaccinated were encouraged to do so.

Goal 2: Increase Availability of Testing and Therapeutics

Access to testing for COVID-19 was improved during this period. The Biden Administration increased the supply of diagnostic tests to aid in identifying infected individuals. By spring 2022, there were free testing sites at 21,500 locations in the country. In January 2021, there were no rapid, at-home tests on the market for Americans, but by January 2022, there were more than 480 million at-home tests available. The administration also created the website COVIDtests.gov where tests could be ordered online and shipped directly to homes—for free. During this phase, private insurance, Medicare, and Medicaid covered rapid at-home tests (The White House, 2022).

In addition, therapeutics were made widely available. The Biden Administration prioritized developing, manufacturing, and procuring COVID-19 treatments. Several effective therapies—including antiviral medications and monoclonal antibody antibodies—developed during the pandemic were effective in preventing severe disease and death. By January 2022, the first doses of monoclonal antibodies were distributed within 48 hours of FDA authorization. By spring 2022, the Administration had secured 20 million doses of Pfizer's antiviral pills, which reduced the risk of hospitalization or death by 89% (The White House, 2022).

Goal 3: Prepare for COVID-19 Endemicity

"An epidemic refers to the rapid spread of a pathogen in a population, while the endemic state refers to the stable maintenance of the pathogen, typically at a lower prevalence" (Antia & Halloran, 2021, p. 2172).

By mid-2021, many public health officials began to speculate that COVID-19 herd immunity through vaccination and prior infection would be an unattainable goal. Rather, they believed that vaccination would save lives, but it would not eradicate the disease. Thomson (2021) summarized this view:

> To appreciate why, first we need to understand herd immunity at its simplest: it is the point at which each person with COVID-19 infects less than one other susceptible individual. This causes infections to decrease, with only sporadic cases that don't spread widely. In theory, you can reach this goal through vaccination or past infection, as both provide some immunity from future infection. In reality, we have only reached herd immunity for other viruses, such as smallpox, through vaccination. . . . The road to herd immunity gets more complex when you consider other influencing factors, including how much social contact communities have, the age at which someone first gets infected, how people's immune systems differ, how influential pre-existing immunity is and the potential impact of genetics. (Thomson, 2021, p. 17)

Similarly, in spring 2022, Dr. Anthony Fauci, Chief Medical Advisor to President Biden, and his colleagues expressed belief about the likelihood of endemicity and the unlikelihood of achieving herd immunity:

> . . . achieving classical herd immunity against SARS-CoV-2 is unlikely, due to a combination of factors that include features of the virus as well as current societal dynamics. These include the virus' ability to continually mutate to new variants; asymptomatic virus transmission, which complicates public health control strategies; the inability of prior infection or vaccination to provide durable protection against reinfection; suboptimal vaccination coverage; and adherence to non-pharmacologic interventions. (National Institutes of Health [NIH], 2022, para. 3)

Instead of seeking herd immunity, Dr. Fauci and others advocated controlling COVID-19 without major disruptions to society through traditional pandemic practices:

- Vaccinating the unvaccinated;
- Boosting those who were vaccinated;
- Providing the best available therapeutics for those who became ill; and
- Reducing community transmission during COVID-19 surges through testing, masking, social distancing, and so forth.

They promoted research to develop pan-coronavirus vaccines to protect against multiple coronaviruses or at least multiple SARS-CoV-2 variants. They concluded that, "living with COVID is best considered not as reaching a numerical threshold of immunity, but as optimizing population protection without prohibitive restrictions on our daily lives" (NIH, 2022, para. 5). The CDC began preparing for endemicity by tailoring guidance for variability in outbreaks. For example, following the omicron surge, the CDC created community-level guidance to inform community mitigation measures. See Table 9.3. Guidance assumed that a high percent of the population was protected from severe COVID-19 due to either natural immunity after COVID-19 infection, vaccination, or both. Community risk (low, medium, or high) was determined using new case rates, as well as COVID-19 hospital admissions and the percent of hospital beds occupied by COVID-19 patients. Communities that had low and medium risk levels could consider discontinuing masking and social distancing in public venues. However, even when communities relaxed masking and social distancing measures, the guidance recommended that unvaccinated individuals or those who were immunosuppressed continued using mitigation measures when in public.

To facilitate additional research needed to reduce COVID-19, the CDC developed the *Public Health Science Agenda for COVID-19*. This agenda would guide future public health efforts "to strengthen public health actions, guidance, and policy essential to limit the spread and impact of SARS-CoV-2 and ultimately end the COVID-19 pandemic" (NCIRD, 2022a, para. 2). See Table 9.4.

Table 9.3. COVID-19 Community Levels, Indicators, and Thresholds

New COVID-19 Cases per 100,000 People in the Past 7 Days	Indicators	Low	Medium	High
Fewer than 200	New COVID-19 admissions per 100,000 population (7-day total)	<10	10.0–19.9	≥20
	Percent of staffed inpatient beds occupied by COVID-19 patients (7-day average)	<10%	10.0%–14.9%	≥15%
200 or more	New COVID-19 admissions per 100,000 population (7-day total)	NA	<10	≥10
	Percent of staffed inpatient beds occupied by COVID-19 patients (7-day average)	NA	<10%	≥10%

Source: National Center for Immunization and Respiratory Diseases, Division of Viral Diseases, & Centers for Disease Control and Prevention. (2022). *COVID-19 community levels, indicators, and thresholds. Science brief: Indicators for monitoring COVID-19 community levels and making public health recommendations.* https://www.cdc.gov/coronavirus/2019-ncov/science/science-briefs/indicators-monitoring-community-levels.html

Table 9.4. Priority COVID-19 Public Health Science Questions

Topic	Questions
Health equity	1. How can the public health community effectively identify and address health inequities to protect populations disproportionately affected by COVID-19?
Vaccines	2. What are the effectiveness and duration of protection afforded by COVID-19 primary series and booster vaccines?
	3. What interventions, programs, and communication approaches are most effective at increasing equitable COVID-19 vaccination access and coverage?
	4. What are the risks and benefits associated with COVID-19 primary series and booster vaccines?
Variants	5. How can the public health community effectively and efficiently enhance surveillance for known and emerging SARS-CoV-2 variants?
	6. How do SARS-CoV-2 variants affect diagnostics, vaccine effectiveness, clinical outcomes, transmissibility, and public health interventions?

(continued)

Table 9.4. Priority COVID-19 Public Health Science Questions (*continued*)

Topic	Questions
Prevention strategies	7. What effective prevention strategies and non-pharmaceutical interventions should be prioritized to reduce transmissions of SARS-CoV-2 in various populations and settings, including schools and workplaces, particularly where vaccination coverage is low?
	8. When should SARS-CoV-2 prevention strategies and non-pharmaceutical interventions in various populations and settings be adjusted; for example, based on vaccination coverage, variant prevalence, community transmission, or transitioning into an endemic disease control phase?
	9. How effective are at home testing/self-testing, rapid diagnostic testing, point of care testing, routine screening, and serial testing strategies in reducing outbreaks, reducing disease burden, detecting potential surges, evaluating criteria for reopening, and detecting re-introduction of SARS-CoV-2 into low transmission settings?
Natural history, transmission, breakthrough infections, and reinfections	10. How does the public health community effectively and efficiently enhance surveillance for SARS-CoV-2 reinfections, breakthrough infections, vaccination, and various health outcomes?
	11. What factors best inform SARS-CoV-2 transmission dynamics and predict surges of community level infection?
	12. What are reliable immune correlates of protection from SARS-CoV-2 infections and accurate ways to measure this?
Post-COVID-19 conditions and other health impacts	13. How does the public health community effectively conduct epidemiologic research on post-COVID-19 conditions, overall and in various populations and settings?
	14. What short- and long-term impacts from the COVID-19 pandemic are of the greatest public health importance, and what are the best ways to address them?

Source: National Center for Immunization and Respiratory Diseases, Division of Viral Diseases, & Centers for Disease Control and Prevention. (2022a). *CDC public health science agenda for COVID-19: Building the evidence base for ongoing COVID-19 response.* https://www.cdc.gov/coronavirus/2019-ncov/science/science-agenda-covid19.html#he

CDC Public Health Science Agenda for COVID-19: Building the Evidence Base for Ongoing COVID-19 Response

Within these topic areas, **15** priority public health science questions relate to the broad scope of the CDC's scientific work, both in the United States and globally, including public health surveillance, epidemiologic research, implementation science, and evaluation. These questions also relate to ongoing work in the broader scientific community (such as other government agencies, academics, the private sector). Other relevant questions are found in the complementary science agendas of other federal agencies, including the National Institutes of Health (NIH), the Food and Drug Administration (FDA), the Environmental Protection Agency (EPA), and the White House. This Science Agenda is intended to inform efforts by the broader public health research community. (NCIRD, 2022a, para. 3)

A resource for accessing information developed for the *Public Health Science Agenda for COVID-19* was the *COVID-19 Response Strategic Science Unit (SSU)*. This unit systematically collected input from multiple entities across the CDC and from external public health partners to identify and update questions in the *Public Health Science Agenda for COVID-19*. Questions were updated every 4 months beginning in April 2021 to ensure their timeliness, relevance, actionability, and impact. By fall 2022, CDC authors had published over 1,000 scientific articles, indexed by priority topic in the searchable COVID-19 CDC Publications Database, which is available at: https://phgkb.cdc.gov/PHGKB/cdcCovPubStartPage.action

Phase 3 Summary

The goals of Phase 3—respond to new variants and outbreaks of COVID-19, increase availability of testing and therapeutics, and prepare for COVID-19 endemicity—were met.

- The remarkable achievements of scientists developing vaccines and boosters to control COVID-19 variants continued successfully throughout Phase 3.
- Public health policies and logistics planning made COVID-19 vaccines, boosters, therapies, and testing widely and equitably available to those in need, particularly in locales with a robust and supported public health effort. This was another outstanding public health achievement during the pandemic.
- The CDC and its partners began the planning needed to treat COVID-19 as endemic and ensure continuing development of knowledge to prevent pandemic-level morbidity and mortality.

LESSONS FROM THE COVID-19 PANDEMIC

KEY IDEA

Public health successes during the COVID-19 pandemic are instructive in how to manage such events. Just as important, however, is learning from oversights and missteps.

Persistent resistance to public health measures—even though these measures were helping to control the pandemic—was a hallmark of the pandemic. And although public health professionals and their partners were successful in achieving their goals to reduce transmission and mitigate serious illness and death, resistance to their work and practices reduced the effectiveness of the response throughout. This section briefly discusses misinformation and its targets, the consequences of resistance, and roots of resistance and its long-term consequences.

Misinformation and Mistrust

Misinformation about the effectiveness of public health methods proliferated, resulting in mistrust and an antipathy for the measures employed to control the COVID-19 pandemic. This hostility was supported and inflamed by widely disseminated accounts on social media. Vaccines and therapies were especially targeted even though scientific investigations had demonstrated their remarkable effectiveness. A sampling of myths about the vaccines were:

- COVID-19 vaccines cause people to be magnetic.
- COVID-19 vaccines prevent getting pregnant.
- COVID-19 vaccines alter DNA.
- COVID-19 vaccines cause one to test positive for COVID-19 on a viral test (CDC, 2021d).

COVID-19 therapies were also targets of misinformation. Several prominent politicians, celebrities, and social media persons disseminated misinformation about a variety of ineffective and potentially dangerous COVID-19 treatments including hydroxychloroquine, ivermectin, bleach, ultraviolet light, and others. These persons often claimed that public health and health care professionals inappropriately suppressed the use of these medications for COVID-19 patients. One example is the ivermectin story:

> But one drug in particular has become the center of many alternative therapies: ivermectin. Originally used to treat parasitic worms, ivermectin has developed an enormous following over the course of the pandemic—especially in politically conservative circles. That's, in part, because of a small cadre of licensed doctors who promote it as an alternative to vaccination against COVID. Among the most prominent is Dr. Pierre Kory, whose group, the Front Line COVID-19 Critical Care Alliance, has become a major force promoting ivermectin.
>
> "Ivermectin is effectively a 'miracle drug' against COVID-19," Kory told a Senate committee in December of 2020. (National Public Radio, 2022, para. 4)

Remarkably, a report on research into the origins of such myths found a limited number of people promoting them. According to a report on National Public Radio: "These figures are well-known to both researchers and the social networks. They include antivaccine activists, alternative health entrepreneurs and physicians. Some of them run multiple accounts across the different platforms. They often promote 'natural health.' Some even sell supplements and books" (Bond, 2021). Many others, including politicians and media figures, contributed to the misinformation by not directly rejecting it or actually agreeing with misstatements.

DID YOU KNOW?

A Kaiser Family Foundation report assessed the public's awareness of, and belief in, a range of "myths" about COVID-19 and the vaccines. The most common misconceptions included:

- Most (60%) adults say they've heard that the government is exaggerating the number of COVID-19 deaths by counting deaths due to other factors and either believe it to be true (38%) or aren't sure if it is true or false (22%).
- Four in 10 (39%) say they've heard pregnant women should not get the COVID-19 vaccine and believe it to be true (17%) or aren't sure (22%).
- Three in 10 (31%) say they've heard that the vaccine has been shown to cause infertility and either believe it (8%) or aren't sure if it's true (23%). (Kaiser Family Foundation, 2021)

The authors of the report noted that misinformation spread quickly, whether inadvertently or deliberately, through social media, polarized news sources, and other outlets. The report concluded that false and ambiguous information was a major challenge for efforts to communicate the evolving science about the COVID-19 pandemic accurately.

Resistance and Its Short-Term Consequences

As a result of persistent misinformation and growing mistrust, public health policies were widely opposed. Strategies to reduce transmission were contested including masking, social distancing, and closures of schools, businesses, and other social gatherings. Many people refused to be vaccinated even though vaccines were shown to be effective in preventing serious illness and death. Ineffective therapies such as ivermectin were demanded by people with COVID-19 in place of proven therapeutics such as Paxlovid and monoclonal antibody antibodies. Public health statistics, which the CDC had reliably produced for decades, were mistrusted. Death rates derived from death certificates were questioned, as were COVID-19 hospitalization rates from hospital reports. In both instances, the preeminent National Center for Health Statistics within the CDC provided these numbers in accordance with well-established standard processes. Misinformation and suspicion decreased the public's acceptance of public health measures.

Inconsistent adherence to public health measures, particularly the recommendation to get vaccinated, had an adverse effect on mortality and morbidity. For example, between January 2021 and June 2022, COVID-19-associated hospitalization rates were 4.6 times higher among unvaccinated adults compared to those who were fully vaccinated (CDC, 2022a). Death rates, too, were higher among the unvaccinated. Age-standardized incidence of COVID-19 cases and deaths in 2021 illustrate the effectiveness of vaccination and boosters. Throughout the study period, both cases and deaths were higher among the unvaccinated. Among the vaccinated and boosted, COVID-19 cases rose somewhat from the delta and omicron variants, but the increase was much less than for the unvaccinated.

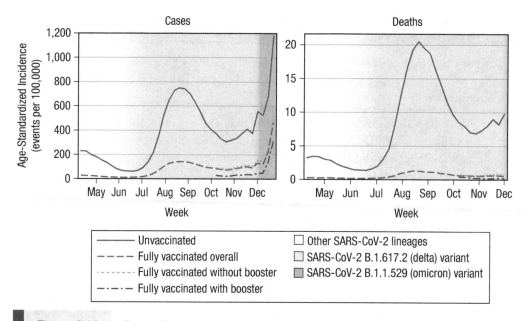

Figure 9.10.   Death Rates by Vaccination Status Among Adults, United States

Source: Scobie, H. M., Johnson, A. G., Amin, A. B., Ali, A. R., DeSantis, A., Shi, M., Adam, C., Armstrong, B., Armstrong, B., Asbell, M., Auche, S., Bayoumi, N. S., Bingay, B., Chasse, M., Christofferson, S., Cima, M., Cueto, K., Cunningham, S., Delgadillo, J., . . . Silk, B. J. (2022). COVID-19 incidence and death rates among un-vaccinated and fully vaccinated adults with and without booster doses during periods of delta and omicron variant emergence—25 U.S. Jurisdictions, April 4–December 25, 2021. *Morbidity and Mortality Weekly Report, 71*(4), 132–138. https://doi.org/10.15585/mmwr.mm7104e2

And even though there was an increase in cases among the vaccinated and boosted from the delta and omicron variants, deaths in this group remained close to zero (Scobie et al., 2022). See **Figure 9.10**. There was also inconsistent adherence to other COVID-19 control measures, such as masking, social distancing, school and business closings, and so forth. However, it would be difficult to calculate the effect of non-adherence to these measures on the rates of cases, hospitalization, and death, particularly after vaccines were available.

Another adverse outcome of resistance to public health practices during the COVID-19 pandemic was demoralization and loss of many in the public health workforce. The effect of the pandemic on health care workers has been discussed, but the impact on public health workers is less well-known. The public's suspicion and mistrust of public health's handling of the pandemic undermined the well-being of the workforce and its ability to implement policy. In addition, mistrust and dissatisfaction with public health's pandemic response led to citizen violence against public health workers. Ward and her colleagues reported on a survey they conducted from March 2020 to January 2021:

> At least 1,499 harassment experiences were identified by Local Health
> Department survey respondents, representing 57% of responding

departments. We also identified 222 position departures by public health officials nationally, 36% alongside reports of harassment. Public health officials described experiencing structural and political under-mining of their professional duties, marginalization of their expertise, social villainization, and disillusionment. (Ward et al., 2022, p. 736)

The experience of violence and threats of violence exacerbated the dissatisfaction and mistrust, and resulted in loss of public health workers. Freeman writes, "Significant numbers of health officials have stepped down, making tough choices to leave long-term positions and careers to protect themselves and their loved ones rather than continue to endure actual or perceived threats and relentless pressure" (Freeman, 2022, p. 731).

Roots of Mistrust and Resistance

The roots of mistrust and resistance to COVID-19 policies went deeper than misinformation. Resistance was partially rooted in the challenges of communicating science-based information during a disaster such as the pandemic. Understandably, the public wanted certainty, which was not always possible, particularly during the early phase of discovery. Public health officials developed policies and advised the public based on the knowledge they had at a point in time, but this often changed as new information became available. In addition, there is always uncertainty inherent in applying scientific knowledge to development of public policies. As has been said, "There aren't always right answers, but some answers are clearly wrong" (Baron & Ejnes, 2022). This truism needed to be communicated clearly to the public. Parasidis and Fairchild (2022) describe this problem:

During the COVID-19 pandemic, public health decision makers haven't always been transparent with the public, often failing to adequately explain the reasoning behind their decisions about interventions such as mask mandates, quarantine and isolation policies, mandatory testing, and transitions to remote work and learning. In many cases, public health leaders simply stated that they were "following the science," without acknowledging that the data models they were relying on have varying degrees of accuracy and reliability, that the available evidence would evolve and require reevaluation, and that reasonable people could disagree about how to translate data into policy. (Parasidis & Fairchild, 2022, p. 961)

These communication problems had the effect of furthering suspicion about COVID-19 policies—policies that had a tremendous impact on the lives of most Americans. This was no localized event; every American felt the impact of COVID-19 and the policies implemented to control it.

Resistance to public health's COVID-19 policies was also partially rooted in a general resistance to collective action undertaken by government. There is a long-standing American preference, among many people, for small government

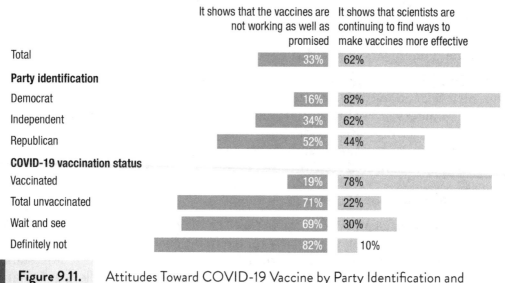

Figure 9.11.   Attitudes Toward COVID-19 Vaccine by Party Identification and Vaccination Status, 2021

Note: Vaccinated adults are those who have received at least one dose of a COVID-19 vaccine. See topline for full question wording.

Source: Hamel, L., Lopes, L., Sparks, G., Kirzinger, A., Kearney, A., Stokes, M., & Brodie, M. (2021). *KFF COVID-19 vaccine monitor: September 2021.* https://www.kff.org/coronavirus-covid-19/poll-finding/kff-covid-19-vaccine-monitor-september-2021/

and self-reliance over collective action. These views are held by people who lean conservative, politically, and include most Republicans, Libertarians, some Independents, and a few others. An example of differences in COVID-19 beliefs by political party is displayed in **Figure 9.11.**

Support for conservative political views varies from place to place, aided by federalism, the American form of government in which power is shared by the national and state governments. State differences in vaccination rates provide an indication of their effect on resistance to public health's COVID-19 policies. The proportion of fully vaccinated persons in September 2022 ranged from 85% in Rhode Island to 52% in Wyoming. **Table 9.5** compares vaccination rates and party affiliation of office holders in each state—governors, state senators, and state representatives. Using majority Republicans in state legislatures as a proxy for conservative-leaning states, **Table 9.5** indicates that states with Republican majorities in state legislatures were likely to have lower vaccination rates. With few exceptions, states in which 70% or more of residents were fully vaccinated had Democratic majority legislatures, while states in which less than 70% were fully vaccinated had Republican majority legislatures. See **Table 9.5.**

Table 9.5. COVID-19 Vaccination Rates by Political Party Affiliation of Elected State Officials, September 2022

State (September 15, 2022)	Fully Vaccinated	With Booster	Party of Governor	Senate Members: Republican/Democrat[a]	House Members: Republican/Democrat[a]	Majority Political Party in Legislature
U.S. total[a]	68%	33%	–	–	–	
Rhode Island	85%	48%	D	5/33	10/65	
Vermont	83%	53%	R	7/21	46/93	
Maine	81%	48%	D	13/22	63/77	
Massachusetts	81%	44%	R	3/37	27/125	
Connecticut	81%	43%	D	13/23	54/97	
Hawaii	80%	46%	D	1/24	4/47	
Washington, DC	79%	35%	D	–	–	
New York	79%	37%	D	20/42	43/106	
Maryland	78%	42%	R	15/32	42/99	
New Jersey	77%	39%	D	16/23	33/46	
Virginia	75%	38%	R	19/21	**52/47**	Mixed
Washington	74%	41%	D	20/29	41/57	
California	74%	41%	D	9/31	19/60	
New Mexico	73%	38%	D	15/26	24/45	
New Hampshire	73%	35%	R	**13/10**	**202/178**	Majority Republican
Colorado	72%	40%	D	14/21	24/41	

(continued)

Table 9.5. COVID-19 Vaccination Rates by Political Party Affiliation of Elected State Officials, September 2022 *(continued)*

State (September 15, 2022)	Fully Vaccinated	With Booster	Party of Governor	Senate Members: Republican/Democrat[a]	House Members: Republican/Democrat[a]	Majority Political Party in Legislature
Delaware	71%	34%	D	7/14	15/26	
Oregon	71%	40%	D	11/18	23/36	
Pennsylvania	71%	32%	D	28/21	113/89	Majority Republican
Minnesota	70%	43%	D	34/31	63/69	Mixed
Illinois	70%	38%	D	18/41	45/73	
Florida	68%	29%	R	23/16	76/42	Majority Republican
Wisconsin	67%	39%	D	21/12	57/38	Majority Republican
Utah	65%	31%	R	23/6	57/17	Majority Republican
Nebraska	65%	35%	R	a	32/17	Majority Republican
South Dakota	64%	28%	R	32/3	62/8	Majority Republican
North Carolina	64%	18%	D	28/22	68/51	Majority Republican
Alaska	63%	30%	R	13/7	21/15	Majority Republican
Kansas	63%	30%	D	29/11	86/38	Majority Republican
Arizona	63%	29%	R	16/14	31/28	Majority Republican
Iowa	63%	35%	R	32/18	60/40	Majority Republican
Texas	62%	23%	R	18/13	83/65	Majority Republican
Nevada	62%	25%	D	9/11	16/25	
Michigan	61%	35%	D	22/16	56/53	Majority Republican

(continued)

Ohio	59%	32%	R	25/8	64/35	Majority Republican
Oklahoma	59%	23%	R	39/9	82/18	Majority Republican
West Virginia	59%	28%	R	23/11	78/22	Majority Republican
Kentucky	58%	27%	D	30/8	75/25	Majority Republican
South Carolina	58%	25%	R	30/16	81/43	Majority Republican
Montana	58%	29%	R	31/19	67/33	Majority Republican
Missouri	57%	26%	R	24/10	107/48	Majority Republican
Indiana	57%	28%	R	39/11	71/29	Majority Republican
North Dakota	57%	26%	R	40/7	80/14	Majority Republican
Georgia	56%	23%	R	34/22	103/76	Majority Republican
Arkansas	56%	23%	R	27/7	78/22	Majority Republican
Tennessee	55%	26%	R	26/6	72/24	Majority Republican
Idaho	55%	25%	R	27/7	58/12	Majority Republican
Louisiana	54%	23%	D	26/11	68/34	Majority Republican
Mississippi	53%	21%	R	36/16	76/42	Majority Republican
Alabama	52%	20%	R	27/8	73/28	Majority Republican
Wyoming	52%	24%	R	28/2	51/7	Majority Republican

[a]Numbers do not include legislators identified as Libertarian, Independent, or Progressive. However, adding these numbers would not change the majority party status in any state.

Sources: Ivory, D., Smith, M., Lee. J. C., Walker, A. S., Shaver, J. W., Collins, K., Gamio, L., Holder, J., Lu, D, Watkins, D., Hassan, A., Allen, J., Lemonides, A., Bao, B., Brown, E., Burr, A, Cahalan, S., Craig, M., Jesus, Y. D., . . . Williams, J. (2022). See how vaccinations are going in your county and state. *The New York Times.* https://www.nytimes.com/interactive/2020/us/covid-19-vaccine-doses.html; and Ballotpedia. (2022, September 15). *Current partisan composition.* https://ballotpedia.org/Historical_partisan_composition_of_state_legislatures#Wyoming

Moreover, political differences had hardened by the time of the pandemic, and the United States was deeply polarized. As discussed earlier, misinformation about COVID-19 and public health measures to control it was ubiquitous. Intensive and successful media campaigns undermined public health messages with misinformation. Unfortunately, there seemed to be no spokespersons who were trusted by most Americans. Thus, political polarization exacerbated the communications problem.

Long-Term Consequences of Resistance

Public discontent with mask mandates and school and business closures catalyzed a backlash against public health authority. Conservative groups characterized COVID-19 policies as overreach. By November 2021, almost every state legislature had seen the introduction of a bill to weaken or remove the emergency powers of governors and/or local or state health officials (Fraser, 2022). Public health officials warned of the danger of limiting public health powers.

> All told, the COVID-era litigation has altered not just the government response to this pandemic. Public health experts say it has endangered the fundamental tools that public health workers have utilized for decades to protect community health: mandatory vaccinations for public school children against devastating diseases like measles and polio, local officials' ability to issue health orders in an emergency, basic investigative tactics used to monitor the spread of infectious diseases, and the use of quarantines to stem that spread. . . . Just as concerning, said multiple public health experts interviewed, is how the upended legal landscape will impact the nation's emergency response in future pandemics. "This will come back to haunt America," said Lawrence Gostin, faculty director of Georgetown University's O'Neill Institute for National and Global Health Law. "We will rue the day where we have other public health emergencies, and we're simply unable to act decisively and rapidly." (Weber & Barry-Jester, 2022, paras. 12–14)

Antidotes to Antipathy

The mistrust and resistance to public health measures that occurred during the COVID-19 pandemic are important to understand, but even more important, to address in a practical way. Antidotes to the antipathy must be developed to preserve the American capacity to respond successfully to pandemics and other public health emergencies. This must be a major effort of public health professionals—current and incoming—in the future. Restoring American's trust and confidence in public health will require communicating effectively, engaging communities fully, and developing leaders with adaptive leadership skills (see Chapters 7 and 8).

CHAPTER SUMMARY

Throughout the COVID-19 pandemic, public health acted to "fulfill society's interest in assuring conditions in which people can be healthy." These efforts were based on the belief that science must inform public health policies and strategies. Thus, in collaboration with scientists across disciplines and in the private and public sectors, public health professionals applied science to the COVID-19 pandemic and developed strategies to meet the challenge. Their efforts included:

- Investigating the nature of SARS-COV-2 virus including its means and ease of transmission;
- Determining COVID-19 health effects and morbidly and CFRs;
- Monitoring the spread and investigating the epidemiology of COVID-19—including persons at risk and their environment;
- Adopting and implementing well-tested infectious disease practices to stem the spread of COVID-19, including testing, quarantine, and social distancing;
- Supporting the development of COVID-19 vaccines to prevent disease, booster shots for the already vaccinated, and testing and therapeutics for those who become ill; and
- Planning and implementing policies to make vaccines and therapies widely and equitably available.

Public health had undeniable successes during the COVID-19 pandemic. As Ashish Jha, COVID-19 Response Coordinator for the Biden Administration, said:

> We are two years into this pandemic, and think about what science has already delivered: lots of effective treatments, multiple powerful vaccines that continue to prevent serious illness. In the coming years, we will have vaccines that are more durable, that prevent transmission, that need to be taken infrequently. We're going to get more therapeutics. Our ability to manage this virus is going to get better and better. (Jha quoted by Khullar, 2022, p. 13)

Similarly, the Editor of *The Lancet* wrote that the COVID-19 pandemic had caused an unprecedented explosion of research activity, which dominated the biomedical research publications. "The vast research effort that has gone into COVID-19 over the past 2 years should be celebrated as a great human achievement—it has given us the tools to turn a pandemic disease into a manageable, endemic one" (Editor, *The Lancet*, 2022, p. 297).

Thus, there are two stories to tell about the American response to COVID-19. The first is a story of tremendous effort and success. Public health officials worked immediately to slow the spread of COVID-19 through application of proven epidemiologic tools. Under often grave conditions, health care workers applied their professional skills unstintingly to save those who became seriously ill with

COVID-19. Scientists quickly came together and developed vaccines and booster doses, diagnostic tests, and therapies to fight the disease.

Yet by September 2022, over a million Americans had died from COVID-19, many unnecessarily; health care and public health workers were burned out and leaving their professions; and the public health field was under siege and facing legislatively imposed loss of authority. Poor communications under uncertainty, public mistrust and misunderstanding of science, and extreme political polarization wounded the COVID-19 response in the United States and, in the end, left public health weakened for the next pandemic.

Going forward, there are immense opportunities for the next generation of public health professionals to recreate the trust and confidence needed to retain public health's ability to "fulfill society's interest in ensuring conditions in which people can be healthy." Understanding the past is essential, and imagination is the key. In the case of COVID-19, imagine how the response could have been better—for example, timely and consistent data collection to inform policy-making, and skillful communications between public health and the general public about what was known and what was unknown, and how "knowns" can change as science evolves. Imagine the future with a fully supported public health system and the trust of citizens. Imagine the successes that would ensue—in the tradition of the historic public health achievements—through study of the past and imagining a better future.

DISCUSSION QUESTIONS

Q: What is the virus that causes COVID-19, how is it transmitted, and what are the ways to prevent transmission?

Q: What were the health impacts of COVID-19, and what groups were most affected?

Q: Why was endemicity considered a likelihood by Phase 3 of the pandemic?

Q: What were the public health successes during the COVID-19 pandemic?

Q: What factors generated mistrust of public health practices and resistance to them?

DATA SOURCE

Surveillance, data collection, and data analysis are essential to understanding how to control an infectious disease outbreak. For Chapter 5, the COVID Data Tracker makes the surveillance data from the CDC publicly available. The information obtained from the COVID Data Tracker can provide a deeper understanding of the pandemic in the United States. On the main page, information can be obtained about cases, testing, deaths, hospitalizations, and vaccinations by county or state. You can begin your investigation here: https://covid.cdc .gov/covid-data-tracker/#datatracker-home

A robust set of instructor resources designed to supplement this text is located at **http://connect.springerpub.com/content/book/978-0-8261-8615-7**. Qualifying instructors may request access by emailing **textbook@springerpub.com**.

REFERENCES

Antia, R., & Halloran, M. E. (2021). Transition to endemicity: Understanding COVID-19. *Immunity, 54*(10), 2172–2176. https://doi.org/10.1016/j.immuni.2021.09.019

Baron, R. J., & Ejnes, Y. D. (2022). Physicians spreading misinformation on social media – do right and wrong answers still exist in medicine? *New England Journal of Medicine, 387*(1), 1–3. https://doi.org/10.1056/NEJMp2204813

Becker, J. H., Lin, J. J., Doernberg, M., Stone, K., Navis, A., Festa, J. R., & Wisnivesky, J. P. (2021). Assessment of cognitive function in patients after COVID-19 infection. *JAMA Network Open, 4*(10), e2130645. https://doi.org/10.1001/jamanetworkopen.2021.30645

Binnicker, M. J. (2020). Challenges and controversies to testing for COVID-19. *Journal of Clinical Microbiology, 58*(11), e01695-e20. https://doi.org/10.1128/JCM.01695-20

Bond, S. (2021). Just 12 people are behind most vaccine hoaxes on social media, research shows. *National Public Radio.* https://www.npr.org/2021/05/13/996570855/disinformation-dozen-test-facebooks-twitters-ability-to-curb-vaccine-hoaxes

Brower, K. J. (2021). Professional stigma of mental health issues: Physicians are both the cause and solution. *Academic Medicine, 96*(5), 635–640. https://doi.org/10.1097/ACM.0000000000003998

Campbell, M., & Gavett, G. (2021). What Covid-19 has done to our well-being, in 12 charts. *Harvard Business Review.* https://hbr.org/2021/02/what-covid-19-has-done-to-our-well-being-in-12-charts.

Centers for Disease Control and Prevention. (2021a). *Delta variant: What we know about the science.* https://www.cdc.gov/coronavirus/2019-ncov/variants/deltavariant.html

Centers for Disease Control and Prevention. (2021b). *Disease burden of influenza.* https://www.cdc.gov/flu/about/burden/index.html

Centers for Disease Control and Prevention. (2021c, February 16). *Interim clinical guidance for management of patients with confirmed Coronavirus Disease (COVID-19).* https://www.cdc.gov/coronavirus/2019-ncov/hcp/clinical-guidance-management-patients.html

Centers for Disease Control and Prevention. (2021d). *Myths and facts about COVID-19 vaccines.* https://www.cdc.gov/coronavirus/2019-ncov/vaccines/facts.html

Centers for Disease Control and Prevention. (2022a, September 10). *Age-adjusted rates of COVID-19-associated hospitalization by vaccination status in patients ages 18 and older, January 2021–June 2022.* https://covid.cdc.gov/covid-data-tracker/#covidnet-hospitalizations-vaccination

Centers for Disease Control and Prevention. (2022b). *COVID-19 weekly cases and deaths per 100,000 population by age, race/ethnicity, and sex.* https://covid.cdc.gov/covid-data-tracker/#demographicsovertime

Centers for Disease Control and Prevention. (2022c). *New admissions of patients with confirmed COVID-19, United States, August 1, 2020–September 7, 2022.* https://covid.cdc.gov/covid-data-tracker/#new-hospital-admissions

Centers for Disease Control and Prevention. (2022d). *Trends in number of COVID-19 cases and deaths in the US Reported to CDC, by State/Territory.* https://covid.cdc.gov/covid-data-tracker/#trends_dailydeaths_select_00

Centers for Disease Control and Prevention. (2023). *COVID-19 testing: What you need to know.* https://www.cdc.gov/coronavirus/2019-ncov/symptoms-testing/testing.html

Cohen, J., & Rodgers, Y. V. M. (2020). Contributing factors to personal protective equipment shortages during the COVID-19 pandemic. *Preventive Medicine, 141*, 106263. https://doi.org/10.1016/j.ypmed.2020.106263

Cooney, E. (2022). *'I'm deeply concerned': Francis Collins on trust in science, how Covid communications failed, and his current obsession.* STAT. https://www.statnews.com/2022/09/19/francis-collins-trust-science-covid-communication-failures/

Douaud, G., Lee, S., Alfaro-Almagro, F., Arthofer, C., Wang, C., Lange, F., Andersson, J. L. R., Griffanti, L., Duff, E., Jbabdi, S., Taschler, B., Winkler, A., Nichols, T. E., Collins, R., Matthews, P. M., Allen, N., Miller, K. L., & Smith, S. M. (2021). Brain imaging before and after COVID-19 in UK Biobank. *MedRxiv.* https://doi.org/10.1101/2021.06.11.21258690

Du, Z., Xu, X., Wu, Y., Wang, L., Cowling, B. J., & Meyers, L. A. (2020). Serial interval of COVID-19 among publicly reported confirmed cases. *Emerging Infectious Diseases, 26*, 1341–1343. https://doi.org/10.3201/eid2606.200357

Editor. (2021). Understanding long COVID: A modern medical challenge. *The Lancet, 398*, 725. https://www.thelancet.com/pdfs/journals/lancet/PIIS0140-6736(21)01900-0.pdf

Editor. (2022). Transitioning to endemicity with COVID-19 research. *The Lancet Infectious Diseases, 22*(3), 297. https://doi.org/10.1016/S1473-3099(22)00070-6

Faust, J. S., & del Rio, C. (2020). Assessment of deaths from COVID-19 and from seasonal influenza. *JAMA Internal Medicine, 180*(8), 1045–1046. https://jamanetwork.com/journals/jamainternalmedicine/fullarticle/2766121

Fraser, M. R. (2022). Harassment of health officials: A significant threat to the public's health. *American Journal of Public Health, 112*(5), 728–730. https://doi.org/10.2105/ajph.2022.306797

Freeman, L. T. (2022). Unanticipated pandemic outcomes: The assault on public health. *American Journal of Public Health, 112*(5), 731–733. https://doi.org/10.2105/AJPH.2022.306810

Gottesman, B. L., Yu, J., Tanaka, C., Longhurst, C. A., & Kim, J. J. (2022). Incidence of new-onset type 1 diabetes among US children during the COVID-19 global pandemic. *JAMA Pediatrics, 176*(4), 414–415. https://doi.org/10.1001/jamapediatrics.2021.5801

Hu, B., Guo, H., Zhou, P., & Shi, Z. (2020). Characteristics of SARS-CoV-2 and COVID-19. *Nature Reviews, Microbiology, 19*, 141–154. https://www.nature.com/articles/s41579-020-00459-7

Khullar, D. (2022). We have to get out of this phase: Ashish Jha on the future of the pandemic. *The New Yorker*. https://www.newyorker.com/news/the-new-yorker-interview/we-have-to-get-out-of-this-phase-ashish-jha-on-the-future-of-the-pandemic

Lauer, S. A., Grantz, K. H., Bi, Q., Jones, F. K., Zheng, Q., Meredith, H. R., Azman, A. S., Reich, N. G., & Lessler, J. (2020). The incubation period of Coronavirus Disease 2019 (COVID-19) from publicly reported confirmed cases: Estimation and application. *Annals of Internal Medicine, 172*, 577–582. https://doi.org/10.7326/M20-0504

Lipsitch, M., Cohen, T., Cooper, B., Robins, J. M., Ma, S., James, L., Gopalakrishna, G., Chew, S. K., Tan, C. C., Samore, M. H., Fisman, D., & Murray, M. (2003). Transmission dynamics and control of severe acute respiratory syndrome. *Science, 300*(5627), 1966–1970. https://doi.org/10.1126/science.1086616

Logue, J. K., Franko, N. M., McCulloch, D. J., McDonald, D., Magedson, A., Wolf, C. R., & Chu, H. Y. (2021). Sequelae in adults at 6 months after COVID-19 infection. *JAMA Network Open, 4*(2), e210830. https://doi.org/10.1001/jamanetworkopen.2021.0830

Maragakis, L. L. (2020). *COVID-19 vs the flu*. Johns Hopkins Medicine. https://www.hopkinsmedicine.org/health/conditions-and-diseases/coronavirus/coronavirus-disease-2019-vs-the-flu

Marvaldi, M., Mallet, J., Dubertret, C., Moro, M. R., & Guessoum, S. B. (2021). Anxiety, depression, trauma-related, and sleep disorders among healthcare workers during the COVID-19 pandemic: A systematic review and meta-analysis. *Neuroscience & Biobehavioral Reviews, 126*, 252–264. https://doi.org/10.1016/j.neubiorev.2021.03.024

National Center for Immunization and Respiratory Diseases, Division of Viral Diseases, & Centers for Disease Control and Prevention. (2021). *Managing healthcare operations during COVID-19*. https://www.cdc.gov/coronavirus/2019-ncov/hcp/facility-planning-operations.html?CDC_AA_refVal=https%3A%2F%2Fwww.cdc.gov%2Fcoronavirus%2F2019-ncov%2Fhcp%2Fguidance-hcf.html

National Center for Immunization and Respiratory Diseases, Division of Viral Diseases, & Centers for Disease Control and Prevention. (2022a, May 17). *CDC public health science agenda for COVID-19: Building the evidence base for ongoing COVID-19 response*. https://www.cdc.gov/coronavirus/2019-ncov/science/science-agenda-covid19.html#he

National Center for Immunization and Respiratory Diseases, Division of Viral Diseases, & Centers for Disease Control and Prevention. (2022b). *Covid-19: Data tracker weekly review*. https://www.cdc.gov/coronavirus/2019-ncov/covid-data/covidview/past-reports/04222022.html

National Center for Immunization and Respiratory Diseases, Division of Viral Diseases, & Centers for Disease Control and Prevention. (2022c). *COVID-19 testing: What you need to know*. https://www.cdc.gov/coronavirus/2019-ncov/symptoms-testing/testing.html

National Center for Immunization and Respiratory Diseases, Division of Viral Diseases, & Centers for Disease Control and Prevention. (2022d). *SARS-CoV-2 variant classifications and definitions*. https://www.cdc.gov/coronavirus/2019-ncov/variants/variant-classifications.html#anchor_1632150752495

National Center for Immunization and Respiratory Diseases, Division of Viral Diseases, & Centers for Disease Control and Prevention. (2022e). *Underlying medical conditions associated with higher risk for severe COVID-19: Information for healthcare professionals.* https://www.cdc.gov/coronavirus/2019-ncov/hcp/clinical-care/underlyingconditions.html

National Institutes of Health. (2022). *NIH experts discuss controlling COVID-19 in commentary on herd immunity.* https://www.nih.gov/news-events/news-releases/nih-experts-discuss-controlling-covid-19-commentary-herd-immunity

National Public Radio. (2022). *Doubting mainstream medicine, COVID patients find dangerous advice and pills online.* https://www.npr.org/sections/health-shots/2022/07/19/1111794832/doubting-mainstream-medicine-covid-patients-find-dangerous-advice-and-pills-onli

Naylor, B. (2021). Biden says goal of 200 million COVID-19 vaccinations in 100 days has been met. *National Public Radio.* https://www.npr.org/2021/04/21/989487650/biden-says-goal-of-200-million-covid-19-vaccinations-in100-days-has-been-met

Nishiura, H., Linton, N. M., & Akhmetzhanov, A. R. (2020). Serial interval of novel coronavirus (COVID-19) infections. *International Journal of Infectious Diseases, 93,* 284–286. https://doi.org/10.1016/j.ijid.2020.02.060

Our World in Data. (2022a). *Coronavirus (COVID-19) vaccinations.* https://ourworldindata.org/covid-vaccinations?country=OWID_WRL

Our World in Data. (2022b). *United States: COVID-19 weekly death rate by vaccination status, all ages.* https://ourworldindata.org/grapher/united-states-rates-of-covid-19-deaths-by-vaccination-status?country=~All+ages

Parasidis, E., & Fairchild, A. L. (2022). Closing the public health ethics gap. *New England Journal of Medicine, 387,* 961–963. https://doi.org/10.1056/NEJMp2207543

Pettengill, M. A., & McAdam, A. J. (2020). Can we test our way out of the COVID-19 pandemic? *Journal of Clinical Microbiology, 58*(11). https://doi.org/10.1128/JCM.02225-20

Piroth, L., Cottenet, J., Mariet, A. S., Bonniaud, P., Blot, M., Tubert-Bitter, P., & Quantin, C. (2020). Comparison of the characteristics, morbidity, and mortality of COVID-19 and seasonal influenza: A nationwide, population-based retrospective cohort study. *The Lancet Respiratory Medicine, 9,* 251–259. https://www.thelancet.com/article/S2213-2600(20)30527-0/fulltext

Rezel-Potts, E., Douiri, A., Sun, X., Chowienczyk, P. J., Shah, A. M., & Gulliford, M. C. (2021). Differential impact of Covid-19 on incidence of diabetes mellitus and cardiovascular diseases in acute, post-acute and long Covid-19: Population-based cohort study in the United Kingdom. *medRxiv.* https://doi.org/10.1101/2021.12.13.21267723

Sahebi, A., Nejati-Zarnaqi, B., Moayedi, S., Yousefi, K., Torres, M., & Golitaleb, M. (2021). The prevalence of anxiety and depression among healthcare workers during the COVID-19 pandemic: An umbrella review of meta-analyses. *Progress in Neuro-Psychopharmacology & Biological Psychiatry, 107,* 110247. https://doi.org/10.1016/j.pnpbp.2021.110247

Scobie, H. M., Johnson, A. G., Amin, A. B., Ali, A. R., DeSantis, A., Shi, M., Adam, C., Armstrong, B., Armstrong, B., Asbell, M., Auche, S., Bayoumi, N. S., Bingay, B., Chasse,

M., Christofferson, S., Cima, M., Cueto, K., Cunningham, S., Delgadillo, J., . . . Silk, B. J. (2022). COVID-19 incidence and death rates among unvaccinated and fully vaccinated adults with and without booster doses during periods of delta and omicron variant emergence—25 U.S. Jurisdictions, April 4–December 25, 2021. *Morbidity and Mortality Weekly Report, 71*(4), 132–138. https://doi.org/10.15585/mmwr.mm7104e2

Spencer, J., & Jewett, C. (2021). Lost on the frontline. *Kaiser Health News.* https://khn .org/news/article/us-health-workers-deaths-covid-lost-on-the-frontline/

Stokes, E. K., Zambrano, L. D., Anderson, K. N., Marder, E. P., Raz, K. M., Felix, S. B., Tie, Y., & Fullerton, K. E. (2020). Coronavirus disease 2019 case surveillance – United States, January 22–May 30, 2020. *Morbidity and Mortality Weekly Review, 69*(24), 759–765. https://www.cdc.gov/mmwr/volumes/69/wr/mm6924e2.htm

The White House. (2022, March). *National COVID-19 preparedness plan.* https://www .whitehouse.gov/wp-content/uploads/2022/03/NAT-COVID-19-PREPAREDNESS -PLAN.pdf

Thomson, H. (2021). Herd immunity to Covid-19 may not be attainable in the UK a high vaccination rate will save many lives, but it probably won't be enough to stop Covid-19 becoming a seasonal disease, finds Helen Thomson. *New Scientist, 251*(3348), 17. https://doi.org/10.1016/S0262-4079(21)01448-2

U.S. Food and Drug Administration. (2021). *Coronavirus (COVID-19) update: FDA authorizes first oral antiviral for treatment of COVID-19.* https://www.fda.gov/news-events/ press-announcements/coronavirus-covid-19-update-fda-authorizes-first-oral-antiviral -treatment-covid-19

Ward, J. A., Stone, E. M., Mui, P., & Resnick, B. (2022). Pandemic-related workplace violence and its impact on public health officials, March 2020–January 2021. *American Journal of Public Health, 112,* 736–746. https://doi.org/10.2105/AJPH.2021.306649

Weber, L., & Barry-Jester, A. M. (2022). Conservative blocs unleash wave of litigation to curb public health powers. *Kaiser Health News.* https://khn.org/news/article/ conservative-blocs-litigation-curb-public-health-powers/

10

The Prospects for Public Health

> **LEARNING OBJECTIVES**
>
> **Students will learn . . .**
>
> 1. Current health problems that public health must address.
> 2. Impact that preference for structural changes requiring political action may have on public health strategies.
> 3. Potential impact of privatization on public health.
> 4. Importance of trust to public health success and how mistrust of public health was revealed during the COVID-19 pandemic.
> 5. Importance of scientific literacy to trust in public health.

For public health practitioners, the public health system in the United States is a source of great pride, as well as a cause for humility. On one hand, the system has a substantial public health infrastructure, a rigorous process for assessing and improving the organizational components of the system, and processes that have led to highly successful programs, policies, and services in a great many areas. On the other hand, long-standing health disparities within the United States as well as unfavorable population health indicators compared to peer countries, indicate the need for public health to revitalize its efforts "to fulfill society's interest in assuring conditions in which people can be healthy" (Institute of Medicine [IOM], 1988, p. 17). This chapter identifies problems and issues that public health must address in order to achieve its goals. This current situation provides opportunities for public health professionals to "reinvent" the field in order that public health can achieve its overarching mission. First, a brief summary of the state of public health.

THE STATE OF PUBLIC HEALTH

Public Health Infrastructure

The public health infrastructure—provided and supported by both government and private entities—is substantial.

Government Sector

The federal government funds a considerable part of the public health infrastructure, including the U.S. Department of Health and Human Services (DHHS) and the U.S. Department of Agriculture (USDA). The DHHS contains most government public health agencies, but of particular importance is the Centers for Disease Control and Prevention (CDC), the leading public health organization in the world. The CDC conducts premier research into the causes, prevention, and remedies of health problems in all areas—infectious disease, injury, and noninfectious disease. Especially through the National Center for Health Statistics (NCHS), the CDC is a leader in health information systems, which are essential for evidence-based research and policy development.

In addition to the federal government, every state has a **public health department**, and there are about 2,800 local health departments. These government agencies identify health problems in their communities, implement solutions, evaluate results, and share their findings with other public health entities. The CDC provides public health leadership to state and local public health organizations, as well as funding. Due to federalism, state and local public health agencies have a great deal of autonomy.

The USDA is another large government funder of public health services and research, addressing hunger, housing, and lack of health care. Most importantly, the Food, Nutrition, and Consumer Services division has 15 nutrition assistance programs including the Supplemental Nutrition Assistance Program (SNAP) and child nutrition programs, including the National School Lunch Program (NSLP) and the Special Supplemental Nutrition Program for Women, Infants, and Children (WIC).

Funding from the federal government for public health is sizable. Funding for the CDC in 2022 was $16.1 billion. The DHHS 2020 budget was $1.7 trillion, or about $4,857/person, and includes the CDC budget amount (DHHS, 2022). The USDA's Food, Nutrition, and Consumer Services division had a $163 billion budget in 2022. See **Figure 10.1**.

Nonprofit Sector

The nonprofit sector providing support to the public health system includes funders, professional organizations, and think tanks.

Nongovernment Funders. There are numerous organizations that support the public health system through funding of demonstration projects and evaluation

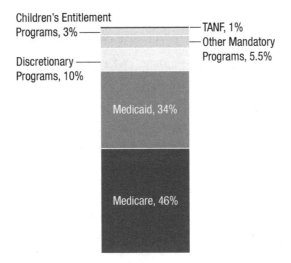

Figure 10.1.   The Department of Health and Human Services Fiscal Year 2022 Budget—$1.7 Trillion in Outlays

TANF, Temporary Aid to Needy Families.

Source: Department of Health and Human Services. *Fiscal year 2022: Budget in brief.* https://www.hhs.gov/sites/default/files/fy-2022-budget-in-brief.pdf

and assessment of policies and programs that impact the health of populations. They include giants like the Robert Wood Johnson Foundation, with total assets in 2020 of over $13 billion and charitable disbursements of about $645 million. They also include smaller organizations like the Trust for America's Health, which had over $14 million in assets in 2020 (Suozzo et al., 2021).

The United Health Foundation (UHF) is an example. Founded in 1999 by the UnitedHealth Group, the UHF is a philanthropic entity "committed to developing and supporting innovative and evidence-based activities that help the health system work better. The foundation identifies meaningful partnerships and initiatives that have the potential to be scaled—leading to improved access to care, better health outcomes and healthier communities" (UnitedHealth Group, 2022, para. 1). Among their partners are the American Academy of Family Physicians, American Indian College Fund, Any Baby Can, Asian and Pacific Islander American Scholars, Congressional Black Caucus Foundation, Congressional Hispanic Caucus Institute, Health Care Center for the Homeless, and more.

Notably, the UHF produces America's Health Rankings reports, which evaluate a wide-ranging set of health, environmental, and socioeconomic data for each state. The UHF has generated reports on women's and children's health, health disparities, senior health, and women serving in the military (UnitedHealth Group, 2022). The UHF had total assets in 2020 of more than $265 million and charitable disbursements of over $74 million (Suozzo et al., 2021).

Professional Organizations. The nonprofit sector also includes many professional organizations that keep their members current with the field, provide an outlet and voice for public health research and policy, and assist in setting standards and guidelines for public health practice. As examples, they include:

- American Public Health Association (APHA),
- American College of Epidemiology,
- American School Health Association,
- Association of Schools and Programs of Public Health (ASPPH),
- Society for Public Health Education (SOPHE),
- National Association of County and City Health Officials (NACCHO), and
- Association of State and Territorial Health Officials (ASTHO).

Think Tanks. One of the most influential nonprofit organizations for public health is the IOM—now the National Academy of Medicine within the National Academies of Sciences, Engineering, and Medicine—which sponsored *The Future of Public Health* (1988) and other advisory reports. The goal of the IOM remains to be an independent, evidence-based scientific advisor—"to carry out our work, we harness the talents and expertise of accomplished, thoughtful volunteers and undertake meticulous processes to avoid and balance bias. Our foundational goal is to be the most reliable source for credible scientific and policy advice on matters concerning human health" (IOM, 2022, para. 3).

Public Health Evaluation and Oversight

There is a rigorous process for assessing and improving the organizational components of the public health system. The following bodies address the qualifications and competency of public health educational programs, health departments, and individual public health practitioners:

- Council on Education for Public Health (CEPH), which accredits schools and programs in public health;
- Public Health Accreditation Board (PHAB), which accredits state, local, tribal, and territorial public health departments; and
- National Board of Public Health Examiners, which credentials public health practitioners.

In addition, there is monitoring and oversight of public health practices. An example is the vaccine monitoring programs, which ensure that vaccine benefits outweigh risks for individuals and populations. Vaccine standards are high since vaccines are generally given to healthy individuals, adults and children, as a primary prevention measure. The process includes clinical trials, the licensure process, the post-licensure surveillance, and causality assessments.

The processes put in place by these organizations serve to improve public health practice.

Public Health Practices

By applying scientific principles to solve health problems, the public health system has achieved success in preventing mortality, morbidity, disability, and premature death in many areas. Evidence-based solutions are continually identified, implemented, and their results shared throughout the public health community. Best practices are proposed and replicated.

The array of problems tackled by public health is astonishing—obesity, hunger, physical inactivity, heart disease, foodborne diseases, unsafe workplaces, lack of housing, motor vehicle injuries, suicide, and much more. The Ten Great Public Health Achievements: United States, 1900 to 1999 is a dazzling list of accomplishments (see Chapter 2):

1. Vaccination against infectious diseases,
2. Motor vehicle safety,
3. Safer workplaces,
4. Control of infectious diseases through medicine and environmental means,
5. Decline in deaths from coronary heart disease and stroke,
6. Safer and healthier foods,
7. Healthier mothers and babies,
8. Family planning,
9. Fluoridation of drinking water, and
10. Recognition of tobacco use as a health hazard.

For contemporary examples of public health system successes, *Healthy People 2020* provides evidence. Of the 985 *Healthy People 2020* trackable objectives, 26 were Leading Health Indicators. Of these 26, 19.2% were met or exceeded, 34.6% improved, and only 15.4% got worse. Among the objectives that were met or exceeded were improvements in air quality, decline in infant deaths, increase in physical activity among adults, decrease in adolescent cigarette smoking, and decrease in exposure of children to secondhand smoke. See Table 10.1 for the status of all 26 indicators.

Public Health Performance

Despite a considerable infrastructure, rigorous oversight processes, and significant success in tackling many health problems, at least two realities indicate the need for improvement in public health performance. These are:

- Health disparities within the United States, and
- Poor health outcomes in the United States compared to peer countries.

Table 10.1. Status of *Healthy People 2020* Leading Health Indicators

Leading Health Indicators (Partial Listing)

Legend: ☑ Target Met or Exceeded ✚ Improved ◯ Little or No Detectable Change ▬ Got Worse ▬ Baseline Only ■ Informational

Final Progress Status (1)	Objective Description	Baseline Value (year)	Final Value (year)	Target	Movement statistically significant
✚	AHS-1.1. Persons with medical insurance (%, under age 65)	83.2 (2008)	89.0 (2018)	100.0	Yes
◯	AHS-3. Persons with a usual primary care provider (%)	76.3 (2007)	76.4 (2016)	83.9	No
✚	AH-5.1. Students graduating from high school within 4 years of starting 9th grade (%)	79 (2010–2011)	85 (2016–2017)	87	…
✚	C-16. Adults receiving colorectal cancer screening based on the most recent guidelines (age-adjusted percent, ages 50–75)	52.1 (2008)	65.2 (2018)	70 5	Yes
◯	D-5.1. Persons with diagnosed diabetes whose A1c value is >9% (age-adjusted percent, ages 18 and over)	18.0 (2005–2008)	18.7 (2013–2016)	16.2	No
◥	EH-1. Air Quality Index >100 (number of days, weighted by population and Air Quality Index value)	7,603,280,922 (2006–2008)	4,295,962,018 (2016–2018)	6,842,952,850	…
◯	FP-7.1. Sexually active females receiving reproductive health services (%, ages 15–44)	78.6 (2006–2010)	78.0 (2015–2017)	86.5	No

Source: National Center for Health Statistics. *Healthy people 2020 progress table.* https://www.cdc.gov/nchs/healthy_people/hp2020/progress-tables.htm

Health Disparities Within the United States

"Health disparities are differences in the incidence, prevalence, and mortality of a disease and the related adverse health conditions that exist among specific population groups. These groups may be characterized by gender, age, race or ethnicity, education, income, social class, disability, geographic location, or sexual orientation" (CDC, 2020b, para. 1). Health disparities are identified as "preventable differences in the burden of disease, injury, violence, or opportunities to achieve optimal health that are experienced by socially disadvantaged populations" (CDC, 2020a, para. 1).

Preventing health disparities promotes health equity—one of public health's foundational beliefs. Health equity is achieved when every person has the opportunity to "attain his or her full health potential" and no one is "disadvantaged from achieving this potential because of social position or other socially determined circumstances" (CDC, 2022b, para. 1).

KEY IDEA

Health disparities by race and ethnicity are often the focus of public health, but as the CDC reminds us, disadvantaged groups may be characterized by gender, age, race or ethnicity, education, income, social class, disability, geographic location, or sexual orientation.

Food insecurity is an example of a health problem that impacts a disadvantaged group and has not been adequately addressed. Insufficient food is inextricably linked to poor health. Food insecurity plagues many Americans, but usually results from the uncertain circumstances of low wage work when the loss of a job, a health emergency, or another crisis leaves no money for food. Through its Food, Nutrition, and Consumer Services, the USDA provides food and nutrition "to ensure that children and low income citizens have sufficient food to support nutritious diets"—an outlay of over $160 billion or 74% of the USDA budget in 2022. Over the course of a year, one in four Americans is served by one of USDA's 15 nutrition assistance programs. These include SNAP; child nutrition programs, including the NSLP, the School Breakfast Program (SBP), the Summer Food Service Program (SFSP), and the Child and Adult Care Food Program (CACFP); the Special Supplemental Nutrition Program for WIC; The Emergency Food Assistance Program (TEFAP); the Food Distribution Program on Indian Reservations (FDPIR); and several similar programs targeted to specific needs (USDA, 2023).

Yet, despite these USDA programs and many others provided by the nonprofit sector, hunger and food insecurity are problems for many Americans. "Most U.S. households have consistent, dependable access to enough food for active, healthy living—they are food secure. However, some households experience food insecurity at times during the year, meaning their access to adequate food is limited by a lack of money and other resources" (Coleman-Jensen et al., 2022, p. 1). Figure 10.2 indicates that food insecurity has been a problem for many years.

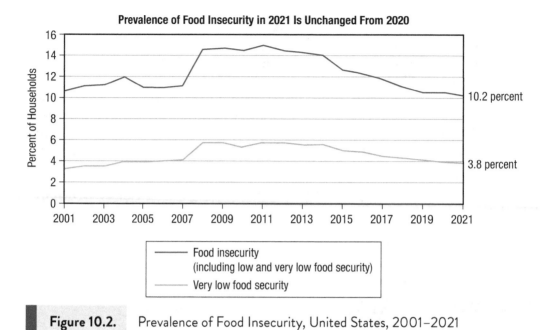

Figure 10.2.   Prevalence of Food Insecurity, United States, 2001–2021

Source: Coleman-Jensen, A., Rabbitt, M. P., Gregory, C. A., & Singh, A. (2022). *Household food security in the United States in 2021.* Economic Research Service. https://www.ers.usda.gov/webdocs/publications/104656/err-309_summary.pdf?v=1837

In addition, other findings about food insecurity are provided from the USDA's annual, nationally representative survey:

- The typical (median) food-secure household spent 16% more for food than the typical food-insecure household of the same size and composition. These estimates include food purchases made with Supplemental Nutrition Assistance Program (SNAP) benefits.

- About 56% of food-insecure households in the survey reported that in the previous month, they participated in one or more of the three largest federal nutrition assistance programs: SNAP; the Special Supplemental Nutrition Program for Women, Infants, and Children (WIC); and the National School Lunch Program. (Coleman-Jensen et al., 2022, p. 2)

U.S. Health Outcomes Compared to Peer Countries

Although the United States has the highest Gross Domestic Product (GDP) of any nation in the world—almost $23 trillion in 2021 (World Bank, 2022)—we compare unfavorably to our peers in health outcomes. Our comparison group is a fair one—countries in the Organization for Economic Cooperation and Development (OECD). The OECD is comprised of 38 democracies with market-based economies. It is a forum for the governments of these countries to collaborate and develop policy standards that promote sustainable economic growth. Yet the United States was ranked close to the bottom of the OECD countries in all major measures of population health—life expectancy, healthy life expectancy (HALE), infant mortality, and maternal mortality. As discussed in Chapter 9:

- Only four countries had a lower life expectancy for women than the United States—Lithuania, Mexico, Latvia, and Hungary.
- Only seven countries had a lower life expectancy for men than the United States—Poland, Slovakia, Hungary, Lithuania, Mexico, Latvia, and Estonia.
- Americans have, on average, fewer years of healthy life compared to most of countries in the OECD. For example, healthy life expectancy at birth for men is highest in Japan at 72.6 years, while the United States is ranked 33 out of 38 with 65.2 years of healthy life, on average. Only four countries had a lower HALE than the United States—Hungary, Lithuania, Mexico, and Latvia.
- For women, Japan is also ranked first with 75.5 years of healthy life expected, and the United States is ranked last of the 38 OECD countries with a HALE of 65 years.
- In 2020, the U.S. infant mortality rate (IMR) was 5.4 per 1,000 live births. Although this rate is low, it is among the highest of the 38 peer countries. Only Mexico, Colombia, Turkey, Costa Rica, and Chile had higher IMR rates.
- Maternal mortality in the United States was among the highest of the OECD countries at 20.1/100,000 live births in 2019 and 23.8/100,000 live births in 2020. The lowest rates were under 11/100,000 live births. Only nine of the 38 countries in 2019 and 10 countries in 2020 had maternal mortality rates higher than 11/100,000 live births.

CREATING A HEALTHY SOCIETY: PROSPECTS FOR PUBLIC HEALTH

The number of issues that affect the health of populations in the United States and the world is daunting. The foundational public health services that provide clean water, air, and food supply; workplace safety; infectious and noninfectious disease prevention, as well as injury control must be maintained. These and other traditional public health endeavors are essential for healthy populations. Particular issues are pressing, and they include:

- Future pandemics,
- Gun violence,
- Substance abuse,
- Women's reproductive health,
- Food and water insecurity,
- Climate change and environmental justice,
- Environmental degradation from population growth and industrialization, and
- Consequences of war.

The promise of public health rests on social justice—everyone is entitled to life conditions in which they can be healthy. As we know that this ideal has not been attained, we ask, "What are the prospects for public health achieving this mission?" In the United States, four sets of circumstances will have a significant impact on how this question will be answered:

- Structural changes requiring political action,
- Fragmentation of public health services and policies,
- Drift toward privatization of public functions, and
- Mistrust of public health revealed during the COVID-19 pandemic.

These four issues imply questions—How much will structural changes be pursued by public health? Will the problem of fragmentation of services and policies be addressed effectively? Will privatization of public health services undermine public health's social justice mission? Will public health be able to increase public trust in its purpose and methods? The public health system of the future will look very different, depending upon the answers to these questions.

Structural Changes Requiring Political Action

There is some evidence suggesting that public health practice is on the cusp of change that will return the field to more politically oriented action aimed at changing underlying structures of society that maintain inequalities in morbidity, disability, and premature death between rich and poor, powerful and powerless, and high and low status. The health impact pyramid points in this direction (Frieden, 2010). Marmot (2005) is another strong voice for political action. For example, he writes:

> Health status, therefore, should be of concern to policy makers in every sector, not solely those involved in health policy. As a response to this global challenge, WHO (World Health Organization) is launching a Commission on Social Determinants of Health, which will review the evidence, raise societal debate, and recommend policies with the goal of improving health of the world's most vulnerable people. *A major thrust of the commission is turning public health knowledge into political action.* (Marmot, 2005, p. 1099)

However, this is a more difficult path for public health. The pressure to continue emphasizing interventions that motivate people to change their behavior through traditional health promotion has wide support because it does not challenge existing power structures. As Berridge wrote:

> Public health has been criticized for preferring "technical fixes," short term interventions which help deal with a particular issue, to fundamental reappraisals of society. It is easier to develop vaccination programmes than to initiate wide-ranging measures which deal more fundamentally with poverty and social inequality and consequently to better health for poorer classes. (Berridge, 2016, p. 9)

It is easier to maintain a focus on motivating individuals to change their own behavior, rather than taking on the difficult task of providing, in the broadest sense, the conditions in which people can be healthy. But are these methods as effective as structural change?

The problem is that seeking structural changes to improve health places public health against powerful, entrenched, and well-funded forces. For example, to implement policies and programs to reduce mortality and injury from gun violence, public health faces the powerful gun manufacturing industry. To affect improvement in children's diets, public health confronts the large, sweetened beverage industry and the fast-food establishment. To reduce carbon dioxide in the atmosphere, public health must deal with the oil and gas industry's interests in business as usual. These are truly David versus Goliath encounters. Success will require considerable political capital and political skill on the part of public health leaders.

DID YOU KNOW?

The Dickey Amendment and Gun Violence
The Dickey Amendment is an example of powerful lobbies influencing public health efforts. Passed in 1996, it quashed gun violence research by the Centers for Disease Control and Prevention (CDC) for 25 years. After the National Rifle Association (NRA) accused the CDC of bias against guns and began lobbying to eliminate a proposed injury prevention center, the legislation to create the injury prevention center was amended so that "[n]one of the funds made available in this title may be used, in whole or in part, to advocate or promote gun control." Gun violence prevention funding was directed instead to traumatic brain injury research. This legislation was modified in 2018 when Congress clarified that the Dickey Amendment does not bar all federal support for research on gun issues, and Congress now can appropriate funds for research that informs initiatives to reduce firearm deaths and injuries. Since then, $25 million has been allocated each year for such research—by the CDC and the National Institutes of Health (Rostron, 2018). "It's really important that we understand the root causes of gun violence so we can truly understand what a public health approach can be to effectively prevent gun death and injury in this country," said Christian Heyne, the vice president of policy at Brady, a gun violence prevention organization (Roubein, 2022, para. 5).

Fragmentation of Public Health Services and Policies

In many areas, public health is highly fragmented. Data collection and sharing is one example. In 2021, the National Coordinator for Health IT Micky Tripathi and Dr. Daniel Jernigan, acting deputy director for public health science and surveillance at the CDC, discussed this problem:

> "Our public health system suffers from not really being a system, which is one of the challenges that we have," Tripathi said. "And it's really a loosely cobbled constellation of systems fragmented in a number of different ways."
> Jurisdictionally, where we have federal, state, county, metropolitan, territorial, tribal levels that, you know, that all of you don't have a single line of authority but are all sort of collaborative partners in a way. So we have a value chain of stratification where you have primitive

integration in many ways between massive clinical and administrative IT infrastructures and then a parallel public health system infrastructure that doesn't really integrate very well through all of the other structures. (Comstock, 2021, paras. 5 and 6)

Another example is the fragmented system of support for young children and their families. There are many health and social programs that aid parents and children, but they are not available to all families and not offered consistently. There are gaps in coverage and availability that leave many children and parents without sufficient help throughout early childhood. Yet, there is an abundance of research on the importance of early childhood. In the influential report *From Neurons to Neighborhoods: The Science of Early Childhood Development* (Shonkoff & Phillips, 2000), the case is made that the earliest years of life set the stage for successful, healthy adulthood. The environment in which a child develops from conception through early childhood—the family and its tangible and intangible resources, the quality of childcare, the support and resources of the community—combine to influence a child's intellectual, emotional, and social well-being, for better or worse. Every family needs:

- Access to family planning including abortion and contraception,
- Prenatal and maternity care,
- Maternity and paternity leave,
- Access to health care,
- Stable childcare based on child development principles,
- Adequate nutrition, and
- Adequate housing.

Where the current system helps some families—though not all families and not consistently—through a complex array of programs at the federal, state, and local levels, a coordinated, comprehensive focus on supporting the needs of families and their young children would prevent or reduce many health problems later on.

Drift Toward Privatization of Public Health Functions

Another issue to consider is who will provide public health services. Much of the work of public health is done by the public sector, but as the IOM emphasized in *The Future of the Public's Health in the 21st Century*, public health extends beyond government to encompass the efforts, science, art, and approaches used by all sectors of society (public, private, and civil society) to assure, maintain, protect, promote, and improve the health of the people (IOM, 2003).

Earlier in this chapter, we named a few of the private, but nonprofit actors in the public health sphere. In the United States, they are necessary to supplement funding and provide other resources needed by public health. However, market-based companies, with incentives to produce profits (in addition to "doing good"), are also drifting into public health areas. For example, we, in the United States, where access to clean water is guaranteed by public utilities through environmental-level structures that deliver potable water to individuals in their homes, worksites, and public places, may assume that our system is the only way to achieve the goal of providing water free from disease-producing agents. However, this is not the case. Other models have been developed and are being tried throughout the world, mostly in poor countries and poor communities. They include:

- Water systems developed by the private sector such as in Bolivia, where the government licensed water distribution in the 1990s to private companies, headed by Bechtel (Salzman, 2013);
- Individual-level strategies whereby people are responsible for filtering their own water using small-scale technologies such as the UV Waterworks, a portable, low-maintenance, energy-efficient water purifier, which uses ultraviolet light to render viruses and bacteria harmless (Davidson, 1998); and
- Market-based approaches using private investment without government assistance, such as promoted by Acumen (2023).

These alternative strategies to providing potable water free from water-borne disease agents illustrate the variety of ways that public health problems can be addressed by the private sector.

However, the questions to ask about privatization to achieve public health goals are related to effectiveness, efficiency, and equity. Will privatization result in equitable, efficient, and effective public health policies and services?

Although there has been s a good deal of privatization of government functions, mostly prompted by public budget shortfalls, there are no studies answering these questions definitively. Two studies published in 2002—*The Perceived Impact of Privatization on Local Health Departments* and *Services Privatized in Local Health Departments*—found health department directors divided on the benefits and costs of privatization. There is, however, much interest in these issues. For example, the Harvard T.H. Chan School of Public Health held a panel discussion in 2021: Privatizing Public Health.

> "This privatization of public health, which has taken shape over the past few years and accelerated rapidly during the pandemic, raises challenging ethical and legal questions. What is lost when public health becomes privatized? Are values like scientific rigor, transparency, equity, and accountability upheld? Are the promised efficiencies of the free market realized?" (Harvard, 2021, para. 3)

Mistrust of Public Health

Importance of Trust. We believe at least three conditions are essential to achieve a high-functioning public health system:

- The population's trust in public health's mission, goals, and methods;
- The legal and moral authority to enforce its policies and practices; and
- Sufficient funding to develop, implement, and evaluate its policies and practices.

However, without the public's trust, gaining the legal and moral authority as well as funding needed for success are in doubt. For this reason, we suggest that the most significant problem for public health today may be the mistrust that was exposed during the COVID-19 pandemic.

Basis of Mistrust. What is the basis for the public's mistrust of public health? Three major causes are:

- Ideology,
- Spread of misinformation, and
- Lack of scientific literacy.

First, a fundamental reason there is mistrust of public health is ideological—the conflict between the "common good" and "individual liberty" ideals. The "public health perspective" rests on commitment to the "common good," which Etzioni (2015) describes as:

> The common good (alternatively called "the public interest" or "public goods") denotes those goods that serve all members of a given community and its institutions, and, as such, includes both goods that serve no identifiable particular group, as well as those that serve members of generations not yet born. It is a normative concept with a long and contested history. Philosophers, theologians, lawyers, politicians, and the public have arrived at distinct understandings about what the common good entails, how it should be balanced against individual goods, and if and by whom it should be enforced. Though there are many critics of the notion of the common good . . ., it has survived as a meaningful concept for well over two millennia, and continues to serve as a very significant organizing principle of civic and political life. (Etzioni, 2015, p. 1)

And here lies a major source of the hostility to public health that was revealed during the COVID-19 pandemic. The common good orientation sanctions limiting individual liberty to serve the public interest. This view is antithetical to a small government political ideology whose adherents are guided by the principles of individual rights and liberty. As Berridge (2016) states about public health:

> Another area of fundamental debate has been the tension between the collective benefits to society of public health interventions contrasted with the liberty of individuals. It is seen as unfair for the majority of individuals to sacrifice their individual freedom for a common good which may be illusory. This was a key area of debate during the early public health reforms in the 19th century, and resurfaced in a different form with discussions of the "nanny state" in more recent times. (Berridge, 2016, p. 9)

Weber and Barry-Jester link the opposition to public health practices during the COVID-19 pandemic to the larger, constitutional issue:

> Galvanized by what they've characterized as an overreach of COVID-related health orders issued amid the pandemic, lawyers from the three overlapping spheres—conservative and libertarian think tanks,

Republican state attorneys general, and religious liberty groups—are aggressively taking on public health mandates and the government agencies charged with protecting community health. . . .

"I don't think these cases have ever been about public health," said Daniel Suhr, managing attorney for the Liberty Justice Center, a Chicago-based libertarian litigation group. "That's the arena where these decisions are being made, but it's the fundamental constitutional principles that underlie it that are an issue." (Weber & Barry-Jester, 2022, paras. 1–3)

The opposition to public health during the COVID-19 pandemic illustrates the tension between the public good and individual rights perspectives. Further, it demonstrates that when people perceive public health as a threat to their liberty, they are susceptible to misinformation—and rather easily persuaded that public health goals and methods are not needed, are incorrect, are irrelevant, and can be disregarded.

Second, misinformation fueled the public's mistrust and opposition to public health methods, despite evidence of their effectiveness in reducing death and serious illness from COVID-19. Peter Hotez (2021), Dean of the National School of Tropical Medicine at Baylor University College of Medicine, dates anti-science misinformation directly impacting public health to the anti-vaccine movement that began about 2000. Social media was used by anti-vaccine believers to spread their message, and over 400 websites are estimated to have formed by 2015. Facebook was a major voice for the movement and Amazon a major provider of misinformed books on the subject. Later, political action committees (PACs) were formed to press for favorable legislation, such as increasing the number of exemptions for childhood vaccinations. They are responsible for thousands of children being unvaccinated and the rise of infectious disease outbreaks such as measles. When the pandemic occurred, the anti-vaccine groups enlarged their scope of anti-science activities to include COVID-19—masking, quarantine, later vaccines, and other control practices. It should be noted that supporters of the anti-vaccine movement tend to be guided by the conservative ideology of small government.

Third, a lack of **scientific literacy** among a great many people compounded the problems of ideology and misinformation. Scientific literacy has been defined as the ability to find, make sense of, and use information about science or technology in order to participate in public dialogue about policy choices involving them (Miller, 2016). Since science and the scientific method underly public health practice, the public's scientific literacy is indispensable to policymakers. Scientific literacy requires an understanding of the goals, methods, and nature of scientific inquiry. In his 2016 report, Jon Miller reports on nearly 30 years tracking Civic Scientific Literacy in the United States. He defines this type of literacy as having "the level of understanding of basic scientific constructs that an individual would need to access and make sense of information about public policy issues involving science and technology" (p. 1). In an analysis of national probability samples, he found an increase in Civic Scientific Literacy beginning in 1995, which peaked in 2008. However, the percentage of people who qualified as scientifically literate rose only to about 28%. See **Figure 10.3**. He also found that literacy was highly related to education. See **Table 10.2**.

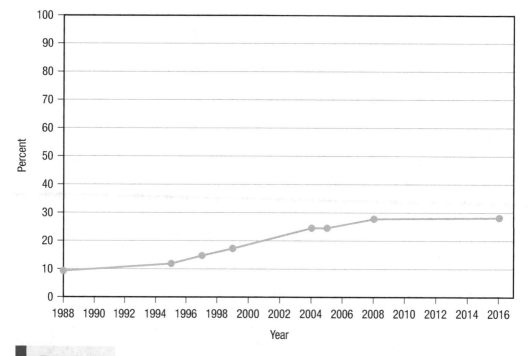

Figure 10.3.   Civic Scientific Literacy in the United States, 1988–2016

Source: Miller, J. D. (2016). *Civic scientific literacy in the United States in 2016.* International Center for the Advancement of Scientific Literacy, Institute for Social Research, University of Michigan. https://smd-cms.nasa .gov/wp-content/uploads/2023/04/NASACSLin2016Report_0_0.pdf

Table 10.2. Factors Associated With Civic Scientific Literacy, 2016

	% CSL	Gamma	N
All adults	28	–	2,835
Gender			
Male	36	–0.37	1,370
Female	20		1,465
Education			
Less than high school	7	0.61	347
High school graduate or GED	17		1,368
Associate degree	27		225
Baccalaureate degree	46		532
Graduate or professional degree	62		361

(continued)

Table 10.2. Factors Associated With Civic Scientific Literacy, 2016 (continued)	% CSL	Gamma	N
College science courses			
None	10	0.74	1,615
1–3 courses	40		631
4 or more courses	62		587
Respondent age			
18–24 years old	32	−0.13	352
25–34 years old	32		487
35–44 years old	30		469
45–54 years old	30		484
55–64 years old	24		503
65 or more years old	21		538

Gamma is a measure of the correlation between ordinal measures. The Gamma coefficient reflects the proportion of the total variance or mutual dependence between two variables that is accounted for by the relationship between the two measures.

Source: Miller, J. D. (2016). *Civic scientific literacy in the United States in 2016*. International Center for the Advancement of Scientific Literacy, Institute for Social Research, University of Michigan. https://smd-cms.nasa.gov/wp-content/uploads/2023/04/NASACSLin2016 Report_0_0.pdf

Given this low level of scientific literacy, it is not surprising that many Americans were suspicious and dismissive of public health messages about COVID-19 and how to control it. And, Carl Sagan's words were prescient when in 1996 he wrote: "We have arranged a global civilization in which most crucial elements—transportation, communications, medicine, agriculture, and so on—profoundly depend on science and technology. We have also arranged things so that almost no one understands science and technology. This is a prescription for disaster" (Sagan, 1996, p. 26).

DID YOU KNOW?

Mistrust of Public Health and COVID-19

The COVID-19 pandemic exacerbated mistrust of public health and resulted in severe challenges to basic methods of pandemic control. The extent of the mistrust of public health that was exposed during the pandemic had not been foreseen. Large numbers of

(continued)

Americans rebelled against every aspect of the public health response to the pandemic—including vaccines—as we described in Chapter 9:

- Strategies to reduce transmission were contested including masking, social distancing, and closures of schools, businesses, and other social gatherings.
- Many people refused to be vaccinated even though vaccines were demonstrated to be effective in preventing serious illness, hospitalization, and death.
- Ineffective treatments such as ivermectin were demanded by people with COVID-19 in place of proven therapeutics such as Paxlovid and monoclonal antibody therapy.
- Public health statistics, which the CDC had reliably produced for decades, were denied. Death rates derived from official death certificates were questioned, as were COVID-19 hospitalization rates from hospital reports. In both instances, the preeminent NCHS within the CDC had provided these numbers in accordance with well-established standard processes.

Addressing the Problem of Mistrust. The COVID-19 pandemic had conflicting impacts on public health in the United States. On one hand, it exacerbated mistrust in public health and the authority of public health science. On the other hand, the pandemic dramatically demonstrated the importance of effective public health.

As the foremost public health organization in the United States, the CDC took the lead in responding to the COVID-19 pandemic. In spring 2022, CDC Director Rochelle Walensky announced two reviews of the agency in response to problems that occurred during the COVID-19 pandemic:

- Scientific and Programmatic Review: To identify ways to improve and institutionalize how CDC develops and deploys its science, both in pandemic and non-emergency times.
- Structural Review: To gather feedback on the agency's current processes, systems, and structure and solicit suggestions for strategic change, with a strong focus on the agency's core capabilities—a diverse public health workforce, data modernization, laboratory capacity, rapid response to disease outbreaks, and preparedness within the United States and around the world. (CDC, 2022a, para. 2)

The recommendations from the reviews were stated as follows in the *CDC Moving Forward Summary Report*:

- Share science and data faster;
- Translate science into practical policy;
- Prioritize public health communications, with a focus on the American public;

- Develop a CDC workforce ready to respond to future threats like COVID-19; and
- Promote results-based internal and external partnerships (CDC, 2022a, para. 7).

In addition, Dr. Walensky conveyed the need to focus on action and impact and align internal CDC incentives to promote them. She also noted that the agency's cross-cutting functions and core capabilities had been underfunded, and their presence within the organization had been de-emphasized in comparison to disease-specific subject matter expertise. She acknowledged problems within the CDC that made it possible for misinformation and mistrust to flourish. Such issues as the speed of CDC's response during the crisis, the difficulty of working across agencies, and overlapping and contradictory public health guidance were cited (CDC, 2022a).

The CDC's actions and leadership are essential, but not sufficient, to deal with the fundamental mistrust of public health. It will take "all hands on deck" to build faith in the public health system and its practitioners that is needed to be highly effective. The COVID-19 pandemic exposed the extent to which Americans subscribe to a small-government ideology, which undermines the trust, authority, and funding that is needed by the public health system to succeed. Deliberate misinformation and lack of scientific literacy aggravated the problems of ideology. Actions needed include:

- Educating the public about the importance of public health and its successes;
- Developing coalitions at every level—federal, state, local, organizational— to help in this effort;
- Training public health professionals to address political conflict effectively;
- Improving public health communications, in general; and
- Countering misinformation.

Also, we must ensure that public health information is credible by strictly adhering to the rules of scientific inquiry. The story of Katherine Flegal (2021) is pertinent. Dr. Flegal and her colleagues conducted research that found a relationship between obesity and excess mortality, although the size of the effect was smaller than previously reported by an established group of researchers, dominant in health promotion. To her surprise, her findings were denigrated over the span of many years, despite her written responses to each charge, and even though her results were similar to those of many other studies. She argues that her findings were challenged because they did not fit the preferred narrative about obesity and mortality held by the challengers. She concludes her account of the story:

> Guidelines and recommendations should be based on objective and unbiased data. Development of public health policy and clinical recommendations is complex and needs to be evidence-based rather than belief-based. This can be challenging when a hot-button topic is involved. Scientific findings should be evaluated on their merits, not on the basis of whether they fit a desired narrative. (Flegal, 2021, p. 78)

Finally, we must educate the public about how scientific advancements are achieved. Science is a process. "Scientific ideas are developed through reasoning. Inferences are logical conclusions based on observable facts" (University of California, Berkeley, 2022, para. 1). Therefore, we must acknowledge uncertainty in the process:

> History has taught us that scientific "truth" is a moving target, that science can be hijacked in ways that jeopardize rather than promote public health and that the authority of science can even be harnessed to justify inhumane policies. As such, fostering open and reasoned critical public discourse about science and health indeed is in the public interest. The challenge before us is how to create online spaces that allow productive, bidirectional communication between influencers from the public sector and communicators from science to advance public health. (Schillinger & Ramirez, 2021, p. E5)

At the same time, we must strive to convince skeptics that, despite uncertainties, evidence-based decisions are preferable to the alternative. And coincidentally, we must remind that:

KEY IDEA

There aren't always right answers, but some answers are clearly wrong. (Baron & Ejnes, 2022)

In the end, the best defense of public health is ". . . a robust, high-functioning and sustainable public health system from which we all benefit. Most important and perhaps hardest of all, however will be reminding all Americans about the importance of our collective good and that the benefit of avoiding future illness and death often means temporarily compromising individual desires to assure the health of many" (Fraser, 2022, p. 729).

DID YOU KNOW?

Carl Sagan on the Nature, Importance, and Practice of Science
The eminent scholar, author, and documentarian—Professor of Astronomy and Space Sciences at Cornell University—has written about science and the scientific method:

- Science is far from a perfect instrument of knowledge. It's just the best we have. (p. 27)
- But the history of science—by far the most successful claim to knowledge accessible to humans—teaches that the most we can hope for is successive improvement in our understanding, learning from our mistakes, an asymptotic approach to the University, but with the proviso that absolute certainly will always elude us. (p. 28)

(continued)

- Advances in medicine and agriculture have saved vastly more lives than have been lost in all the wars in history. (p. 13)
- Science is more than a body of knowledge; it is a way of thinking. (p. 12)
- Science thrives on errors, cutting them away one by one. False conclusions are drawn all the time, but they are drawn tentatively. Hypotheses are framed so they are capable of being disproved. A succession of alternative hypotheses is confronted by experiment and observation. Science gropes and staggers toward improved understanding. Proprietary feelings are of course offended when a scientific hypothesis is disproved, but such disproofs are recognized as central to the scientific enterprise. (p. 21)
- Again, the reason science works so well is partly that built-in error-correcting machinery. There are no forbidden questions in science . . . That openness to new ideas, combined with the most rigorous, skeptical scrutiny of all ideas, sifts the wheat from the chaff. . . . You must prove your case in the face of determined, expert criticism. Diversity and debate are valued. Opinions are encouraged to contend. (p. 31)
- In science we may start with experimental results, data, observations, measurements, "facts." We invent, if we can, a rich array of possible explanations with the facts. In the course of their training, scientists are equipped with a baloney detection kit. The kit is brought out as a matter of course whenever new ideas are offered for consideration. If the new idea survives examination by the tools in our kit, we grant it warm, although tentative acceptance. Tools for skeptical thinking [are] the means to construct, and to understand, a reasoned argument and, especially important, to recognize a fallacious or fraudulent argument. (p. 211)
- The sword of science is double-edged. Its awesome power forces on all of us, including politicians, but of course especially on scientists, a new responsibility—more attention to the long-term consequences of technology, a global and transgenerational perspective, an incentive to avoid easy appeals to nationalism and chauvinism. Mistakes are becoming too expensive. (p. 12)

Source: From Sagan, C. (1996). *The demon-haunted world: Science as a candle in the dark.* Random House Publishing.

Effects on Public Health

As the United States entered the third decade of the 21st century, the cumulative effect on public health of fragmentation and debate over methods, privatization, and public mistrust was apparent.

- Public health workers faced condemnation and even assault from constituents during the pandemic. The people we are trying to protect are attacking us and removing our authority, said a NACCHO official, and many public health workers were leaving the field (Baker & Ivory, 2021).

- Public health authority was being limited by legislators. By 2021, legislators throughout the country had approved more than 100 new laws to reduce state and local public health powers, undermining such practices as vaccination protocols and epidemic control methods like quarantine. Furthermore, there were more legislative actions in progress to limit public health influence (Baker & Ivory, 2021; Warraich, 2022).

- Public health budgets that had been chronically underfunded were targeted for greater decline (Trust for America's Health, 2023; Alfonso et al., 2021). Between 2010 and 2020, public health department spending fell 16% per capita and local health department funding decreased by 18%. The public health system was being "hollowed-out" (Weber, Ungar, Smith, et al., 2020).

- The public's confidence in public health had weakened. In 2021, the Robert Wood Johnson Foundation and Harvard T. H. Chan School of Public Health (2021) conducted a survey of the public's views on the public health system. The survey found generally good support for public health aims. However, positive ratings of the public health system's performance had dropped from 43% to 34% between 2009 and 2021. The CDC's job performance ratings declined, as well. While 59% gave the CDC a positive rating in 2009, that had dropped to 54% in 2021. The Pew Research Center survey (Funk & Tyson, 2022) found poor perceptions of public health officials including "unprepared for the outbreak" (46%), "too slow to respond to changes in the outbreak" (32%), and "too quick to dismiss views that challenged their scientific understanding" (34%).

Public health has gone from being the recipient of benign neglect to intentional neglect and then to outright obstruction.

IMAGINE: PUBLIC HEALTH "REINVENTED"

Public health in the United States has a substantial public health infrastructure, a rigorous process for assessing and improving the organizational components of the system, and processes that have led to highly successful programs, policies, and services in a great many areas. On the other hand, long-standing health disparities within the United States as well as unfavorable population health indicators compared to peer countries, indicate the need for public health to revitalize its efforts "to fulfill society's interest in assuring conditions in which people can be healthy."

This chapter has described issues that need to be addressed in order for public health to achieve its mission and goals. Clearly, public health must continue and strengthen the activities that have led to its greatest successes including control of infectious diseases through scientific discovery of vaccines and therapeutics, provision of clean water and sanitary waste disposal, assurance of a safe food supply and workplace, and continued attention to prevention of intentional and unintentional injuries.

It is just as clear that the public health system must go beyond the traditional to include emerging health issues and reduce health disparities in order to prevent avoidable disease, injury, and disability and premature death. Pressing health problems require a high-functioning public health system that can address them effectively. We need to achieve health equity, prevent violence and deaths of despair, reduce chronic conditions like diabetes and lung diseases, ensure that children are raised in healthy environments, and maintain preparedness against future pandemics. A study of world public health systems by *U.S. News & World Report* (2022) ranked the United States #21. Twenty other nations, including Denmark, Netherlands, Canada, Japan, Norway, and South Korea were judged to have better public health systems. This is especially alarming given that the U.S. GDP is higher than any other nation in the world and our GDP per capita is among the highest.

Achieving the public health system we need will require public trust and the funding and authority that comes with trust. As described in a discussion paper sponsored by the National Academy of Medicine, the decline in funding for public health has been severe:

> Overall funding for foundational capabilities has run dry in the face of long-standing neglect and deprioritization by both local and national leaders, with the expenditures of public health agencies decreasing by approximately 10% (between 2010 and 2018) and the share of health care spending attributable to public health declining by nearly 17% (between 2002 and 2014) . . . Indeed, rather than valuing prevention, the American system has become increasingly biased in favor of reaction, with per capita spending on public health services equivalent to 1–3% of per capita expenditures on medical care. Chronically deprived of resources, the capabilities of health departments have begun to atrophy over several key domains. (DeSalvo et al., 2021)

As professionals who dedicate their careers to creating a healthier world, public health practitioners have been profoundly affected by the mistrust and anger directed at them and disturbed by the shortcomings of public health acutely revealed during the pandemic. As a result, there has been a great deal of introspection, study, and rethinking the practice of public health. Some changes have already been made and are identified in Chapter 3. Others will be made to address the problems recently disclosed. See, for example, Frieden (2021).

Thus, the current situation is an opportunity for public health to "reinvent" itself. And there is every reason to believe that the people who have inherited the values and beliefs of those who ended cholera and other deadly infectious disease epidemics, who worked tirelessly to reduce motor vehicle injuries and death, who brought about a significant decline in deaths from coronary heart disease and stroke, whose efforts led to safer workplaces, and who have ensured safer and healthier foods will do just that. Missteps are not final—they are opportunities to learn and improve. For public health, practices will be reinvigorated and strengthened. Communications and advocacy will be improved. Collaborations with communities, other agencies, and business will be expanded. The *collective public health imagination* will prevail to make the changes necessary to achieve the overarching mission of the field.

As we wrote in Chapter 9:

Going forward, there are immense opportunities for the next generation of public health professionals to recreate the trust and confidence needed to retain public health's ability to "fulfill society's interest in ensuring conditions in which people can be healthy." Understanding the past is essential, and imagination is the key. In the case of COVID-19, imagine how the response could have been better— for example, timely and consistent data collection to inform policy-making, and skillful communications between public health and the general public about what was known and what was unknown and how "knowns" can change as science evolves. Imagine the future with a fully supported public health system and the trust of citizens. Imagine the successes that will ensue—in the tradition of the historic public health achievements—through study of the past and imagining a better future.

DISCUSSION QUESTIONS

Q: What are the most pressing health problems in the United States?

Q: What obstacles and dangers does mistrust in public health pose for the success of the public health system?

Q: How does privatization affect public health?

Q: What are the obstacles to focusing interventions on the bottom levels of the health impact pyramid? What are the benefits?

DATA SOURCES

An important online source of public health information is CDC WONDER, an easy-to-use, menu-driven system available to public health professionals and the public at large. It provides access to a wide array of public health information including death certificates and birth certificates. Its purpose is to promote information-driven decision-making by placing timely, useful facts in the hands of public health practitioners and researchers, and to provide the general public with access to specific and detailed information from the CDC.

With CDC WONDER you can:

- Access statistical research data published by the CDC, as well as reference materials, reports, and guidelines on health-related topics;
- Query numeric data sets on the CDC's computers, via "fill-in-the blank" web pages. Public-use data sets about mortality (deaths), cancer incidence, HIV and AIDS, tuberculosis, vaccinations, natality (births), census data, and many

other topics are available for query, and the requested data are readily summarized and analyzed, with dynamically calculated statistics, charts, and maps.

More information about CDC WONDER and how to access its information are found at: https://wonder.cdc.gov

---

 A robust set of instructor resources designed to supplement this text is located at **http://connect.springerpub.com/content/book/978-0-8261-8615-7**. Qualifying instructors may request access by emailing **textbook@springerpub.com**.

REFERENCES

Acumen. (2023). *Investment sector: Water and sanitation.* https://acumen.org/companies/sectors/water-sanitation/

Alfonso, Y. N, Leider, J. P., Resnick, B., McCullough, J. M., & Bishai, D. (2021). US public health neglected: Flat or declining spending left states ill equipped to respond to COVID-19. *Health Affairs, 40*(4). https://doi.org/10.1377/hlthaff.2020.01084

Baker, M., & Ivory, D. (2021, October 20). Why public health faces a crisis across the U.S. *The New York Times.* https://www.nytimes.com/2021/10/18/us/coronavirus-public-health.html

Baron, R. J., & Ejnes, Y. D. (2022). Physicians spreading misinformation on social media—Do right and wrong answers still exist in medicine? *New England Journal of Medicine, 387*(1), 1–3. https://doi.org/10.1056/nejmp2204813

Berridge, V. (2016). *Public health: A very short introduction.* Oxford University Press.

Centers for Disease Control and Prevention. (2020a). *Health disparities.* https://www.cdc.gov/healthyyouth/disparities/

Centers for Disease Control and Prevention. (2020b). *Health disparities in HIV, viral Hepatitis, STD's and TB.* https://www.cdc.gov/nchhstp/healthdisparities/africanamericans.html

Centers for Disease Control and Prevention. (2022a). *CDC moving forward summary report.* https://www.cdc.gov/about/organization/cdc-moving-forward-summary-report.html

Centers for Disease Control and Prevention. (2022b). *Health equity.* https://www.cdc.gov/chronicdisease/healthequity/index.htm

Coleman-Jensen, A., Rabbitt, M. P., Gregory, C. A., & Singh, A. (2022). *Household food security in the United States in 2021.* Economic Research Service. https://www.ers.usda.gov/webdocs/publications/104656/err-309_summary.pdf?v=1837

Comstock, J. (2021). ONC, CDC want to fix the fragmented public health system COVID-19 exposed. *Healthcare IT News.* https://www.healthcareitnews.com/news/onc-cdc-want-fix-fragmented-public-health-system-covid-19-exposed

Davidson, M. (1998). *Innovative lives: UV waterworks - Ashok Gadgil.* Smithsonian Institute, Lemelson Center for the Study of Invention and Innovation. https://invention.si.edu/innovative-lives-uv-waterworks-ashok-gadgil

DeSalvo, K., Hughes, B., Bassett, M., Benjamin, G., Fraser, M., Galea, S., Gracia, J. N., & Howard, J. (2021). *Public health COVID-19 impact assessment: Lessons learned and compelling needs*. National Academy of Medicine. https://nam.edu/public-health-covid-19-impact-assessment-lessons-learned-and-compelling-needs/

Etzioni, A. (2015). The common good. In M. T. Gibbons (Ed.), *The encyclopedia of political thought* (1st ed.). John Wiley. https://doi.org/10.1002/9781118474396.wbept0178

Flegal, K. M. (2021). The obesity wars and the education of a researcher: A personal account. *Progress in Cardiovascular Diseases, 67*(July-August), 75–79. https://doi.org/10.1016/j.pcad.2021.06.009

Fraser, M. R. (2022). Harassment of health officials: A significant threat to the public's health. *American Journal of Public Health, 112*(5), 728–730. https://doi.org/10.2105/AJPH.2022.306797

Frieden, T. R. (2010). A framework for public health action: The health impact pyramid. *American Journal of Public Health, 100*(4), 590–595.

Frieden, T. R., Rajkumar, R., & Mostashari, F. (2021). We must fix US health and public health policy. *American Journal of Public Health, 111*(4) 623–627. https://doi.org/10.2105%2FAJPH.2020.306125"10.2105/AJPH.2020.306125

Funk, C., & Tyson, A. (2022). *Lack of preparedness among top reactions Americans have to public health officials' COVID-19 response*. Pew Research Center. https://www.pewresearch.org/science/2022/10/05/lack-of-preparedness-among-top-reactions-americans-have-to-public-health-officials-covid-19-response/

Harvard T. H. Chan School of Public Health. (2021). *Privatizing public health: A panel discussion*. https://www.hsph.harvard.edu/event/privatizing-public-health-a-panel-discussion/

Hotez, P. J. (2021). *Preventing the next pandemic: Vaccine diplomacy in a time of anti-science*. Johns Hopkins University Press.

Institute of Medicine. (1988). *The future of public health*. National Academies Press.

Institute of Medicine. (2022). *About the National Academy of Medicine*. https://nam.edu/about-the-nam/

Institute of Medicine of The National Academies. (2003). *The future of the public's health in the 21st century*. The National Academies Press. https://doi.org/10.17226/10548

Marmot, M. (2005). Social determinants of health inequalities. *The Lancet, 365*(9464), 1099–1104. https://doi.org/10.1016/S0140-6736(05)71146-6

Miller, J. D. (2016). *Civic scientific literacy in the United States in 2016*. International Center for the Advancement of Scientific Literacy, Institute for Social Research, University of Michigan.

Robert Wood Johnson Foundation & Harvard T. H. Chan School of Public Health. (2021). The public's perspective on the United States public health system. https://www.hsph.harvard.edu/wp-content/uploads/sites/94/2021/05/RWJF-Harvard-Report_FINAL-051321.pdf

Rostron, A. (2018). The Dickey amendment on federal funding for research on gun violence: A legal dissection. *American Journal of Public Health, 108*(7), 865–867. https://doi.org/10.2105/AJPH.2018.304450

Roubein, R. (2022). Now the government is funding gun violence research, but it's years behind. *Washington Post*. https://www.washingtonpost.com/politics/2022/05/26/now-government-is-funding-gun-violence-research-it-years-behind/

Sagan, C. (1996). *The demon-haunted world: Science as a candle in the dark*. Random House Publishing.

Salzman, J. (2013). Thirst: A short history of drinking water. *Yale Journal of Law and the Humanities, 18*(3), 6. http://hdl.handle.net/20.500.13051/7394

Schillinger, D., & Ramirez, A. S. (2021). Schillinger and Ramirez respond. *American Journal of Public Health, 111*(2), E4–E5. https://doi.org/10.2105/AJPH.2020.306058

Shonkoff, J. P., & Phillips, D. A. (Eds.). (2000). *From neurons to neighborhoods: The science of early childhood development*. National Academies Press. https://doi.org/10.17226/9824

Suozzo, A., Schwencke, K., Tigas, M., Wei, S., Glassford, A., & Roberts, B. (2021). *Nonprofit explorer: Research tax-exempt organizations*. ProPublica. https://projects.propublica.org/nonprofits/

Trust for America's Health. (2023). The impact of chronic underfunding on America's public health system: Trends, risks, and recommendations, 2023. https://www.tfah.org/report-details/funding-2023/

UnitedHealth Group. (2022). *United health foundation*. https://www.unitedhealthgroup.com/what-we-do/building-healthier-communities/our-foundations.html

University of California, Berkeley. (2022). *Understanding evolution*. https://evolution.berkeley.edu/

U.S. Department of Agriculture, Food and Nutrition Service. (2023). *Programs*. https://www.fns.usda.gov/

U.S. Department of Health & Human Services. (2022). *Fiscal year 2022 budget in brief*. https://www.hhs.gov/sites/default/files/fy-2022-budget-in-brief.pdf

U.S. News & World Report. (2022). *These countries have the most well-developed public health systems*. https://www.usnews.com/news/best-countries/rankings/well-developed-public-health-system

Warraich, H. J. (2022). A growing gap in premature deaths along party lines underscores the collision of politics and public health. *STAT*. https://www.statnews.com/2022/06/07/us-death-rates-politicization-public-health/

Weber, L., Ungar, L., Smith, M. R., The Associated Press, Recht, H., & Barry-Jester, A. M. (2020). Hollowed-out public health system faces more cuts amid virus. *KFF Health News*. https://kffhealthnews.org/news/us-public-health-system-underfunded-under-threat-faces-more-cuts-amid-covid-pandemic/

Weber, L., & Barry-Jester, A. M. (2022). Conservative blocs unleash litigation to curb public health powers. *Kaiser Health News*. https://khn.org/news/article/conservative-blocs-litigation-curb-public-health-powers/

World Bank. (2022). *World Bank open data*. https://data.worldbank.org/indicator/NY.GDP.MKTP.CD?locations=LY&most_recent_value_desc=true

Glossary

Adaptive leadership: the ability to guide organizations and individuals through perilous and confusing times by facilitating the organizational community to own their adaptive problems and solutions

Advocacy: the active promotion of a cause or principle involving actions that will lead to a goal

Age-adjusted rates: a value calculated by applying a population's age-specific rates to a standardized age distribution

Agency for Healthcare Research and Quality (AHRQ): the lead federal agency charged with improving the quality, safety, efficiency, and effectiveness of health care

Body Mass Index (BMI): a weight-to-height calculation that provides the most useful population-level measure of weight and obesity

Case surveillance: the foundation of public health practice aimed at controlling infectious diseases in human populations

Centers for Medicare and Medicaid Services: the organization that administers the largest health insurance programs in the country

Child Passenger Safety Program: a major public health initiative developed in the 1970s that focuses on reducing child passenger motor vehicle injuries and death

Community engagement: the facilitation of communities in the process of problem-solving by encouraging them to own their problems and solutions

Contagious: diseases that are spread from person to person

Core State Injury Prevention Program (SIPP): a program that facilitates surveillance and prevention of injuries and death

Coronavirus: a large family of viruses that cause diseases in mammals and birds

Council on Education for Public Health (CEPH): an independent agency recognized by the U.S. Department of Education that accredits schools of public health and certain public health programs offered in settings other than schools of public health

Department of Health and Human Services (DHHS): the central federal agency responsible for public health and health care in the United States

Determinants of health: various factors that affect the health of individuals and communities

Emerging infections: infections that have increased recently or are threatening to increase in the near future

Epidemiology: the study of the distribution and determinants of health-related states or events in specified populations, and the application of this study to the control of health problems

Evidenced-based public health (EBPH): an effort to demonstrate what works and what does not work in public health practice that is based on scientifically valid empirical research

Food and Drug Administration (FDA): the agency charged with regulating drugs and most food products in the United States

Food insecurity: insufficient access to sufficient food of an adequate quality

Health disparities: differences in the incidence, prevalence, and mortality of a disease and the related adverse health conditions that exist among specific population groups

Health impact pyramid: a framework used to integrate behavioral and environmental approaches to public health practice

Healthy People: the health-promotion and disease-prevention agenda for the United States

Herd immunity: the state that occurs when enough people in a community or population are immune to a specific disease to reduce or eliminate transmission among those who are still susceptible to the disease

Incidence: a measure of the proportion of new cases of a disease in a population during a specific time period

Incident management system (IMS): a comprehensive, national approach applicable to all jurisdiction levels that improves coordination and cooperation when responding to any type of incident

Incubation period: the time between exposure of a susceptible person to the development of the infection

Infectious disease: a disease caused by pathogenic microorganisms that can be transmitted from person to person or from other species to persons

Intentional injury: an injury that is self-inflicted or inflicted by a person or persons on others

International Classification of Diseases **(ICD)**: a globally used classification system that allows for analysis of the causes of mortality and morbidity

Life expectancy: the average number of years of life that could be expected if current death rates remain constant

National Center for Health Statistics: the premier organization for the collection, processing, analysis, and dissemination of health data

National Health Expenditure Accounts (NHEA): the official estimates of total health care spending in the United States

National Immunization Survey (NIS): a program that monitors immunization coverage among children in the United States

National Notifiable Diseases Surveillance System (NNDSS): a program developed in the 19th century that focuses on controlling and preventing infectious disease outbreaks

Noninfectious disease: a disease caused by factors that are not communicable or contagious

Nutrition, Physical Activity and Obesity Program (NPAO): a program that develops interventions to prevent and control childhood obesity

Physical environment: the natural and built environments

PRECEDE-PROCEED model: a model used to guide health promotion strategies that focuses on individual behavior change and attributes that hinder behavior change

Prevalence: the proportion of individuals who have a particular disease at a given point in time or during a specified time period

Primary prevention: a type of prevention that intends to prevent the development of disease and the occurrence of injury

Public Health Accreditation Board (PHAB): the board that addresses the quality of policies, services, and programs offered by public health organizations through the accreditation of state and local public health departments

Public Health Data Modernization Initiative: an initiative that focuses on accelerating health-related data that can improve health

Public health department: a government agency that identifies health problems in their communities, implements solutions, evaluates results, and shares their findings with other public health entities

Scientific literacy: the ability to find, make sense of, and use information about science or technology in order to participate in public dialogue about policy choices involving them

Secondary prevention: a type of prevention that focuses on reducing the impact of a disease or injury that has already occurred

Social environment: the context defined by our relationships with other people

Social marketing: the marketing strategies used to influence health-related behaviors

Teen Drivers program: a major public health initiative developed in the 1970s that aims to reduce motor vehicle death and injuries among teens

Tertiary prevention: a type of prevention that aims to treat ongoing illness or injury to slow or stop disease progression

Unintentional injury: an accidental injury that can be self-inflicted or inflicted by others

Variant: a mutation of an original virus

Years of potential life lost (YPLL): the number of years of life lost due to death before the expected age of death in a population during a given time period

Zoonotic diseases: diseases caused by microbes that spread between animals and people

Index

Note: Page numbers followed by *f* and *t* refer to figures and tables.